CEN® EXAM PREP
STUDY GUIDE

CEN® EXAM PREP
STUDY GUIDE

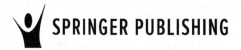 SPRINGER PUBLISHING

Springer Publishing Company, LLC
11 West 42nd Street, New York, NY 10036
www.springerpub.com

Acquisitions Editor: Jaclyn Koshofer
Compositor: diacriTech

ISBN: 978-0-8261-6401-8
ebook ISBN: 978-0-8261-6406-3
DOI: 10.1891/9780826164063

23 24 25 26 / 5 4 3 2 1

The author and the publisher of this Work have made every effort to use sources believed to be reliable to provide information that is accurate and compatible with the standards generally accepted at the time of publication. The author and publisher shall not be liable for any special, consequential, or exemplary damages resulting, in whole or in part, from the readers' use of, or reliance on, the information contained in this book. The publisher has no responsibility for the persistence or accuracy of URLs for external or third-party Internet websites referred to in this publication and does not guarantee that any content on such websites is, or will remain, accurate or appropriate.

CEN® is a registered trademark of the Board of Certification for Emergency Nursing (BCEN). BCEN does not endorse this resource, nor does it have a proprietary relationship with Springer Publishing Company.

Library of Congress Control Number: 2022941905

Contact sales@springerpub.com to receive discount rates on bulk purchases.

Publisher's Note: **New and used products purchased from third-party sellers are not guaranteed for quality, authenticity, or access to any included digital components.**

Printed in the United States of America by Gasch Printing.

CONTENTS

PREFACE

This *Exam Prep Study Guide* was designed to be a high-speed review—a last-minute gut check before your exam day. We created this review to supplement your certification preparation studies. We encourage you to use it in conjunction with other study aids to ensure you are as prepared as possible for the exam.

This book follows the Board of Certification for Emergency Nursing's most recent exam content outlines and uses a succinct, bulleted format to highlight what you need to know. The aim of this book is to help you solidify your retention of information in the month or so leading up to your exam. It is written by certified emergency nurses who are familiar with the exam and the content you need to know. Special features appear throughout the book to call out important information, including:

- **Complications:** Problems that can arise with certain disease states or procedures
- **Nursing Pearls:** Additional patient care insights and strategies for knowledge retention
- **Alerts:** Need-to-know details on how to handle emergency situations or when to transfer care
- **Pop Quizzes:** Critical-thinking questions to test your ability to synthesize what you've learned (answers in the back of the book)
- **Two Full-Length Practice Tests:** One printed in the book, one online
- **Free One-Month Access to ExamPrepConnect:** The digital study platform that guides you confidently through your exam prep journey

We know life is busy. Being able to prepare for your exam efficiently and effectively is paramount, which is why we created this *Exam Prep Study Guide*. You have come to the right place as you continue on your path of professional growth and development. The stakes are high, and we want to help you succeed. Best of luck to you on your certification journey.

PASS GUARANTEE

If you use this resource to prepare for your exam and do not pass, you may return it for a refund of your full purchase price, excluding tax, shipping, and handling. To receive a refund, return your product along with a copy of your exam score report and original receipt showing purchase of new product (not used). Product must be returned and received within 180 days of the original purchase date. Refunds will be issued within 8 weeks from acceptance and approval. One offer per person and address. This offer is valid for U.S. residents only. Void where prohibited. To initiate a refund, please contact Customer Service at csexamprep@springerpub.com.

1 GENERAL EXAMINATION INFORMATION

OVERVIEW

The purpose of the CEN examination is to provide national certification for emergency nurses, allowing for the validation of knowledge, skills, and expertise in the field. This book covers each body system that is presented on the CEN examination.

CEN CERTIFICATION

The Board of Certification for Emergency Nursing (BCEN) seeks to have emergency nurses display their competence in the full array of emergency nursing. The examination is open to all licensed RNs within the United States and to those who hold an equivalent certificate verified through the Commission on Graduates of Foreign Nursing Schools International. While there is no requirement for emergency nursing experience, it is recommended that the applicant have 2 years of nursing experience in the ED before taking the examination.

About the Examination

- There are 175 questions: 150 scored and 25 pretest questions that are not scored. The examinee must answer 106 questions correctly to pass the examination.
- The examinee is allowed 180 minutes to complete the multiple-choice examination.
- 150 questions from the examination are broken down as follows: 19 cardiovascular; 18 respiratory; 18 neurologic; 18 gastrointestinal, genitourinary, gynecology, and obstetric; 11 mental health; 14 medical; 13 musculoskeletal and wound; 11 maxillofacial and ocular; 14 environment/toxicology and communicable diseases; 14 professional issue.
- There are 134 clinical items that are broken down into 32 assessment questions, 34 analysis questions, 43 intervention questions, and 25 evaluation questions.
- The applicant submits an application online or by mail. Once the application is processed and approved, the candidate has a 90-day window to test. The applicant will coordinate with Pearson VUE to schedule the examination. The applicant must wait 90 days to retest if they do not pass the initial examination.

How to Apply

- The application cost is $230 for Emergency Nurses Association (ENA) members to take the initial examination and $200 for a retest of the initial examination.
- The application cost for non–ENA members is $370 for the initial examination and $340 for a retest of the initial examination.

How to Contact BCEN

Website: www.bcen.org
  Email: bcen@bcen.org
  Toll-free phone number: 1-877-302-2236
  Mailing address:
  1900 Spring Road
  Suite 50
  Oak Brook, IL 60523

RESOURCES

Board of Certification for Emergency Nursing. (n.d.). *Certified emergency nurse*. https://bcen.org/cen

2 CARDIOVASCULAR EMERGENCIES

ACUTE CORONARY SYNDROME

Overview

- *Acute coronary syndrome (ACS)* refers to a continuum of unstable coronary artery disease and symptoms associated with myocardial ischemia. ACS may be classified as ST-elevation myocardial infarction (STEMI), non-STEMI (NSTEMI), or unstable angina. Myocardial infarction is diagnosed when abnormal cardiac biomarkers, such as an elevated serum troponin level, are present with clinical evidence of myocardial ischemia. Angina refers to ischemic chest pain and may be classified as stable or unstable.

[ ] **COMPLICATIONS**

Complications of ACS include arrhythmias, cardiogenic shock, and death. Early reperfusion of the myocardium is vital in preventing complications related to myocardial necrosis.

Signs and Symptoms

- Symptoms may vary from mild to severe, including anxiety, arrhythmias, chest pain, diaphoresis, hypertension, hypotension, new systolic murmur, pain radiating down the left arm, sense of impending doom, and shortness of breath.
- Atypical symptoms are more likely to occur in women, people with diabetes, and older adults and include back pain, fatigue, hiccups, jaw pain, neck pain, weakness, and umbilical pain.

Diagnosis
Labs

- Complete blood count (CBC)
- Comprehensive metabolic panel (CMP)
- Coagulation panel
- Creatine kinase–myoglobin binding (CK-MB): serves as a specific indicator of myocardial damage if elevated (reference range may vary across laboratories)
- Lactic acid: elevated lactic acid (greater than 2 mmol/L) in ACS associated with increased risk for poor outcomes
- Troponin: considered elevated if greater than 0.04 ng/mL

Diagnostic Testing

- Chest x-ray
- Coronary angiography
- Echocardiogram

[ ] **NURSING PEARL**

Troponin is an important marker in determining whether cardiac injury has occurred. Serial serum sampling for troponin levels (usually assessed upon initial presentation, and again at 3 and 6 hours later) is routinely indicated for patients who present to the ED for evaluation of chest pain, as troponin usually becomes detectable 2 to 6 hours after symptom onset. Troponin may also be elevated in other conditions, such as burn injuries and sepsis.

Diagnostic Testing (continued)

- Nuclear imaging
- EKG: Patients with myocardial infarction demonstrate EKG changes reflecting cardiac damage. Examples of this progression over time are shown in Figures 2.1 to 2.3.
- Figure 2.1 demonstrates T wave inversion and early cardiac ischemia.
- Figure 2.2 demonstrates ST segment depression and progressive cardiac ischemia.
- Figure 2.3 demonstrates ST segment elevation and cardiac injury; STEMI may be diagnosed if elevation is present in two or more contiguous leads. Other presentations include transient ST segment elevation (occurring for several minutes and then resolving) in Prinzmetal angina and diffuse ST segment elevation in pericarditis.

Treatment

- Rapid assessment and treatment of ACS crucial in improving outcomes. For all patients with chest pain or symptoms of ACS, an EKG should be obtained and interpreted by the provider within 10 minutes of arrival. Continuous cardiac monitoring should be applied as soon as possible to observe for rhythm changes. Proactive application of defibrillator pads may be indicated.

[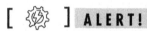]   **ALERT!**

Prompt identification of a STEMI is crucial. An EKG should be obtained within 10 minutes of arrival for any patient presenting with chest pain. "Door to balloon" (PCI) time from arrival to the ED should be 90 minutes or less, and "door to needle" (fibrinolysis medication) is 30 minutes or less.

- Notification of cardiology and catheterization team as soon as acute myocardial infarction (AMI) is identified to expedite "door-to-balloon" percutaneous coronary intervention [PCI] time (aiming to reduce time to PCI to less than 90 minutes)
- If PCI not available: ED administration of fibrinolytics, such as alteplase, for patients with STEMI: Target "door-to-needle" time is less than 30 minutes from arrival. Patients require cardiac consultation and close monitoring before, during, and after administration of fibrinolytics. Assess for contraindications to fibrinolysis, such as history of intracranial hemorrhage. Prepare for interfacility transfer if appropriate cardiac interventions are not available. ▶

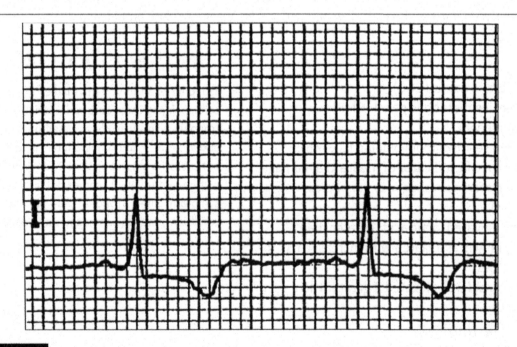

FIGURE 2.1 T wave inversion: early ischemia.

Source: Knechtel, M. A. (2021). *EKGs for the nurse practitioner and physician assistant* (3rd ed.). Springer Publishing Company.

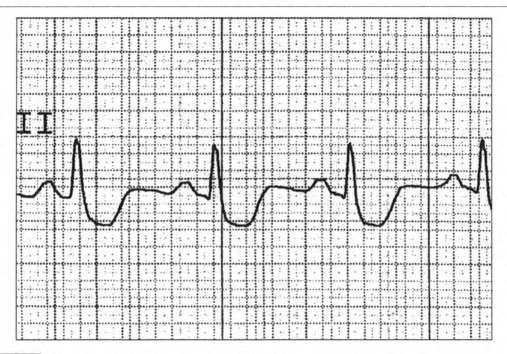

FIGURE 2.2 ST segment depression: progressive ischemia.

Source: Knechtel, M. A. (2021). *EKGs for the nurse practitioner and physician assistant* (3rd ed.). Springer Publishing Company.

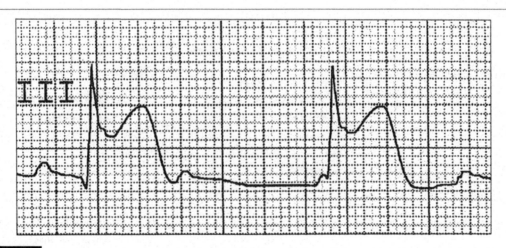

FIGURE 2.3 ST segment elevation: injury pattern.

Source: Knechtel, M. A. (2021). *EKGs for the nurse practitioner and physician assistant* (3rd ed.). Springer Publishing Company.

Treatment *(continued)*

- Administration of supplemental oxygen to maintain SpO_2 above 90% for patients with possible ACS
- Identification of any prehospital medications to determine if patients who have been educated regarding ACS, or those who have been prescribed PRN medication for angina, may have taken medications (e.g., nitroglycerin, and aspirin) prior to arrival
- Aspirin plus an additional antiplatelet agent, such as clopidogrel (see Table 2.1 for medications used for cardiovascular conditions). Immediately administer 162 to 324 mg aspirin unless contraindicated, encouraging patient to chew medication to accelerate absorption. ▶

Treatment *(continued)*

- Administration of nitrates to improve chest pain by causing vasodilation and improving myocardial perfusion (see Table 2.1). Typically, up to three doses of 0.4 mg sublingual nitroglycerin is administered every 5 minutes for continued ischemic chest pain; intravenous (IV) nitrate administration may be considered if chest pain persists. Nitrate administration is contraindicated in patients with inadequate preload (as in inferior myocardial infarction (MI), right ventricle infarction, hypotension, marked tachycardia or bradycardia, or recent phosphodiesterase inhibitor use).
- Possible administration of analgesics (e.g., morphine and fentanyl; see Table A.2 in Appendix A). Morphine may also reduce preload and is contraindicated in patients with inadequate preload.
- Typical during PCI: anticoagulant medications, such as heparin (see Table 2.1)

TABLE 2.1   Medications for Cardiovascular Conditions

INDICATIONS	MECHANISM OF ACTION	CONTRAINDICATIONS, PRECAUTIONS, AND ADVERSE EFFECTS
ACE inhibitors (lisinopril)		
• HTN • HF	• Block conversion of angiotensin I into angiotensin II	• Monitor for angioedema. • Use caution in patients with hyperkalemia.
Antiarrhythmics, class III (amiodarone)		
• Ventricular arrhythmias	• Delay repolarization in the myocardium • Antiarrhythmic and vasodilator	• Do not use in patients with iodine hypersensitivity.
Antiarrhythmics, miscellaneous (adenosine)		
• SVT	• Induce sinus bradycardia by stimulating adenosine-sensitive potassium channels to release potassium from cardiac myocyte membrane	• Administer rapidly and follow with 20-mL saline flush.
Anticholinergics (atropine)		
• To treat bradyarrhythmia	• Inhibit at the postganglionic cholinergic receptor	• Atropine is ineffective in heart transplant patients.
Anticoagulants (heparin, enoxaparin sodium)		
• NSTEMI, PVD, DVT • Bridge therapy for oral anticoagulants • Treatment and prevention of thromboembolic disease (warfarin) • PE	• Enhance activity of antithrombin III (ATIII) to inactivate thrombin (heparin) • Block synthesis of vitamin K coagulation factors (II, VII, IX, X)	• The reversal agent for heparin is protamine. • The reversal agent for warfarin is vitamin K.
Antiplatelets (aspirin)		
• AMI	• Inhibit platelet aggregating	• Monitor for signs of bleeding.

TABLE 2.1 Medications for Cardiovascular Conditions *(continued)*

INDICATIONS	MECHANISM OF ACTION	CONTRAINDICATIONS, PRECAUTIONS, AND ADVERSE EFFECTS
Beta-blockers (esmolol, metoprolol, labetalol)		
• HTN • Reduce blood pressure in patients with aortic dissection (esmolol)	• Inhibit beta-1 and beta-2 stimulation	• Use caution in patients with pulmonary disease, as beta-blockers can inhibit bronchodilation. • Avoid using beta-blockers for hypotensive patients and patients with a bradyarrhythmia.
Calcium channel blockers (diltiazem)		
• Treat angina, HTN, atrial dysrhythmias, SVT	• Inhibit inflow of extracellular calcium across myocardial and vascular smooth muscle	• Avoid bradyarrhythmia, AMI, hypotension, cardiogenic shock, HF, and ventricular dysfunction.
Cardiac dopaminergic agents (dobutamine, dopamine)		
• Treat cardiogenic shock and septic shock • CHF • Can be used after cardiac surgery • Pulmonary edema	• Sympathomimetic • Stimulate dopaminergic receptors; can potentially stimulate beta-1 and alpha receptors depending on dose (dopamine) • Stimulate primary beta-1 receptors, with some stimulation at beta-2 and alpha-1 (dobutamine) • Increase cardiac output and contractility	• Use caution in patients with arrhythmias, as dobutamine can cause ectopy in the ventricles. • Avoid in patients with corn sensitivity. • Infuse medications in a large vessel (e.g., central line). • Dopamine extravasation antidote is phentolamine. • Do not use with hypovolemic patients.
Cardiac glycosides (digitalis)		
• CHF	• Inhibit sodium potassium adenosine phosphate pump, increasing intracellular sodium and calcium, which activates contractile proteins (e.g., actin, myosin)	• Do not use with bradyarrhythmia or ventricular arrhythmias. • Be aware of the signs of digitalis toxicity and the antidote, digoxin immune fab.
Fibrinolytics (tPA)		
• PE • AMI caused by a coronary thromboembolism	• Convert plasminogen to plasmin, which then break down fibrin and fibrinogen to dissolve clot	• Monitor for signs of bleeding.
Diuretics, loop (furosemide)		
• CHF • Pulmonary edema • Edema	• Inhibit sodium and water reabsorption in distal and proximal tubules	• Monitor for electrolyte imbalances. • Loop diuretics are contraindicated in anuric patients. • Use cautiously in patients with renal disease.

TABLE 2.1 Medications for Cardiovascular Conditions *(continued)*

INDICATIONS	MECHANISM OF ACTION	CONTRAINDICATIONS, PRECAUTIONS, AND ADVERSE EFFECTS
Vasodilators (nitroglycerin, nitroprusside)		
• HF • HTN • Nitroglycerin for AMI and angina	• Dilate both venous and arterial blood vessels • Reduce both preload and afterload	• Be aware of signs and symptoms of possible cyanide toxicity and nitroprusside administration. • Monitor blood pressure frequently, as nitroglycerin and nitroprusside can cause hypotension.
Vasopressors (epinephrine, norepinephrine)		
• Anaphylaxis • Hypotension due to shock • Cardiac arrest • Croup (racemic epinephrine) • Severe asthma (epinephrine)	• Sympathomimetic catecholamine • Stimulate alpha-1 receptors, causing increased vascular smooth muscle contraction	• Adverse effects are cardiac arrythmias, anxiety, decreased renal perfusion, and pulmonary edema. • Monitor for skin necrosis at site of extravasation.

ACE, angiotensin-converting enzyme; AMI, acute myocardial infarction; CHF, congestive heart failure; DVT, deep vein thrombosis; HF, heart failure; HTN, hypertension; NSTEMI, non-ST elevation myocardial infarction; PE, pulmonary embolism; PVD, peripheral vascular disease; SVT, supraventricular tachycardia; tPA, tissue plasminogen activator.

Nursing Interventions

- Place the patient on continuous pulse oximetry and cardiac monitoring, observing for any changes in vital signs or cardiac rhythm.
- Apply defibrillator pads, if indicated. Immediately proceed with resuscitation per advanced cardiovascular life support (ACLS) guidelines if cardiac arrest occurs.
- Apply supplemental oxygen if oxygen saturation is lower than 90% or if the patient has signs of respiratory distress.
- Establish IV access, drawing blood for stat lab studies as ordered.
- Administer medications as ordered, such as nitrates and antiplatelet agents.
- Assess PQRST of pain and medicate patient as ordered. Alert provider regarding any changes in quality, severity, or location of chest pain. Continually reassess pain after interventions, aiming to achieve total resolution of chest pain. Additional medications, such as opiates, may be indicated if pain is not controlled with nitroglycerin.
- Prepare the patient for the catheterization lab. Expedite transfer to catheterization lab to minimize door to PCI time.
- If facility is not PCI capable, administer fibrinolytic medication as ordered and closely monitor patient until transfer to higher level of care is complete.

Patient Education

- If at risk for cardiac disease, consider lifestyle modifications to improve cardiovascular health, such as: Adhere to a heart-healthy diet. Control hypertension and hyperlipidemia, adhere to dietary ▶

 NURSING PEARL

Using PQRST to Assess Pain

- **P**rovoking symptoms? What caused the pain? D anything make it better or worse?
- **Q**uality of pain? What does the pain feel like?
- **R**adiation of pain? Where is the pain? Does it go anywh
- **S**everity of pain?
- **T**ime of pain? When did the pain start? How long d last? Is it constant or intermittent?

Patient Education *(continued)*

changes, and take medications as prescribed. Exercise as tolerated. Limit alcohol use and discontinue use of tobacco or other substances.

- If prescribed nitroglycerin sublingual tablets for angina, adhere to medication instructions as follows: Take one sublingual tablet if chest pain occurs; if chest pain does not cease after 5 minutes, take another tablet; if another 5 minutes passes and chest pain continues, take a third tablet. After a total of three tablets have been taken, and if angina is still present, call for emergency medical services (EMS). If dizziness or lightheadedness occurs following medication administration, do not take any additional doses and call EMS.
- Recognize signs and symptoms of ACS and seek emergent care for any recurrence of chest pain.
- Follow up with cardiology as instructed for continued monitoring and treatment of cardiac disease.

ANEURYSM

Overview

An *aneurysm* is a weakened area of the artery, causing dilation of the artery that may lead to a dissection of the aortic wall or rupture of the vessel. This can occur throughout the aorta (e.g., abdominal and thoracic).

- A ruptured or dissecting aneurysm can be lethal and requires immediate treatment.
- There are two classification systems to describe the types of aortic dissections based on location of the dissection: the Stanford system and the DeBakey classification system.

[🧠] **COMPLICATIONS**

Dissection, rupture, and thromboembolism are complications of an aneurysm. During a dissection, the force of blood against the weakened vessel splits the layers of the artery wall, and blood leaks between them. A rupture is caused by a burst in the vessel. A thromboembolism is caused by the dilation of the aneurysm, which gives space for a thrombus to form. The thrombus can break off and cause an occlusion distal to the aneurysm. Both rupture and dissection can cause hemorrhagic shock, pericardial tamponade, and death.

Signs and Symptoms

- Absent pulses on one side of the body
- Anxiety
- Back pain
- Can be asymptomatic until the aneurysm ruptures or dissects
- Chest pain "ripping" and radiating to the back (thoracic aortic aneurysm)
- Diastolic murmur
- Lower extremity numbness
- Pulsating mass (abdominal aortic aneurysm [AAA])
- Tachycardia
- Syncope
- Discrepancy in systolic blood pressure of greater than 20 mmHg in each arm
- Narrow pulse pressure

Diagnosis

Labs

There are no lab tests specific to diagnosing an aortic aneurysm. However, the following may be indicated for a patient with a suspected aortic aneurysm/dissection:

- CBC
- CMP
- Coagulation studies ▶

Labs (continued)

- D-dimer
- Troponin
- Type and screen

Diagnostic Testing

- Chest x-ray: possibly showing a new-onset widening of the mediastinum
- CT chest/abdomen with contrast
- Echocardiogram
- Transesophageal echocardiogram
- Ultrasound

Treatment

- Dependent on size and location of aneurysm and whether dissection or rupture has occurred.
- Medical management focused on strict blood pressure and heart rate control. Beta-blockers and vasodilators such as nitroprusside (see Table 2.1) maintain goal heart rate of 60 bpm and systolic blood pressure of 80 to 90 mmHg. Opioid analgesics may be required to maintain pain control to help prevent associated increases in blood pressure and heart rate (see Table A.2).
- Possible need for immediate surgical intervention for a dissecting or ruptured aneurysm; expedited stabilizing interventions necessary to ensure timely surgical intervention to prevent death associated with aortic rupture.

Nursing Interventions

- Place patient on continuous pulse oximetry and cardiac monitoring, alerting emergency provider to any changes in vital signs or cardiac rhythm. Assist with placement and management of arterial line for continuous blood pressure monitoring.
- Apply supplemental oxygen to maintain SpO_2 greater than 94%.
- Establish at least two large-bore IV lines and obtain stat lab studies as ordered.
- Administer and titrate prescribed medications to maintain systolic blood pressure of 80 to 90 mmHg and heart rate of approximately 60 bpm. Frequently reassess pressure or place an arterial line for continuous monitoring.
- Prepare patient for surgery and expedite transfer to the operating room.

Patient Education

- Seek emergent care if chest pain, severe abdominal pain, lightheadedness, or loss of consciousness occurs.
- If discharged with a medically managed aortic aneurysm, such as an AAA measuring less than 5 mm, adhere to instructions regarding ongoing management of the aneurysm. Take all medications as prescribed. Adhere to activity restrictions as instructed. Follow up with cardiology as instructed, including repeat radiographic imaging to monitor for any expansion of the aneurysm. Seek emergent care for any symptoms that may be related to dissection or rupture of the aneurysm, including pain in the chest, back, or abdomen, or lower extremity numbness/tingling or weakness.

 POP QUIZ 2.1

An adult patient arrives at the ED complaining of chest p
The patient has a history of Marfan syndrome, pancreat
and recent tricuspid valve replacement surgery. Vital si
are blood pressure of 200/120 mmHg on the right arm
160/100 mmHg on the left arm and a heart rate of 100 b
What does the nurse suspect as the origin of the patie
pain?

 COMPLICATIONS

Complications from arrhythmias range from mild to dea
including palpitations, lightheadedness, poor cardiac ou
increased risk for thromboembolism, and increased ris
sudden cardiac arrest.

ARRHYTHMIAS

Overview

- *Arrhythmias* are abnormal cardiac rhythms that are a result of disrupted electrical activity; they may be due to a variety of causes and may vary in severity, with some arrhythmias causing minimal symptoms and some leading to sudden cardiac arrest.
- Sinus rhythms originate in the sinoatrial (SA) node, generating a P wave followed by a QRS complex.
- If the sinus node fails, atrial tissue may generate the cardiac impulse, leading to premature atrial contractions or an atrial or supraventricular arrhythmia.
- In atrioventricular (AV) blocks, the electrical signal is blocked or interrupted while traveling from the atria to the ventricles (Figure 2.4).
- When the SA node and atrioventricular (AV) tissues fail to generate an impulse, it leads to premature ventricular contractions or a ventricular arrhythmia (Figure 2.5).
- Arrhythmias may lead to cardiac arrest, requiring immediate implementation of resuscitation efforts following ACLS protocol. An example of asystole is shown in Figure 2.6.
- Patients may have a pacemaker surgically placed due to arrhythmias, and when this device malfunctions, abnormal rhythms can occur.
- Symptoms typically due to decreased cardiac output associated with rhythm abnormalities
- Possibly asymptomatic with mild or transient arrhythmias
- Symptoms for more concerning arrhythmias: anxiety, chest pain, diaphoresis, dizziness, palpitations, shortness of breath, syncope, weakness

Diagnosis

Labs

- CBC
- CMP: electrolyte abnormalities, such as hypo- and hyperkalemia, associated with significant risk for arrhythmias (see Chapter 9, "Medical Emergencies," for more information regarding the importance of maintaining proper electrolyte balance)
- Magnesium: development of arrhythmias if magnesium falls outside normal parameters (1.3–2.1 mEq/L)
- Lactic acid: increased risk for ventricular arrhythmias with acidosis
- Troponin: possible serial testing (q3h × 3)

Diagnostic Testing

- Chest x-ray
- EKG

Treatment

- ACLS resuscitation protocol for any pulseless arrhythmia, including defibrillation where appropriate, as with pulseless ventricular tachycardia (VT), ventricular fibrillation (VF), and torsades de pointes; synchronized cardioversion where appropriate, as

[⚡] **ALERT!**

Lethal rhythms (leading to cardiac standstill if not immediately corrected) include ventricular fibrillation and ventricular tachycardia, torsades de pointes, idioventricular rhythms, agonal rhythms, pulseless electrical activity (PEA), and asystole. Second-degree Mobitz type II and complete heart block may also be deadly.

[⚡] **ALERT!**

A prolonged QT interval (possibly due to overuse of QT-prolonging medications) and hypomagnesemia carry the risk of developing torsades de pointes, a type of polymorphic VT that can lead to cardiac death. Initial treatment of torsades de pointes is magnesium administration. If the patient remains unresponsive to magnesium administration, advanced cardiovascular life support protocol should be followed.

Treatment (continued)

with unstable supraventricular tachycardia (SVT). Alert patients who require cardioversion should receive sedation/pain management for procedure. If patient becomes pulseless, provide high-quality CPR, limiting interruptions in compressions whenever possible. Unstable patients with shockable rhythms such as VF or VT may require multiple defibrillation attempts at 120 to 360 joules to ▶

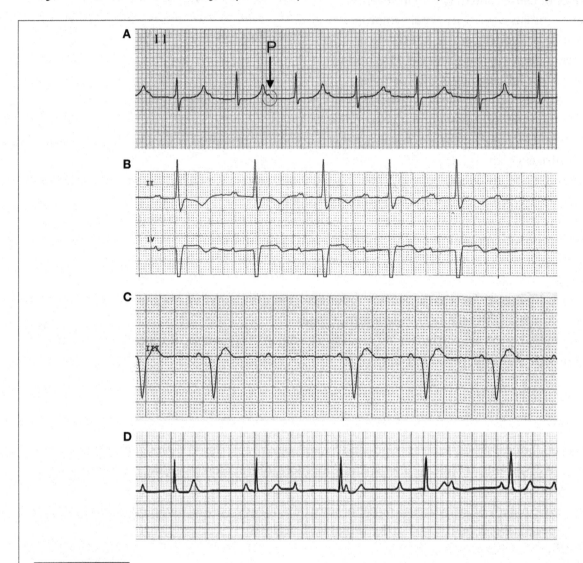

FIGURE 2.4 **(A)** First-degree AV block (PR interval greater than 200 milliseconds). In this image, the PR interval is prolonged to the point that it is nearly hidden by the preceding T wave. **(B)** Second-degree Mobitz type I Wenckebach block (a rhythm with progressively prolonged PR intervals leading to a missed beat). In this image, PR intervals are shown to become progressively longer until the last beat is dropped (final QRS complex is absent). **(C)** Second-degree Mobitz type II block (a dangerous rhythm with a consistent PR interval in which there is a sudden failure in conduction resulting in intermittent missed beats; may progress to third-degree block). In this image, the second P wave shown is missing its corresponding QRS complex. **(D)** Third-degree (or complete) heart block (a potentially lethal rhythm with total loss of electrical communication between the atria and ventricles, leading to a dissociation of P waves from QRS complexes). In this image, P waves have no relationship with QRS complexes; in the first beat, the P wave is hidden within the T wave.

AV, atrioventricular.

Source: Roberts, D. (2020). *Mastering the 12-lead EKG* (2nd ed.). Springer Publishing Company.

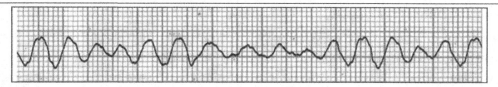

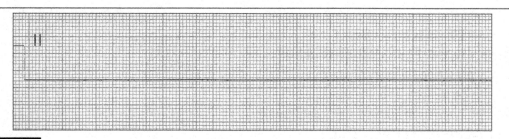

FIGURE 2.5 Ventricular fibrillation (no coordination to generate a heart rate; impulses generated in multiple points throughout ventricular tissue).

Source: Roberts, D. (2020). *Mastering the 12-lead EKG* (2nd ed.). Springer Publishing Company.

FIGURE 2.6 Asystole: the absence of cardiac activity that appears as a "flatline."

Source: Roberts, D. (2020). *Mastering the 12-lead EKG* (2nd ed.). Springer Publishing Company.

Treatment *(continued)*

restore normal rhythm. Patients with organized rhythms such as unstable atrial fibrillation, atrial flutter, or SVT may require synchronized cardioversion to deliver a lower-energy shock (50–20 joules) just after the peak of the R wave.

- Patients experiencing stable SVT: may attempt vagal maneuvers to convert to normal sinus rhythm. Instruct patient to "bear down" for 10 to 15 seconds (may be used in combination with position changes, such as lying supine with lower extremities elevated) to stimulate vagal nerve. If unsuccessful, medications and synchronized cardioversion may be required.
- Transcutaneous or transvenous pacing: may be required for unstable bradycardias
- Urgent cardiology consultation: may be required to determine definitive treatment of arrhythmias, such as placement of a permanent pacemaker for complete heart block or cardiac ablation for SVT
- Medication administration specific to identified conditions (see Table 2.1): antiarrhythmics, atropine, beta-blockers, calcium channel blockers, epinephrine

Nursing Interventions

- Place patient on continuous cardiac monitoring and pulse oximetry. Obtain EKG promptly for interpretation by the emergency provider. Prepare defibrillation pads if indicated.
- If an arrhythmia is noted on cardiac monitoring, palpate pulse, and perform cardiovascular assessment. Alert the emergency provider to any rhythm abnormalities, chest pain, palpitations, or changes in level of consciousness. ▶

[⚡] ALERT!

Synchronized cardioversion precisely times the shock to prevent delivering electricity during cardiac repolarization. If a shock is delivered during repolarization, the patient may go into VF.

[🌐] NURSING PEARL

Implanted devices, such as pacemakers and automatic implantable cardioverter-defibrillators, may be interrogated to transmit valuable information regarding cardiac events and arrhythmias. This allows the ED team to compare the device history with the patient's symptom history.

Nursing Interventions (continued)

- If a pulse is not present, immediately proceed with interventions outlined in ACLS protocol. Attempt to palpate pulse for no more than 10 seconds before proceeding with CPR.
- Establish two large-bore IV lines and administer medications as ordered, such as isotonic crystalloid solutions and antiarrhythmic medications. Draw blood for stat laboratory studies as ordered.
- Assist patient in performing vagal maneuvers, if indicated.
- Frequently reassess vital signs and report any changes in clinical status to the emergency provider.

Patient Education

- Adhere to treatment plan as instructed, including taking all medications as prescribed.
- If arrhythmia is related to an electrolyte disturbance, adhere to any prescribed dietary changes.
- Follow up with cardiology as instructed.
- Seek emergent evaluation if chest pain, palpitations, dizziness, or shortness of breath occur.

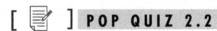

[📝] POP QUIZ 2.2

What is the critical difference when using synchronize cardioversion versus defibrillation?

CARDIOPULMONARY ARREST

Overview

- *Cardiopulmonary arrest* is a sudden disruption in electrical impulses that causes the heart to stop beating.
- Cardiac arrest is often preceded by an abnormal heart rhythm, typically VF or VT.

Signs and Symptoms

- Absence of breathing or pulse
- Agonal breathing
- Lethal cardiac arrhythmia observed on EKG: asystole, VF, pulseless VT, or PEA

Diagnosis

Labs

There are no lab tests specific to diagnosing arrhythmias. However, the following tests may be indicated to determine the underlying pathology leading to the arrest (Table 2.2):

- Arterial blood gas (ABG)/venous blood gas
- CBC
- CMP ▶

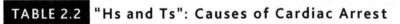

TABLE 2.2 "Hs and Ts": Causes of Cardiac Arrest
• Hypovolemia
• Hypoxia
• Hydrogen ions
• Hypo- or Hyperkalemia
• Hypothermia
• Tension pneumothorax
• Thrombosis, pulmonary
• Thrombosis, coronary
• Tamponade
• Toxins

Labs (continued)
- Coagulation studies
- Drug levels (e.g., digoxin level)

Diagnostic Testing
- Cardiac ultrasound

Treatment

- Resuscitation per ACLS guidelines; attempt to palpate pulse for no more than 10 seconds before initiating compressions; provide high-quality CPR with minimal interruptions in compressions; provide ventilation via bag-valve-mask bag-valve-mask (BVM) until an advanced airway is established to optimize oxygenation during resuscitation.
- Vascular access and labs as ordered; intraosseous access for administration of medications if vascular access not possible
- Medications as ordered/per ACLS protocol, such as epinephrine (repeating dose every 3–5 minutes) and antiarrhythmic agents (such as amiodarone; see Table 2.1)
- Consideration of potential causes of cardiac arrest (see Table 2.2) to determine need for additional therapies. Additional medications, such as magnesium sulfate, sodium bicarbonate, or 50% dextrose, may be indicated to treat reversible causes of cardiac arrest. Emergent procedures may be attempted at the bedside while resuscitation efforts are ongoing, such as needle decompression of pericardial fluid for patients with cardiac tamponade. Further interventions may be required to treat specific conditions, such as PCI for an arrest secondary to coronary thrombosis.
- If resuscitation efforts are successful in restoring cardiac function: Ongoing care and monitoring of hemodynamics and neurologic status required. Post-arrest targeted temperature management to improve neurologic outcomes after cardiac arrest.

Nursing Interventions

- Attempt to palpate carotid pulse for no more than 10 seconds. If pulse is not present, immediately begin chest compressions and call for assistance.
- Continue resuscitation interventions per ACLS protocol, providing high-quality CPR with minimal interruptions.
- Place patient on continuous cardiac monitoring and apply defibrillator pads.
- Provide ventilation via BVM until advanced airway is established. Assist with placement and monitoring of advanced airway.
- Establish vascular or intraosseous access and administer medications as prescribed.
- Draw blood for lab tests as ordered, if possible.
- Assist with bedside procedures, such as needle decompression or chest tube placement, if needed.
- If cardiac function is restored, initiate targeted temperature management and expedite transfer to critical care unit for ongoing care and monitoring.

Patient Education

- Mitigate risk for cardiac arrest by managing any existing disease. Adhere to any prescribed treatment plans, including taking all medications as prescribed. ▶

 POP QUIZ 2.3

An adult patient arrives at the ED via ambulance after a syncopal episode. After transferring to the ED stretcher, the patient becomes unresponsive and the cardiac monitor shows VT. What action should the nurse take first?

 COMPLICATIONS

Complications from endocarditis may occur when infected material breaks off, forming septic emboli. This may then travel throughout the body and cause an abscess in the lungs or brain, meningitis, a pulmonary embolism (PE), or stroke. Endocarditis can also cause arrhythmias and sepsis.

Patient Education (continued)

- Participate in lifestyle changes to reduce risk of cardiac disease, such as maintaining a nutritious diet, increasing physical activity (as tolerated), and quitting smoking.

ENDOCARDITIS

Overview

- *Endocarditis* is a condition in which the heart's lining, chamber, valves, and blood vessels become infected and inflamed.
- Endocarditis may be caused by infectious material clumping on the valves or the lining of the heart.
- Infectious material may be bacterial or fungal.
- Bacterial infection in endocarditis is typically due to *Staphylococcus* or *Streptococcus*.

Signs and Symptoms

- Chest pain
- Chills
- Cough
- Dermatologic changes: Osler nodes—painful lesions on fingertips and toes; Janeway lesions—painless lesions on the palms and soles of feet
- Fever
- Heart murmur
- Night sweats

Diagnosis

Labs

- Blood cultures: may isolate microorganisms responsible for infection. Delay antibiotic administration until at least two sets of blood cultures drawn.
- CBC: possible leukocytosis and anemia
- CMP
- C-reactive protein (CRP): typically elevated and expected to gradually decrease within first week of antibiotic treatment. Persistently elevated CRP is possible indicator of poor outcomes.
- Erythrocyte sedimentation rate (ESR): elevated ESR in endocarditis
- Troponin: may be elevated in endocarditis. Persistent elevation is possible predictor of poor outcomes and heart failure.

Diagnostic Testing

- Cardiac CT angiography
- EKG: increased PR interval, low-voltage QRS, AV blocks, and STEMI
- Echocardiogram

Treatment

- Antibiotic administration for treatment of underlying bacterial infection (see Table A.1)
- Anti-inflammatory medications (e.g., steroids) to help minimize tissue damage by decreasing inflammation (see Table A.4)
- Possible repeat lab testing to reassess troponin, ESR, and CRP to monitor progression
- Surgical intervention: may be required for repair or replacement of the damaged valve

Nursing Interventions

- Perform head-to-toe assessment with focus on cardiac and respiratory assessments.
- Place patient on continuous pulse oximetry and cardiac monitoring. Frequently reassess vital signs and alert provider to any changes in cardiac rhythm, chest pain, or abnormal vital signs.
- Establish IV access and draw blood for cultures and laboratory studies as ordered. Placement of a peripherally inserted central catheter (PICC) line may be indicated for continued administration of IV antibiotics.
- Administer medications as ordered, such as antibiotics and corticosteroids.
- Assess pain and medicate patient as ordered, alerting provider to any development of, or changes in, chest pain.
- Monitor temperature and administer antipyretic as needed.
- Prepare patient for surgical valve repair or replacement.

Patient Education

- Manage risk factors for endocarditis. Know that bacteria may be introduced into the bloodstream by contaminated needles used for injection of IV drugs. Explore resources for substance use cessation and harm reduction, if needed. Maintain good dental hygiene practices to prevent endocarditis. Take any prophylactic antibiotics prior to future dental procedures, if ordered.
- Understand that a PICC line may remain in place upon discharge for continued antibiotic therapy. Use PICC line exclusively as directed. Inspect site and dressing daily and keep area clean to prevent serious infection. Follow up with home care resources as instructed to continue prescribed antibiotic treatment and facilitate ongoing care of the PICC line. Follow up for reevaluation and PICC removal.
- Follow up with cardiology as instructed.
- Seek emergent care if severe chest pain, shortness of breath, fevers, or altered mental status occur.

HEART FAILURE

Overview

- *Heart failure (HF)* is the result of left, right, or biventricular failure to maintain adequate cardiac output, whether due to a functional issue, such as arrhythmias, or a structural problem, such as valvular stenosis. Left HF often leads to right HF. Left ventricular failure may be further classified as systolic or diastolic dysfunction. Systolic dysfunction results in poor pumping action of the left ventricle, leading to decreased ejection fraction, while diastolic dysfunction refers to poor ventricular filling, causing ejection fraction to remain normal.

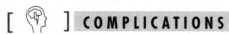 **COMPLICATIONS**

Complications that can arise from HF include arrhythmias, malnutrition, peripheral edema, and pulmonary hypertension.

- HF may present as an acute or a chronic problem. Acute presentation could be the result of an infection, damage from ACS, or a PE. Chronic presentation is the result of chronic medical conditions that affect the heart, such as cardiomyopathy, chronic hypertension, or valvular heart disease. Acute decompensated HF, whether a new-onset HF or an acute exacerbation of chronic failure, is life threatening, and treatment with ventilatory support and diuretic medications is vital in preventing onset of cardiogenic shock. Inotropic agents may be required for management of hypotension and poor ejection fraction.

Signs and Symptoms

- Abdominal discomfort/swelling due to ascites or hepatic congestion in right HF
- Bilateral rales (usually occurring in biventricular/left-sided HF)

Signs and Symptoms (continued)

- Cough
- Dependent edema
- Fatigue
- Fluid retention/weight gain (generally greater than 2–3 lb in 24 hours)
- Jugular venous distention
- Orthopnea
- S3 gallop
- Shortness of breath
- Weakness

Diagnosis

Labs

- Brain natriuretic peptide (BNP): degree of elevation may reflect severity of HF
- CBC
- CMP
- Troponin

Diagnostic Testing

- Chest x-ray
- EKG
- Nuclear stress test

[⚡] **ALERT!**

BNP is a hormone released by the heart when ventricul... stretching occurs. Diagnosis of CHF may be general... excluded if serum BNP is below 100 pg/mL.

Treatment

- Largely dictated by course of disease (compensated vs. uncompensated) and whether uncompensated congestive heart failure (CHF) is acute or chronic. Compensated chronic CHF treatment focused on lifestyle modification and long-term adherence to the therapeutic plan, including compliance with sodium and fluid restrictions as well as medication administration (see Table 2.1). Uncompensated CHF may occur in acute or chronic presentations of HF and requires more aggressive treatment to achieve and maintain hemodynamic stability.
- Possible cardiac surgical intervention to achieve hemodynamic stability necessary to treat underlying cause. Coronary artery bypass grafting or angioplasty may be indicated to revascularize cardiac tissue in patients with ischemic disease. An intra-aortic balloon pump or ventricular assist device may be used to maintain adequate cardiac output while awaiting further surgical intervention, such as valve repair or replacement or cardiac transplant.

Nursing Interventions

- Adhere to fluid and sodium restrictions as ordered, monitoring both oral and parenteral intake.
- Administer medications as ordered, titrating infusions as prescribed.
- Administer supplemental oxygen for treatment of hypoxia. Trial of high-flow oxygen via non-rebreather mask or noninvasive ventilation may be attempted. Prepare for intubation if SpO$_2$ greater than 90% is not achieved with noninvasive measures.
- Assist patient to rest in high-Fowler's position to promote adequate ventilation.
- Establish IV access, drawing blood for lab studies as ordered.
- Place patient on continuous pulse oximetry and cardiac monitoring, frequently reassessing vital signs and alerting emergency provider to any concerning changes in heart rate, blood pressure, or cardiac ▶

Nursing Interventions *(continued)*

rhythm. Placement of an arterial line for continuous blood pressure monitoring may be indicated. Assist to obtain an EKG for prompt interpretation by the emergency provider.

- Place a urinary catheter, if ordered, and monitor intake/output (I/O).

Patient Education

- Manage risk factors for development of CHF. Explore resources for detox or cessation of habits that increase risk, such as smoking and alcohol or substance use. Maintain a nutritious diet and exercise as tolerated. Manage chronic disease, which may lead to the development or worsening of CHF, such as atrial fibrillation, coronary artery disease, or valve issues.
- Adhere to any prescribed sodium and/or fluid restrictions.
- Take all medications as prescribed.
- Seek emergent evaluation if shortness of breath, chest pain, palpitations, increase in swelling (particularly to lower extremities), lightheadedness, or altered mental status occur.
- Monitor weight daily if advised to do so, and return for evaluation if weight increases by more than 3 lb.
- Follow up with cardiology for continued monitoring and disease management.

HYPERTENSION

Overview

- *Hypertension* is one of the most common chronic conditions; it is chronically elevated blood pressure defined by systolic pressure above 130 mmHg and diastolic pressure above 80 mmHg. Primary hypertension is thought to be largely related to lifestyle factors, such as high salt intake, sedentary lifestyle, and smoking. Secondary hypertension refers to elevated blood pressure due to other medical conditions, such as renal disease and pregnancy.
- Chronic hypertension places patients at increased risk for other conditions, such as HF, renal failure, stroke, and MI. Table 2.3 outlines the stages of hypertension. ▶

[ ] **COMPLICATIONS**

Untreated hypertensive emergency may result in serious complications, such as neurologic deficits, aortic dissection, chest pain, myocardial infarction, pulmonary edema, and stroke.

TABLE 2.3 Stages of Hypertension	
CATEGORY	**BLOOD PRESSURE VALUES (mmHg)**
Normal	Systolic less than 120
	Diastolic less than 80
Elevated	Systolic 120–129
	Diastolic less than 80
Stage 1 hypertension	Systolic 130–139
	Diastolic 80–89
Stage 2 hypertension	Systolic greater than 140
	Diastolic greater than or equal to 90
Stage 3 hypertension (hypertensive crisis)	Systolic greater than 180
	Diastolic greater than or equal to 120

Source: Data from the American Heart Association. (n.d.). *The facts about high blood pressure.* https://www.heart.org/en/health-topics/high-blood-pressure

Overview (*continued*)

- *Hypertensive crisis* is defined as a sudden increase in blood pressure with a systolic pressure of 180 mmHg or greater and a diastolic pressure of 120 mmHg or greater. It is categorized as hypertensive urgency or hypertensive emergency. *Hypertensive urgency* usually develops over the course of days or weeks, does not typically require hospitalization, and occurs without signs of end-organ damage. *Hypertensive emergency* is a sudden significant elevation in blood pressure in which signs of organ damage are present, such as renal failure, pulmonary edema, or neurologic compromise. It requires close monitoring and interventions to decrease blood pressure to prevent further organ damage.

Signs and Symptoms

- Anxiety
- Blurry vision
- Epistaxis
- Headache
- With progression to hypertensive emergency, signs of possible end-organ damage: Cardiovascular: angina, HF, and shortness of breath; neurologic: altered mental status, hypertensive encephalopathy, intracerebral hemorrhage, seizures, and stroke; ocular: retinal hemorrhage and papilledema; renal: acute kidney failure and acute kidney injury.

Diagnosis

Labs

- CBC
- CMP
- Coagulation panel
- BNP
- Troponin

Diagnostic Testing

There are no tests specific to diagnosing hypertensive crises. However, the following may be used in establishing a differential diagnosis and investigating associated conditions:

- Chest x-ray
- CT (head, chest)
- EKG
- Eye examination and visual acuity test (if ocular symptoms are present)

Treatment

- Management focused on reducing blood pressure with antihypertensive medications, such as nitrates and beta-blockers (see Table 2.1)
- Possible placement of an arterial line for continuous blood pressure monitoring
- Varied treatment goals depending on whether organ damage has occurred and which body system is affected. If possible per patient condition, treatment goal should be to lower blood pressure by no more than 25% within the first hour, then achieve blood pressure of 160/100 mmHg within the following 2 to 4 hours, then return to baseline within 24 to 48 hours. If aortic dissection is suspected, patients require more aggressive management to lower blood pressure.
- Possible additional treatment depending on suspected cause of hypertensive emergency. Noncompliance with prescribed medication regimen is the leading cause of hypertensive crises in patients with chronic hypertension. Patients may require treatment for conditions such as thyroid dysfunction and renal disease, which may precipitate a hypertensive crisis.

Nursing Interventions

- Administer supplemental oxygen as indicated.
- Establish IV access and administer medications as prescribed, titrating antihypertensive therapy to parameters as ordered.
- Place patient on continuous pulse oximetry and cardiac monitoring, alerting emergency provider to changes in vital signs or cardiac rhythm. Reassess blood pressure frequently, assisting to place and monitor arterial line if needed. Assist to quickly obtain an EKG for interpretation by the emergency provider.
- Perform thorough head-to-toe assessment, noting any changes or deficits that may indicate organ damage, such as visual disturbances or crackles upon lung auscultation.
- Monitor I/O, placing indwelling urinary catheter if indicated.
- Monitor patient condition as blood pressure decreases. Alert provider and adjust medications appropriately if symptoms of poor coronary, cerebral, or renal perfusion occur, such as altered mental status/loss of consciousness or decreased urinary output.

Patient Education

- Recognize signs and symptoms of elevated blood pressure and hypertensive crisis.
- Decrease risk for hypertension and cardiovascular disease with lifestyle changes such as smoking cessation and reduced-sodium diet.
- If advised to monitor blood pressure at home using an automatic blood pressure cuff, follow instructions regarding use of automatic cuff, logging record of pressures, and reporting changes in blood pressure to primary care provider or cardiologist upon follow-up.
- If chronic hypertension, adhere to medication regimen as prescribed to prevent hypertensive crisis.
- If hypertensive crisis is related to substance use, explore resources for substance use disorder treatment.
- Return for emergent evaluation if symptoms such as chest pain, shortness of breath, blurred vision, or severe headache occur.

> **[📝] POP QUIZ 2.4**
>
> An adult patient is being treated for hypertensive emergency in the ED. The initial blood pressure reading was 220/120 mmHg. The patient was given one sublingual nitrogen tablet and placed on a nitroglycerin infusion. Fifteen minutes later, the patient appears confused with altered mental status. Upon reassessment, blood pressure is now 140/88 mmHg. What is the most likely cause of the change in mental status?

PERICARDIAL TAMPONADE

Overview

- *Pericardial tamponade*, or cardiac tamponade, is an increase in fluid in the pericardial sac, which can compress the chambers of the heart and lead to decreased cardiac output.

> **[ ] COMPLICATIONS**
>
> Complications from pericardial tamponade include obstructive shock and death.

- Fluid may fill the pericardial sac quickly or accumulate slowly over time; fluid may be classified as hemorrhagic, serosanguineous, or exudative. Hemorrhagic pericardial effusion often occurs secondary to penetrating or blunt cardiac trauma, with rapid fluid accumulation requiring emergent intervention to control bleeding and relieve compression of the heart to restore adequate cardiac output. Serosanguineous or exudative effusion may occur secondary to infection or malignancy, and fluid often accumulates more gradually.

- Emergent intervention is required to remove fluid and reduce pressure on the heart, restoring cardiac output.

Signs and Symptoms

- Beck's triad: hypotension; jugular venous distention (JVD); muffled or absent heart tones
- Chest pain
- Dyspnea
- Pulsus paradoxus: a decrease in systolic pressure upon inspiration of 10 mmHg or more
- Abnormal cardiac rhythm: may initially present with tachycardia as the heart attempts to compensate for reduced cardiac output; may progress to cardiac arrest/PEA as pumping action of the heart becomes increasingly impaired

Diagnosis

Labs

Varied based on clinical presentation:

- Antinuclear antibody titers, if autoimmune disease is suspected
- CBC
- CMP
- Troponin
- Type and screen

Diagnostic Testing

- Chest x-ray
- EKG
- Echocardiogram

Treatment

- Possible emergent needle aspiration of pericardial fluid at bedside
- Surgical management if pericardiocentesis is needed to create pericardial window (pericardiectomy)
- Emergent resuscitative thoracotomy possible in patients with cardiac tamponade with traumatic cardiac arrest

Nursing Interventions

- Place patient on continuous pulse oximetry and cardiac monitoring, alerting emergency provider to changes in vital signs or cardiac rhythm. If a pulse is not present, proceed immediately with resuscitation per ACLS guidelines. Reassess blood pressure frequently, assisting to place and monitor arterial line if needed. Assist to quickly obtain an EKG for interpretation by the emergency provider.
- Perform head-to-toe assessment with focus on cardiovascular evaluation, noting any JVD or muffled heart sounds. If traumatic chest injury is suspected, perform complete trauma assessment, noting further injuries and maintaining spinal immobilization if indicated.
- Establish IV access and administer medications as prescribed.
- Assist emergency provider with pericardiocentesis, if needed. Elevate head of bed to 30 to 45 degrees to place patient in semi-Fowler's position; Prepare necessary equipment, such as bedside ultrasound, 16- to 18-G needle, guidewire, and sterile drapes. A drainage catheter may remain in place; assess site and monitor output, alerting provider to changes in output quantity or quality of drainage. Closely monitor cardiac rhythm and vital signs throughout procedure, proceeding with resuscitation interventions per ACLS guidelines if cardiac arrest occurs.
- Expedite transfer to operating room for surgical intervention.

Patient Education

- Learn about risk factors for pericardial effusion and cardiac tamponade.
- Return for emergent evaluation if experiencing chest pain, shortness of breath, and distended neck veins.
- Adhere to treatment plans, including taking all medications as prescribed and following up with cardiology.

PERICARDITIS

Overview

- *Pericarditis* refers to inflammation of the pericardial sac, which most often occurs secondary to infection (viral or bacterial), although this condition may also occur secondary to a variety of causes such as chest trauma, radiation, malignancy, or autoimmune conditions.

Signs and Symptoms

- Chest pain with inspiration
- Chills
- Dyspnea
- Fever
- Pain with lying flat; sitting up and forward can ease pain
- Pleural friction rub
- Tachycardia

Diagnosis

Labs

- Blood cultures
- CBC: patients likely to develop leukocytosis
- CMP
- CRP: typically elevated in pericarditis
- ESR: typically elevated in pericarditis; elevation may be associated with increased risk for prolonged inflammation and disease recurrence
- Troponin

Diagnostic Testing

- Cardiac CT
- Cardiac MRI
- EKG: ST segment elevation of 1 to 3 mm noted in all leads except aVR and V1
- Echocardiogram

[📝] **POP QUIZ 2.5**

An adult patient presents to the ED complaining of chest and abdominal pain and stating that they are currently receiving chemotherapy for lung cancer. Upon assessment, the patient is noted to have distant heart tones, distended neck veins, and shortness of breath, with a blood pressure of 89/60 mmHg. What concerning triad of symptoms is this patient exhibiting?

[🧠] **COMPLICATIONS**

Complications of pericarditis include pericardial effusion, cardiac tamponade, and chronic constrictive pericarditis.

[⚡] **ALERT!**

Troponin levels may be elevated in pericarditis because pericardial inflammation may progress to perimyocardial inflammation, leading to necrosis of myocardial tissue.

Treatment

- Anti-inflammatory drug: benefits for all patients
- Further treatment guided by suspected etiology: Otherwise healthy patient, suspected bacterial infection—antibiotics. Autoimmune pericarditis—may benefit from IV immunoglobulin. Immunocompromised patients, those experiencing signs of hemodynamic instability or systemic infection, those with large pericardial effusions or signs of cardiac tamponade, and those with an elevated troponin level require hospital admission for continued treatment and monitoring.
- Medical management: focused on reducing inflammation using nonsteroidal anti-inflammatory drugs (NSAIDs) and colchicine (see Table 2.1)
- Consult to cardiology for continued management

Nursing Interventions

- Administer medications as prescribed.
- Assess pain and administer medications as ordered.
- Assist with patient positioning; patients may feel most comfortable in high-Fowler's position.
- Establish IV access and draw blood for lab tests and blood cultures as ordered.
- Perform head-to-toe assessment with focused cardiovascular and respiratory evaluation, alerting emergency provider to any abnormal heart sounds, chest pain, or shortness of breath.
- Place patient on continuous pulse oximetry and cardiac monitoring, alerting emergency provider to changes in vital signs or cardiac rhythm. Apply supplemental oxygen if needed to maintain SpO_2 greater than 95%. Assist to quickly obtain an EKG for interpretation by the emergency provider.

Patient Education

- Adhere to activity restrictions as prescribed, avoiding strenuous activity until symptoms resolve and biomarkers return to normal.
- Adhere to treatment plan, including taking all medications as prescribed and following up with cardiology as ordered.
- Expect to experience some pain for up to 3 months, although pleuritic chest pain should improve within the first week of treatment. Return for evaluation if no symptom improvement occurs within 1 week or if worsening symptoms, such as severe chest pain or shortness of breath, occur.
- Follow up with specialist providers to address the etiology of pericarditis, such as treatment with oncology or rheumatology to manage underlying disease.
- If biomarkers are elevated upon diagnosis (such as an elevated CRP level), return for repeat serum testing as ordered to ensure that elevations normalize over time.

[ ] **POP QUIZ 2.6**

An adult patient presents to the ED complaining midsternal chest pain, stating that the pain is worst wh[en] supine and improves upon sitting up and leaning sligh[tly] forward. What condition would the nurse suspect?

PERIPHERAL VASCULAR DISEASE

Overview

- *Peripheral vascular disease (PVD)* is a chronic condition in which blocked or narrowed vessels cause impaired circulation that progressively worsens over time. *Atherosclerosis*, or the buildup of plaque that causes narrowing of the vessels, is the most common cause of PVD.

[ ] 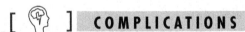   **COMPLICATIONS**

Complications of PVD include AMI, coronary artery dise[ase,] decreased mobility, infections, limb ischemia, sores, stroke.

Signs and Symptoms

Patients with PVD may be asymptomatic initially but experience worsening symptoms as the disease progresses, such as:

- Cool skin temperature
- Decreased or absent pulses in one or both feet
- Intermittent claudication (lower extremity pain/ cramping with activity that resolves with rest)
- Lack of toenail or leg-hair growth
- Pale or discolored leg or foot
- Shiny skin
- Poor wound healing

Diagnosis

Labs

There are no lab tests specific to diagnosing PVD. However, the following may be helpful in investigating symptoms:

- CBC
- CMP
- D-dimer
- Lipid panel

Diagnostic Testing

- Ankle-brachial index (ABI) assessment
- CT angiogram
- Doppler ultrasound
- MRA

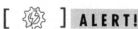

[🌐] NURSING PEARL

The 6 Ps of Limb Ischemia:

- Pain, usually located distal to ischemia; can be severe initially followed by absent pain due to sensory loss
- Pallor
- Paralysis
- Paresthesia
- Poikilothermia
- Pulselessness

[⚡] ALERT!

ABI assessment evaluates discrepancies in blood pressure between upper and lower extremities. While this testing is not often conducted in the ED, it can provide valuable insight regarding diagnosis and progression of vascular disease. ABI normal range is between 1.0 and 1.4, with a value of 0.9 or below considered to be diagnostic of peripheral arterial disease (PAD). Values below 0.5 are indicative of severe PAD.

Treatment

- Emergent management not likely in ED due to chronic condition. Possible treatment of acute exacerbations of lower extremity pain or other PVD-related concerns, such as poor peripheral pulses, pallor, paresthesia, or poor wound healing. Evaluation vital to rule out conditions that present similarly (e.g., deep vein thrombosis [DVT]).
- Risk factors addressed. Lifestyle changes, such as smoking cessation and routine exercise, to reduce risk of worsening condition. Management of chronic diseases that contribute to development of PVD—such as diabetes, hypertension, and hyperlipidemia—to reduce vascular damage.
- Medications to control symptoms and progression (see Table 2.1). Platelet-aggregation inhibitors (e.g., cilostazol) to relieve symptoms of intermittent claudication. Antiplatelet drugs (e.g., clopidogrel) to help prevent blood clotting. Statins (e.g., atorvastatin) to treat hyperlipidemia and prevent worsening atherosclerosis.
- Depending on severity of PVD, possible surgical intervention. Angioplasty to dilate sclerosed vessels; stents may be placed to maintain vascular patency; peripheral vascular bypass possible to divert blood flow around an occluded vessel.

Nursing Interventions

- Administer medications as prescribed.
- Assess skin color, temperature, and moisture, noting any wounds or ulcerations, and discuss wound history with patient. ▶

Nursing Interventions (continued)

- Establish IV access, if needed, and draw blood for lab tests as ordered.
- Perform thorough head-to-toe assessment, paying particular attention to assessment of peripheral pulses. Doppler ultrasound may be used to assess pulses if not easily palpable.
- Perform wound care as needed.

Patient Education

- Manage risk factors to prevent development or worsening of PVD. Seek support for smoking cessation, if applicable. Adopt healthy habits, such as routine exercise and heart-healthy diet. Manage chronic conditions that increase risk for PVD, such as diabetes and hyperlipidemia.
- Take all medications as prescribed. If prescribed anticoagulant or antiplatelet therapy, be aware of increased risk for bleeding, and seek emergent evaluation if uncontrolled bleeding occurs.
- Follow up with cardiology as instructed.

[📝] **POP QUIZ 2.7**

An adult patient with a history of PVD, chronic obstructiv pulmonary disease, and hyperlipidemia presents to the E complaining of intermittent cramping calf pain with activit that improves with rest. What condition does the nurs suspect?

SHOCK

Overview

- *Shock* is a state of inadequate perfusion in which oxygen delivery cannot meet oxygen demand, which can lead to multiorgan dysfunction, failure, and death.
- Shock may be classified as cardiogenic, hypovolemic, distributive, or obstructive. *Cardiogenic shock* is decreased cardiac output secondary to ineffective pumping action of the heart; it may occur secondary to an AMI, arrhythmias, or a structural issue such as a valve problem. *Hypovolemic shock* is caused by severe body fluid or blood loss that reduces circulating blood volume; it may be caused by hemorrhage, severe vomiting or diarrhea, or fluid loss from burn injuries. *Distributive shock* occurs when systemic vasodilation leads to inadequate perfusion of vital organs; it may occur secondary to sepsis or anaphylaxis. *Obstructive shock* is impairment of circulation due to a physical obstruction of the heart's vessels; it may be caused by an issue with diastole, as in cases of tension pneumothorax, or an issue with systolic flow, as in left ventricular outflow obstruction or PE.
- Shock progresses through four stages: In initial nonprogressive shock, cardiac output decreases, and tissue perfusion becomes compromised. In the compensatory phase, the body attempts to maintain cardiac output to maintain adequate perfusion. In the progressive stage, compensatory mechanisms begin to fail, and normal metabolism is disrupted. If shock progresses to the refractory stage, the process is considered to be irreversible, and the patient is no longer responsive to therapies.

[🧠] **COMPLICATIONS**

Complications of shock include organ damage and death.

Signs and Symptoms

Symptoms evolve as shock progresses through each phase, initially demonstrating few symptoms, then progressing as compensatory mechanisms fail.

- Compensatory phase: flash capillary refill; normal blood pressure to mild hypotension (mean arterial pressure [MAP] 10–15 mmHg below baseline); tachycardia; tachypnea; slight elevation in serum lactic acid.   ▶

Signs and Symptoms *(continued)*

- Progressive phase: altered mental status/loss of consciousness; cool, clammy skin/pallor; hypotension (MAP 20 mmHg below baseline); oliguria; tachycardia with weak pulse; marked increase in serum lactic acid.
- Refractory phase: multiorgan failure; profound hypotension (systolic less than 70 mmHg); shock persistent (as evidenced by bradycardia, bradypnea, and high serum lactic acid) despite correction of hemodynamic issues (e.g., sufficient volume replacement).

Diagnosis

Labs

The following lab tests may be indicated, although diagnostic evaluation may vary depending on suspected etiology of shock.

- ABG
- Blood cultures
- CBC
- CMP
- Lactic acid
- Troponin
- Type and screen

Diagnostic Testing

- Chest x-ray
- Echocardiogram
- Ultrasound

Treatment

- Varied treatment depending on suspected etiology of shock
- Fluid resuscitation with isotonic crystalloid bolus likely in all cases
- Likely to require increasingly supportive interventions, such as mechanical ventilation, renal dialysis, and extracorporeal membrane oxygenation (ECMO), to sustain life as shock progresses
- Hypovolemic shock: fluid administration primary means of correcting hemodynamic changes. Hypovolemia due to uncontrolled hemorrhage: bleeding controlled and blood products administered to restore hemodynamic stability. Fluid losses related to vomiting or diarrhea: medications such as antiemetics possible to control symptoms (see Table A.2). Burn injuries with combination of hypovolemic and distributive shock: fluid resuscitation per facility's burn fluid replacement protocol to maintain hemodynamic stability without causing fluid overload.
- Distributive shock: fluid resuscitation, although more likely to require vasopressor support to maintain adequate circulation. Septic shock: often requires aggressive fluid resuscitation with vasopressors such as norepinephrine to maintain tissue perfusion. Anaphylactic shock: relies on removal of the allergen, if possible, and immediate administration of epinephrine (intramuscular administration followed by additional intramuscular or IV administration if needed) (see Table 2.1).
- Cardiogenic shock: fluid administration more conservative, more likely to require vasopressors to improve pumping action of the heart. Antiarrhythmic medications (see Table 2.1) to correct abnormal rhythms. Anticoagulants and antiplatelet medications (see Table 2.1) to relieve/prevent further coronary blockages. PCI or bypass grafting possible to restore normal circulation.
- Obstructive shock: primary treatment goal to identify and remove obstruction; interventions specific to the cause. Cardiac tamponade: needle aspiration to clear some fluid to restore cardiac function, although pericardial window likely needed. Tension pneumothorax: immediate needle decompression to relieve obstruction before chest tube placement possible.

Nursing Interventions

- Establish IV access, drawing blood for lab tests as ordered, and administer medications as prescribed. Placement of at least two large-bore peripheral IV lines is required initially to begin shock resuscitation. Assist provider with central line placement; monitor site and dressing. Administer IV fluids per orders or per appropriate algorithm (sepsis algorithm, burn fluid resuscitation protocol). Administer blood products as ordered. Alert blood bank immediately if emergency release blood/mass transfusion protocol is required.
- Expedite transfer for surgical intervention/PCI if needed.
- Expedite transfer to critical care unit for continued treatment and monitoring.
- Perform head-to-toe assessment with focus on cardiovascular and respiratory evaluation. Administer supplemental oxygen to maintain SpO_2 greater than 90%. Mechanical ventilation is often required; assist with placement and management of endotracheal tube (ETT) or noninvasive ventilation if needed.
- Place patient on continuous pulse oximetry and cardiac monitoring, alerting emergency provider to changes in vital signs or cardiac rhythm. If pulse is not present, proceed immediately with resuscitation per ACLS guidelines. Reassess blood pressure frequently, assisting to place and monitor arterial line if needed. Assist to quickly obtain an EKG for interpretation by the emergency provider.

Patient Education

- If known cardiac condition, follow up with cardiology for ongoing disease management. Seek emergent evaluation if chest pain, shortness of breath, sudden weight gain, or swelling occurs.
- If prescribed an epinephrine auto-injector, follow instructions regarding how and when to administer the medication. Keep two auto-injectors available at all times, and always seek emergent care after using epinephrine.
- If prescribed anticoagulant therapy, be aware of risk for bleeding and seek emergent evaluation if uncontrolled bleeding occurs. Monitor for signs of gastrointestinal bleeding, such as abdominal discomfort; coffee-ground emesis; and dark, tarry stools.
- Maintain adequate nutrition and hydration. Seek treatment if prolonged vomiting or diarrhea occurs.
- Seek emergent care of any suspected allergic reaction with airway involvement, as evidenced by facial or oral lesions or swelling, throat or chest tightness, or shortness of breath.
- Take general safety precautions to prevent traumatic injury, such as wearing a seat belt and removing trip hazards within the home.

[📝] **POP QUIZ 2.8**

An older adult patient presents to the ED via ambulan[ce] after having been found unresponsive by a family memb[er]. The patient appears pale with shallow, rapid respiratio[ns]. The patient is tachycardic with a heart rate of 136 bpm a[nd] a blood pressure of 72/50 mmHg. The patient's adult ch[ild] states that the patient has a history of congestive he[art] failure and coronary artery disease. EKG shows an AMI. [In] addition to the MI, what condition would the nurse suspe[ct]?

THROMBOEMBOLIC DISEASE

Overview

- *Thrombosis* refers to the formation of a blood clot within an artery or vein, leading to ischemia. Thrombosis can occur anywhere in the body, leading to events such as ischemic stroke, MI, PE, and DVT. It may occur as a result of venous or arterial stasis, vascular damage, or hypercoagulability.
- Many factors place patients at increased risk for venous thromboembolism (VTE; e.g., DVT and PE), such as decreased mobility due to activity restrictions, injury, or paralysis; use of medications such as birth control or estrogen therapy; hypercoagulable states such as those of pregnant and postpartum (up to 6 weeks) patients; and some chronic conditions, such as coronary artery disease and metastatic disease. Acute ▶

Overview *(continued)*

injuries, such as lower limb fracture, major trauma, or hip/knee replacements, also increase risk for VTE. *DVT*, a clot within the deep veins of the pelvis or upper or lower extremities, impairs blood return from the affected extremity. When a clot dislodges, it often travels to pulmonary vasculature, referred to as a PE; PE is a leading cause of sudden cardiac arrest because the clot causes an acute obstruction of pulmonary circulation that may impair right ventricular outflow, leading to obstructive shock.

Signs and Symptoms

Symptoms related to thrombosis are specific to the affected organ:

- MI
- PE
- Ischemic stroke
- DVT: unilateral limb pain, tenderness upon palpation; unilateral limb edema, erythema, and/or warmth

Diagnosis

Labs

- Coagulation panel
- D-dimer

Diagnostic Testing

There are no tests specific to diagnosing thromboembolic disease. However, diagnostic tests may be required to rule out further complications of thromboembolic disease, such as the following to rule out DVT:

- Duplex ultrasound
- MRI

Treatment

- Anticoagulation: primary therapy for VTE. Hospitalized patients may receive IV heparin before transitioning to oral therapy (see Table 2.1). Preferred oral therapy for DVT uses direct-acting anticoagulants such as apixaban or rivaroxaban (see Table 2.1). Duration of anticoagulant therapy varies depending on suspected etiology of the thrombus; patients with no known inciting factor may remain anticoagulated indefinitely to reduce risk of recurrence.
- Patients who are poor candidates for anticoagulation: possible surgical placement of an inferior vena cava filter to prevent embolization to the lungs
- Patients at risk for thrombosis or with known DVT: monitoring for complications such as PE and ischemic stroke

Nursing Interventions

- Administer medications, such as anticoagulants, as ordered. Provide patient with teaching regarding anticoagulant therapy.
- Draw labs as ordered. Placement of a peripheral IV may also be necessary, depending on patient condition. ▶

[ ]   **ALERT!**

Serious complications are associated with thromboembolic disease. Clots that mobilize to the brain can lead to ischemic stroke, and clots within cardiac vasculature can lead to MI. Pulmonary hypertension, pulmonary vascular disease, and sudden cardiac arrest may occur as a result of PE. Patients who have experienced DVT are at increased risk for post-thrombotic syndrome, characterized by recurrent DVT and chronic pain and swelling in the affected extremity. Patients may also experience complications related to anticoagulation required after a thromboembolic event.

[ ]   **NURSING PEARL**

D-dimer, a product of fibrinolysis, serves as a sensitive indicator of DVT, although it is not very specific. An elevated D-dimer may be found in other conditions, such as heart disease and malignancy.

Nursing Interventions *(continued)*

- If indicated, place patient on continuous pulse oximetry and cardiac monitoring, alerting provider to any change in vital signs or cardiac rhythm. If indicated, assist to quickly obtain an EKG for interpretation by the emergency provider.
- Perform frequent neurologic and respiratory assessments. Alert provider to any changes in patient condition.
- Perform thorough head-to-toe assessment, with particular attention to circulatory assessment, noting quality of peripheral pulses, as well as any edema, erythema, or tenderness to extremity. Use Doppler ultrasound to assess pulses, if needed.
- Take prophylactic measures to prevent VTE in hospitalized patients. Apply sequential compression device or compression stockings as ordered. Assist patient to perform range-of-motion exercises, or assist to ambulate, if possible. Administer prophylactic medications as ordered for prevention of VTE.

Patient Education

- Adhere to activity restrictions as prescribed. If a DVT is present, know that a period of bed rest may be prescribed to reduce the risk of mobilizing the clot.
- If prescribed anticoagulant therapy, adhere to treatment plan as instructed, including taking all medications as prescribed and following up for additional blood tests, if needed.
- Manage factors that increase risk for VTE. If prescribed medications that increase risk for VTE, such as oral contraceptives or hormone replacement medications, be aware of this potential adverse effect. Seek support for smoking cessation, if applicable. Maintain healthy habits and exercise routinely, as tolerated. Wear compression stockings as directed.
- Monitor for signs and symptoms of PE, stroke, and MI. Seek emergent evaluation if symptoms such as chest pain, shortness of breath, altered mental status, unilateral weakness or numbness/tingling, changes in speech or vision, or abnormal gait occur.
- Seek emergent care for any uncontrolled bleeding. Monitor for signs of occult bleeding, such as abdominal discomfort, dark/tarry stools, and coffee-ground emesis. Take precautions to reduce risk for injury, including removing trip hazards within the home and limiting activity as prescribed (e.g., no contact sports).

[📝] **POP QUIZ 2.9**

An adult patient presents with calf tenderness and swelli[ng]. The patient states that they recently flew from Europe [to] the United States and developed lower extremity swell[ing] shortly after returning. The patient also reports bein[g a] cigarette smoker. What condition would the nurse suspec[t is] responsible for this patient's complaints?

TRAUMA

Overview

- Chest trauma is associated with significant mortality risk and may be the result of blunt or penetrating trauma. Blunt cardiac injury is the result of blunt impact to the chest. This may cause arrhythmias and injuries such as myocardial contusions or blunt pericardial rupture, which may lead to arrhythmia, cardiogenic shock, and death. Penetrating trauma is often more deadly than blunt injury and includes high-velocity injuries, such as gunshot wounds, and low-impact injuries, such as stabbings. Thoracic penetrating injuries may cause direct injury to cardiac tissue or the great vessels, pneumothorax or hemothorax, pericardial tamponade, hypovolemic or obstructive shock, and death.

[ ] **COMPLICATIONS**

Blunt cardiac injury can result in sudden cardiac arrest in [the] absence of structural damage to the heart, a phenome[non] referred to as *commotio cordis*. In this condition, a di[rect] blow to the chest disrupts the normal cardiac rhyt[hm,] causing ventricular fibrillation. This rare complica[tion] of blunt cardiac injury most often occurs in young a[nd] athletes with undiagnosed cardiomyopathy or conge[nital] cardiac defects.

Signs and Symptoms

The following symptoms may be present as a result of thoracic trauma, although presentation varies depending on mechanism of injury:

- Arrhythmias
- Cardiac structural damage, such as cardiac contusions and damage to chambers or valves
- Chest pain
- Shortness of breath
- Hemorrhage: external or internal (hemothorax and hemopericardium)
- Thoracic contusions, lacerations, or penetrating/puncture injuries, with or without foreign body
- Signs of shock

Diagnosis

Labs

Indications for lab testing may vary depending on injury severity; however, the following tests may be valuable when caring for a patient with chest trauma:

- CBC
- CMP
- Lactic acid
- Troponin (serial testing to assess for delayed elevation)
- Type and screen
- Toxicology (ethyl alcohol, urine drug screen)

Diagnostic Testing

- Focused assessment with sonography in trauma (FAST) examination prioritized for any trauma patient; performed after provider completes the primary survey to quickly identify internal injuries in any patient presenting with blunt or penetrating trauma. Includes bedside ultrasound of the heart, right upper quadrant, left upper quadrant, and pelvis. If severe injury/uncontrolled bleeding identified with initial FAST, and patient hemodynamically compromised, further imaging may be deferred to expedite surgical intervention.
- If patient hemodynamically stable, the following tests may be ordered to further investigate injuries: chest x-ray; CT; EKG; echocardiogram.

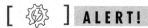 **ALERT!**

The FAST examination reviews four areas: the hepatorenal recess (Morrison's pouch), the pelvis, the pericardium, and the splenorenal fossa. This bedside ultrasound exam assesses the presence of free fluid but does not entirely rule out internal bleeding. The FAST examination is not able to detect injuries to hollow organs, small amounts of fluid, or retroperitoneal injuries.

[ ] **ALERT!**

In trauma patients with acute blood loss, administer IV fluids cautiously to prevent hemodilution. Replace volume with blood products as soon as they become available. Permissive hypotension may be indicated if appropriate for patient condition.

Treatment

- Primary trauma survey by provider, with trauma team immediately proceeding with stabilizing interventions if complications of thoracic trauma, such as tension pneumothorax or flail chest, are present. Assess pulse and cardiac rhythm. If pulse is not present, immediately proceed with resuscitation per ACLS guidelines. Administer supplemental oxygen to maintain SpO_2 greater than 94%. Patients with chest trauma are likely to require noninvasive ventilation or mechanical ventilation.
- Unstable chest trauma: Address any uncontrolled hemorrhage. Manage airway, breathing, and circulatory concerns alongside emergency provider. When external hemorrhage noted or provider notes concern for hemorrhage, perform FAST examination. ▶

Treatment *(continued)*

■ Administration of medications and IV fluids by patient condition: antiarrhythmic medications (see Table 2.1); blood products; fluid resuscitation with isotonic crystalloid solution; pain medications, such as opiate analgesics (see Table A.2).

Nursing Interventions

■ Place patient on continuous pulse oximetry and cardiac monitoring, alerting emergency provider to changes in vital signs or cardiac rhythm. Maintain spinal immobilization with cervical collar and backboard, if applicable. If pulse is not present, proceed immediately with resuscitation per ACLS guidelines. Reassess blood pressure frequently, assisting to place and monitor arterial line if needed. Assist to quickly obtain an EKG for interpretation by the emergency provider. Obtain repeat EKGs as needed.

■ Perform head-to-toe assessment with focus on cardiovascular and respiratory evaluation. Administer supplemental oxygen to maintain SpO_2 greater than 94%. Mechanical ventilation is often required; assist with placement and management of ETT or noninvasive ventilation if needed. If a foreign body is present, such as a weapon embedded in the chest, do not remove object. Instead, secure object to limit movement, if possible, and expedite transfer for surgical removal.

■ Establish IV access, drawing blood for lab tests as ordered, and administer medications as prescribed. Initiate at least two large-bore peripheral IV lines. Assist provider with central line placement if needed; monitor site and dressing. Administer IV fluids judiciously, as ordered, to prevent fluid overload/ hemodilution. Administer blood products as ordered. Alert blood bank immediately if emergency release blood/mass transfusion protocol is required.

■ Expedite transfer to operating room for surgical intervention, if needed, or transfer to critical care unit for continued treatment and monitoring.

Patient Education

■ Return for emergent evaluation if worsening chest pain or shortness of breath occurs, or if signs of infection occur, such as fever, chills, or productive cough.

■ Practice deep breathing and use incentive spirometer as directed to prevent atelectasis and pneumonia.

■ Adhere to activity restrictions as prescribed.

RESOURCES

Adler, Y., Charron, P., Imazio, M., Badano, L., Barón-Esquivias, G., Bogaert, J. , Brucato, A., Gueret, P., Klingel, K., Lionis, C., Maisch, B., Mayosi, B., Pavie, A., Ristic, A. D., Sabaté Tenas, M., Seferovic, P., Swedberg, K., Tomkowski, W., & ESC Scientific Document Group. (2015). 2015 ESC Guidelines for the diagnosis and management of pericardial diseases: The Task Force for the diagnosis and management of pericardial diseases of the European Society of Cardiology (ESC) endorsed by: The European Association for Cardio-Thoracic Surgery (EACTS). *European Heart Journal*, *36*(42), 2921–2964. https://doi.org/10.1093/eurheartj/ehv318

American Heart Association. (n.d.-a). *Acute coronary syndrome*. https://www.heart.org/en/health-topics/ heart-attack/about-heart-attacks/acute-coronary-syndrome

American Heart Association. (n.d.-b). *Hypertensive crisis: When you should call 911 for high blood pressure*. https:// www.heart.org/en/health-topics/high-blood-pressure/understanding-blood-pressure-readings/ hypertensive-crisis-when-you-should-call-911-for-high-blood-pressure

American Heart Association. (n.d.-c). *Infective endocarditis*. https://www.heart.org/en/health-topics/ infective-endocarditis

American Heart Association. (n.d.-d). *Lifestyle changes for heart attack prevention*. https://www.heart.org/en/ health-topics/heart-attack/life-after-a-heart-attack/lifestyle-changes-for-heart-attack-prevention

American Heart Association. (n.d.-e). *Prevention and treatment of pericarditis*. https://www.heart.org/en/ health-topics/pericarditis/prevention-and-treatment-of-pericarditis

American Heart Association. (n.d.-f). *Symptoms and diagnosis of pericarditis*. https://www.heart.org/en/health-topics/pericarditis/symptoms-and-diagnosis-of-pericarditis

American Heart Association. (n.d.-g). *What is pericarditis?* https://www.heart.org/en/health-topics/pericarditis/what-is-pericarditis

Bacidore, V. (2020). Abdominal and genitourinary trauma. In V. Sweet & A. Foley (Eds.), *Sheehy's emergency nursing: Practice and principles* (7th ed., p. 465–476). Elsevier.

Centers for Disease Control and Prevention. (n.d.-a). *Aortic aneurysm*. U.S. Department of Health and Human Services. https://www.cdc.gov/heartdisease/aortic_aneurysm.htm

Centers for Disease Control and Prevention. (n.d.-b). *Diagnosis and treatment of venous thromboembolism*. U.S. Department of Health and Human Services. https://www.cdc.gov/ncbddd/dvt/diagnosis-treatment.html

Centers for Disease Control and Prevention. (n.d.-c). *Heart failure*. U.S. Department of Health and Human Services. https://www.cdc.gov/heartdisease/heart_failure.htm

Centers for Disease Control and Prevention. (n.d.-d). *Peripheral arterial disease (PAD)*. U.S. Department of Health and Human Services. https://www.cdc.gov/heartdisease/PAD.htm

Centers for Disease Control and Prevention. (n.d.-e). *What is venous thromboembolism?* U.S. Department of Health and Human Services. https://www.cdc.gov/ncbddd/dvt/facts.html

de Alencar Neto, J. N. (2018). Morphine, oxygen, nitrates, and mortality reducing pharmacological treatment for acute coronary syndrome: An evidence-based review. *Cureus, 10*(1), Article e2114. https://doi.org/10.7759/cureus.2114

Fadel, R., El-Menyar, A., ElKafrawy, S., & Gad, M. G. (2019). Traumatic blunt cardiac injuries: An updated narrative review. *International Journal of Critical Illness and Injury Science, 9*(3), 113–119. https://doi.org/10.4103/IJCIIS.IJCIIS_29_19

Gomes, R. T., Tiberto, L. R., Bello, V. N., Lima, M. A., Nai, G. A., & Abreu, M. A. (2016). Dermatologic manifestations of infective endocarditis. *Anais Brasileiros de Dermatologia, 91*(5 Suppl. 1), 92–94. https://doi.org/10.1590/abd1806-4841.20164718

Guo, W., Su, Y., Chen, L., Zhou, Y., Li, Y., Liu, Q., & Guo, H. (2020). Effects of nursing methods for emergency PCI and non-emergency PCI on the treatment of patients with acute myocardial infarction. *Journal of the Pakistan Medical Association, 70* [Special issue](9), 31–37. PMID: 33177725.

Hirai, T., & Koster, M. (2013). Osler's nodes, Janeway lesions and splinter haemorrhages. *BMJ Case Reports, 2013*, bcr2013009759. https://doi.org/10.1136/bcr-2013-009759

InformedHealth.org. (2018, January 25). *Types of heart failure*. Institute for Quality and Efficiency in Health Care. https://www.ncbi.nlm.nih.gov/books/NBK481485

Jones, D. E., Braun, M., & Kassop, D. (2020). Acute coronary syndrome: Common complications and conditions that mimic ACS. *FP Essentials, 490*, 29–34. https://www.aafp.org/cme/subscriptions/fp-essentials/editions/490-ed.html

Knechtel, M. A. (2021). *EKGs for the nurse practitioner and physician assistant* (3rd ed., pp. 83–108). Springer Publishing Company.

Mayo Foundation for Medical Education and Research. (2019, November 13). *Supraventricular tachycardia*. Mayo Clinic. https://www.mayoclinic.org/diseases-conditions/supraventricular-tachycardia/symptoms-causes/syc-20355243

MedlinePlus. (2019, September 23). *Hypovolemic shock*. National Library of Medicine. https://medlineplus.gov/ency/article/000167.htm

Mitchell, M., & Carpenter, J. (2020). Clinical features and diagnosis of acute lower extremity ischemia. *UpToDate*. https://www.uptodate.com/contents/clinical-features-and-diagnosis-of-acute-lower-extremity-ischemia

National Heart, Lung, and Blood Institute. (n.d.-a). *Arrhythmias*. U.S. Department of Health and Human Services, National Institutes of Health. https://www.nhlbi.nih.gov/health-topics/arrhythmia

National Heart Lung and Blood Institute. (n.d.-b). *Cardiogenic shock*. U.S. Department of Health and Human Services, National Institutes of Health. https://www.nhlbi.nih.gov/health-topics/cardiogenic-shock

National Heart, Lung, and Blood Institute. (n.d.-c). *Heart failure*. U.S. Department of Health and Human Services, National Institutes of Health. https://www.nhlbi.nih.gov/health-topics/heart-failure

National Heart, Lung, and Blood Institute. (n.d.-d). *Heart inflammation*. U.S. Department of Health and Human Services, National Institutes of Health. https://www.nhlbi.nih.gov/health-topics/heart-inflammation

National Heart, Lung, and Blood Institute. (n.d.-e). *Peripheral artery disease*. U.S. Department of Health and Human Services, National Institutes of Health. https://www.nhlbi.nih.gov/health-topics/peripheral-artery-disease

National Heart, Lung, and Blood Institute. (n.d.-f). *Sudden cardiac arrest*. U.S. Department of Health and Human Services, National Institutes of Health. https://www.nhlbi.nih.gov/health-topics/sudden-cardiac-arrest

National Heart, Lung, and Blood Institute. (n.d.-g). *Venous thromboembolism*. U.S. Department of Health and Human Services, National Institutes of Health. https://www.nhlbi.nih.gov/health-topics/venous-thromboembolism

Panchal, A. R., Bartos, J. A., Cabañas, J. G., Donnino, M. W., Drennan, I. R., Hirsch, K. G., Kudenchuk, P. J., Kurz, M. C., Lavonas, E. J., Morley, P. T., O'Neil, B. J., Peberdy, M. A., Rittenberger, J. C., Rodriguez, A. J., Sawyer, K. N., & Berg, K. M. (2020). Part 3: Adult basic and advanced life support: 2020 American Heart Association guidelines for cardiopulmonary resuscitation and emergency cardiovascular care. *Circulation, 16*(142), S366–S468. https://doi.org/10.1161/CIR.0000000000000916

Prescribers' Digital Reference. (n.d.-a). *Adenosine* [Drug information]. https://www.pdr.net/drug-summary/Adenosine-adenosine-24200

Prescribers' Digital Reference. (n.d.-b). *Alteplase* [Drug information]. https://www.pdr.net/drug-summary/Activase-alteplase-1332.3358

Prescribers' Digital Reference. (n.d.-c). *Amiodarone* [Drug information]. https://www.pdr.net/drug-summary/Amiodarone-Hydrochloride-Injection-amiodarone-hydrochloride-3234.8358

Prescribers' Digital Reference. (n.d.-d). *Aspirin* [Drug information]. https://www.pdr.net/drug-summary/Durlaza-aspirin-3789.4184

Prescribers' Digital Reference. (n.d.-e). *Atropine sulfate* [Drug information]. https://www.pdr.net/drug-summary/Atropine-Sulfate-Injection-atropine-sulfate-684.4376

Prescribers' Digital Reference. (n.d.-f). *Diltiazem hydrochloride* [Drug information]. https://www.pdr.net/drug-summary/Cardizem-diltiazem-hydrochloride-2077.8341

Prescribers' Digital Reference. (n.d.-g). *Dobutamine hydrochloride* [Drug information]. https://www.pdr.net/drug-summary/Dobutamine-dobutamine-hydrochloride-3534#10

Prescribers' Digital Reference. (n.d.-h). *Esmolol hydrochloride* [Drug information]. https://www.pdr.net/drug-summary/Brevibloc-esmolol-hydrochloride-1159

Prescribers' Digital Reference. (n.d.-i). *Furosemide* [Drug information]. https://www.pdr.net/drug-summary/Lasix-furosemide-2594

Prescribers' Digital Reference. (n.d.-j). *Heparin sodium* [Drug information]. https://www.pdr.net/drug-summary/Heparin-Sodium-in-0-45--Sodium-Chloride-Injection-heparin-sodium-737.107

Prescribers' Digital Reference. (n.d.-k). *Lisinopril* [Drug information]. https://www.pdr.net/drug-summary/Prinivil-lisinopril-376

Prescribers' Digital Reference. (n.d.-l). *Nitroglycerin* [Drug information]. https://www.pdr.net/drug-summary/Nitroglycerin-in-5--Dextrose-nitroglycerin-1148.3324

Prescribers' Digital Reference. (n.d.-m). *Sodium nitroprusside* [Drug information]. https://www.pdr.net/drug-summary/Nitropress-sodium-nitroprusside-3404.1125

Prescribers' Digital Reference. (n.d.-n). *Warfarin sodium* [Drug information]. https://www.pdr.net/drug-summary/Warfarin-warfarin-sodium-3720.4534

Sherman Jollis, M. M., & Jollis, J. G. (2018). Time to reperfusion, door-to-balloon times, and how to reduce them. In T.J. Watson, P. J. L. Ong, & J.E. Tcheng (Eds.), *Primary angioplasty: A practical guide* (pp. 289–306). Springer. https://www.ncbi.nlm.nih.gov/books/NBK543575

Verhagen, D. W. M., Hermanides, J., Korevaar, J. C., Bossuyt, P. M. M., van den Brink, R. B. A., Speelman, P., & van der Meer, J. T. M. (2008). Prognostic value of serial C-reactive protein measurements in left-sided native valve endocarditis. *Archives of Internal Medicine, 168*(3), 302–307. doi:10.1001/archinternmed.2007.73

Windecker, S., Kolh, P., Alfonso, F., Collet, P., Cremer, J., Falk, V., Filippatos, G., Hamm, C., Head, S. J., Jüni, P., Kappetein, A. P., Kastrati, A., Knuuti, J., Landmesser, U., Laufer, G., Neumann, F., Richter, D. J., Schauerte, P., Uva, M. S. . . . Witkowski, A. (2014). 2014 ESC/EACTS guidelines on myocardial revascularization: The Task Force on Myocardial Revascularization of the European Society of Cardiology (ESC) and the European Association for Cardio-Thoracic Surgery (EACTS) developed with the special contribution of the European Association of Percutaneous Cardiovascular Interventions (EAPCI). *European Heart Journal, 35*(37), 2541–2619. https://doi.org/10.1093/eurheartj/ehu278

3 RESPIRATORY EMERGENCIES

ACUTE RESPIRATORY DISTRESS SYNDROME

Overview

- *Acute respiratory distress syndrome (ARDS)* is an acute inflammatory lung response causing capillary leakage into the alveoli, deactivation of the surfactant in the alveoli, and damage to the alveolar-capillary permeability.
- The result is impaired oxygen exchange causing hypoxemia. Patients often have persistent low oxygen levels despite receiving supplemental oxygen.
- ARDS is a life-threatening condition that develops from many different causes. Fluid buildup makes the lungs heavy and stiff.
- The Berlin definition of ARDS requires that all of the following criteria be present for diagnosis: The onset of respiratory symptoms beginning within 1 week of a known clinical insult, or new or worsening symptoms during the past week; the presence of bilateral opacities on either chest x-ray or chest CT scan consistent with pulmonary edema that are not explained by pleural effusions, lobar collapse, lung collapse, or pulmonary nodules; respiratory failure that cannot be fully explained by cardiac failure or fluid overload (consider echocardiogram or cardiac assessment if no other ARDS risk factors); the presence of a moderate to severe impairment of oxygenation, as defined by PaO_2/FIO_2 ratio of less than or equal to 300.

[ ] **COMPLICATIONS**

Complications of ARDS include ventilator-associated pneumonia, barotrauma, atelectasis, pulmonary hypertension, lung scarring, multiorgan failure, and death. ARDS often presents with multiple other comorbidities and diagnoses (e.g., sepsis, multisystem trauma, acute pancreatitis); thus, collaborative care and management is essential to prevent permanent lung damage and death.

Signs and Symptoms

- Abnormal breath sounds: crackles, wheezes, or rales
- Accessory muscle use
- Altered mental status
- Anxiety
- Chest pain
- Cyanosis
- Cough
- Decreased lung compliance
- Diaphoresis
- Dyspnea
- Fatigue
- Fever
- Hypotension ▶

Signs and Symptoms *(continued)*

- Hypoxia
- Pulmonary consolidation
- Retractions
- Tachycardia
- Tachypnea

Diagnosis

Labs

- Arterial blood gases (ABGs)
- Cardiac enzymes
- Complete blood count (CBC)
- Comprehensive metabolic panel (CMP)
- Sputum culture

Diagnostic Testing

- Bronchoscopy
- Chest CT scan
- Chest x-ray
- Echocardiogram
- Lung biopsy

[⚡] ALERT!

ARDS can be a complication of COVID-19, which is caused by the SARS-CoV-2 virus. Care parameters are continually evolving. For current information on caring for patients with COVID-19, consult the National Institutes of Health (www.covid19treatmentguidelines.nih.gov) and the Centers for Disease Control and Prevention (www.cdc.gov/coronavirus/2019-nCoV/index.html).

Treatment

- No specific medication to treat ARDS; treatment focused on identifying and treating underlying cause(s)
- Extracorporeal membrane oxygenation (ECMO): may be considered if all other measures fail
- Implementation of supportive care: nutrition and intravenous (IV) hydration
- Medications to treat diseases/potential causes: antibiotics (see Table A.1); bronchodilators (see Table 3.1 for medications used for respiratory conditions); diuretics to optimize fluid status; steroids (see Table 3.1) ▶

TABLE 3.1 Medications for Respiratory Conditions		
INDICATIONS	**MECHANISM OF ACTION**	**CONTRAINDICATIONS, PRECAUTIONS, AND ADVERSE EFFECTS**
Anticholinergics (ipratropium bromide)		
• ARDS • Asthma • Bronchospasm • Bronchoconstriction • COPD	• Block the effects of acetylcholine to help relax the muscles causing bronchoconstriction • Reduce the production of mucus • Inhibit cholinergic receptors in bronchial smooth muscle	• Medication is contraindicated in cross sensitivity to atropine or bromide. • Inhaled anticholinergics can produce a paradoxical bronchospasm, which can be life-threatening in some patients; however, it is rare and usually occurs with first use of new canister. • Use caution in soy or peanut allergy, in patients with known arrhythmia, or in BPH or urinary obstructions.

TABLE 3.1   Medications for Respiratory Conditions (*continued*)

INDICATIONS	MECHANISM OF ACTION	CONTRAINDICATIONS, PRECAUTIONS, AND ADVERSE EFFECTS
		• Adverse effects include hypotension, GI irritation, allergic reaction, headache, nervousness, arrhythmia, and urinary retention.
Beta-2 agonists/bronchodilators (albuterol)		
• Asthma • COPD	• Relax smooth muscle (e.g., lungs) by stimulating beta-2 receptors • Allow airways to open for increased air movement; reduce bronchospasms	• Paradoxical asthma can occur, which can be deadly. • Use caution in patients who have seizures, hyperthyroidism, or pheochromocytoma, and in those who have a unique response to other sympathomimetic medications. • Possible arrhythmias can occur, so monitor QT interval.
Decongestant (pseudoephedrine)		
• Cough • Sinus congestion • Pneumonia	• Sympathomimetic • Vasoconstriction of the nasal mucosa	• Discontinue if tachycardia, syncope, or vomiting develops. • Medication is contraindicated with diabetes and glaucoma.
Expectorants (dextromethorphan, guaifenesin)		
• COPD • Pneumonia	• Thin and loosen mucus and secretions in bronchi	• Do not give for persistent or chronic cough due to smoking, asthma, or COPD. • Medication is contraindicated in alcohol intolerance. • Use caution in prolonged cough accompanied by fever, rash, or headache, and in diabetic patients. • Adverse effects include dizziness, headache, nausea, vomiting, diarrhea, and rash.
Magnesium sulfate		
• Severe asthma • Status asthmaticus	• Smooth muscle relaxer • Bronchodilation by competing with calcium-mediated, smooth muscle binding sites	• Medication is contraindicated in kidney failure and atrioventricular block.
Mucolytics (acetylcysteine solution)		
• Reduce COPD exacerbation	• Decrease over secretion and thickness of mucus in the lungs	• To decrease the risk of bronchospasm, administer acetylcysteine solution after a bronchodilator.

ARDS, acute respiratory distress syndrome; BPH, benign prostatic hyperplasia; COPD, chronic obstructive pulmonary disease; GI, gastrointestinal.

Treatment *(continued)*

- Physical therapy services referral
- Prone positioning to improve ventilation of dorsal lung regions, which allows better ventilation/perfusion matching
- Respiratory therapy consult to maintain adequate respiratory status
- Supplemental oxygenation with continuous positive airway pressure (CPAP), bilevel positive airway pressure (BIPAP), or mechanical ventilation. Mechanical ventilation: can be crucial to ARDS management. Paralytic initiation considered.

Nursing Interventions

- All intubated patients should be in prone position for at least 12 hours per day with continuous monitoring of oxygenation status and tube placement. Awake patients should be in prone position if they are able to tolerate.
- Administer fluid and nutrition therapy as ordered.
- Ensure adequate sedation for intubated patients (increased if patients are in prone position).
- Establish IV access, laboratory draws, and repeat ABGs as needed.
- Monitor and document CPAP, BIPAP, or ventilator settings.
- Monitor strict intake and output (I/O).
- Obtain frequent ABGs and adjust ventilator settings as needed.
- Provide frequent respiratory assessments.
- Titrate medication drips to maintain mean arterial pressure (MAP) goals.

Patient Education

- Continue using incentive spirometry. To use incentive spirometer, place the mouthpiece facing the mouth. Exhale deeply, make a tight seal around the mouthpiece with mouth and lips, and inhale as deeply as possible. Repeat 10 times every 1 to 2 hours.
- Engage in physical activity. Start small and work up to regain baseline functioning.
- Follow up with outpatient appointments, diagnostic tests, and laboratory draws.
- Participate in pulmonary rehabilitation.
- Stay up to date on current situation and plan of care. Family should stay up to date if patient is ventilated and sedated.
- Supplemental home oxygen may be required at time of discharge. Engage in safe oxygen therapy practices by avoiding smoking, open flames, flammable products, and heat sources. Avoid products with oil or petroleum, and keep a fire extinguisher close by.
- Take medication as prescribed.

ASTHMA

Overview

- *Asthma* is a chronic inflammatory disorder characterized by narrowing of the lower airways, bronchospasm, increased mucus production, and increased airway reactivity.

[📝] **POP QUIZ 3.1**

A 42-year-old patient has been intubated and placed in the prone position. A few hours later, the patient's pulse oximetry drops, and end-tidal readings go up. What is the nurse's next step in correcting this situation?

[🧠] **COMPLICATIONS**

Status asthmaticus is a severe form of acute asthma exacerbation that does not respond to medications. It is a medical emergency that requires early intervention to avoid respiratory failure and death.

Overview (continued)

- Symptoms range from mild and well-controlled to severe and life-threatening attacks.
- Asthma affects both children and adults but is commonly diagnosed before age 10 years.
- Patient education should emphasize maintenance and prevention of exacerbation. Chronic asthma leads to permanent changes in airway structures. Asthma may become more complicated with comorbidities (e.g., chronic obstructive pulmonary disease [COPD] and emphysema). Asthma exacerbations must be treated urgently; exacerbations may be triggered by viral respiratory infections, exercise, or irritants such as allergens, cold or dry air, and smoke. *Acute severe asthma*, or *status asthmaticus*, is a severe asthma exacerbation in which interventions to reduce airway edema and hyperresponsiveness are minimally effective; the condition is characterized by hypoxia, hypercarbia, and respiratory failure and is associated with significant mortality risk.

Signs and Symptoms

Patients with well-controlled asthma often experience minimal respiratory symptoms. During an asthma exacerbation, patients are likely to present to the ED with the following complaints:

- Anxiety
- Chest tightness
- Cough
- Diaphoresis
- Hypercarbia
- Hypoxemia
- Low peak expiratory flow rate (PEFR)
- Nasal flaring
- Pulsus paradoxus
- Retractions
- Shortness of breath
- Tachycardia
- Tachypnea
- Tripod position
- Wheezing

Diagnosis

Labs

There are no lab tests specific to diagnosing asthma. However, the following tests may be indicated for patients experiencing an asthma exacerbation:

- ABG: reflects hypoxemia and hypercarbia
- CBC: elevated eosinophils
- Immunoglobulin E (IgE): levels elevated
- Sputum specimen

Diagnostic Testing

- Usually diagnosed in outpatient setting with pulmonary function testing
- Used in ED to assess patients with acute asthma presentations: chest x-ray, PEFR.
- Pulse oximetry

[ ] **ALERT!**

During auscultation, asthmatics typically have wheezing on inspiration and expiration. As bronchospasm progresses, breath sounds will become severely diminished or absent. This is sometimes referred to as a silent chest and requires immediate intervention.

[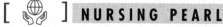] **NURSING PEARL**

PEFRs are useful in assessing lung function and predicting asthma exacerbations. Many asthmatic patients are instructed to monitor their peak flow daily and to take action if the value falls below 80% of their personal best peak flow reading (a value that is established over the course of several weeks during a period in which asthma is well controlled). The patient may then be instructed to administer medications as needed (PRN), such as a rescue inhaler, and may be advised to proceed to the ED if symptoms persist.

Treatment

- Medication management focused on relaxing bronchial smooth muscle, controlling inflammation, and reducing bronchospasm (see Table 3.1): anticholinergic medication such as ipratropium; beta$_2$ adrenergic agonists such as albuterol; epinephrine (may be indicated for asthma induced by allergy); heliox therapy; magnesium sulfate (may be used for patients who present with a life-threatening exacerbation that is refractory to initial therapy).
- Oxygen therapy: systemic glucocorticoids such as methylprednisolone (see Table A.4)
- Referral to specialty consulting services (e.g., pulmonology) for continued monitoring and ongoing disease maintenance; improved awareness, removal of triggers, and control of symptoms to help prevent future asthma exacerbations
- Supplemental oxygen to patients who are hypoxemic (SpO$_2$ less than 90%). Possible trial of noninvasive ventilation, such as CPAP or BIPAP, for certain patients. More severe presentations may require ventilatory support. Intubation if patient is unable to maintain a patent airway. If available, heliox, a mixture of helium and oxygen, to reduce airway resistance.

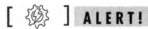

ALERT!

Wheezing in status asthmaticus patients may be absent because of a significant decrease in alveolar airflow. Although these patients are not wheezing, they are in severe respiratory distress and often require ventilatory support.

Nursing Interventions

- Administer nebulized medications as ordered.
- Assess mental status and patient's ability to maintain airway. Prepare for intubation if indicated and gather appropriate equipment and supplies.
- Assess PEFR. If the patient monitors PEFR at home, compare with established personal best value.
- Establish IV access and obtain laboratory tests as ordered. Closely trend ABG results.
- Maintain Richmond agitation sedation scale (RASS) and pain goal as ordered with sedation and anxiety and pain medications.
- Monitor for worsening signs of respiratory distress, including the following: hypoxemia, as evidenced by SpO$_2$ less than 90%; increasing oxygen requirements with minimal response to initial therapy; new inability to complete sentences or communicate verbally due to shortness of breath; patient seated in the tripod position; retractions.
- Place patient on continuous pulse oximetry and provide supplemental oxygen if needed.
- Perform a thorough head-to-toe assessment with focus on respiratory and cardiac evaluation. Auscultate lung sounds and note respiratory rate and work of breathing. Alert provider to any increase in respiratory effort, such as accessory muscle use.
- Place patient on cardiac monitoring and/or obtain an EKG. Alert emergency provider of abnormal vital signs or changes in cardiac rhythm.
- Position patient appropriately for maximum ventilation and pressure ulcer prevention.
- Reassess patient's airway, breathing, circulation, mental status, vital signs, and monitoring. Auscultate breath sounds after medication administration. Monitor patient for 30 to 60 minutes after last treatment.

Patient Education

- Review asthma control plan.
- Change occupation if allergen or trigger exposure is occupational.
- Control asthma triggers by self-monitoring symptoms and removing sources of allergen if possible. This may include avoiding tobacco, dust mites, animals, or pollen. ▶

Patient Education *(continued)*

- Engage in smoking cessation protocol.
- Ensure proper inhaler use. To use most inhalers, use thumb and fingers to hold the inhaler upright with the mouthpiece down, pointing toward mouth. Remove the mouthpiece cover and gently shake. Hold the mouthpiece away from mouth and exhale deeply. Use the inhalation method recommended by provider (open mouth versus closed mouth) and breathe in slowly (3–5 seconds) while pressing down at the top of the canister to dispense medication. Hold breath for 10 seconds before removing the mouthpiece and exhaling slowly. Repeat this process for the recommended number of puffs. Once finished, wipe the mouthpiece and reapply the cap.
- Have allergy testing done if the cause is unknown.
- Keep rescue inhalers on hand in case of acute attack.

CHRONIC OBSTRUCTIVE PULMONARY DISEASE

Overview

- *COPD* is an irreversible, progressive, and chronic inflammatory disease of the lungs; it causes breathing and airway difficulties due to obstructed airflow.
- COPD consists of both chronic bronchitis and emphysema. Patients with chronic bronchitis (inflammation of the bronchioles) may be described as "blue bloaters," due to their characteristic cyanosis and edema as a result of right-sided heart strain. Patients with emphysema may be described as "pink puffers," due to their characteristic thin, barrel-chested appearance. These patients often experience shortness of breath with pursed-lip breathing due to destruction of the alveoli secondary to exposure to irritants such as cigarette smoke or particulates.
- COPD causes chronic hypercapnia because of air being trapped in the alveoli leading to acidosis.
- Providing too much oxygen to a COPD patient creates hyperoxia-induced hypercapnia, reducing or eliminating respiratory drive.

[ ]   **COMPLICATIONS**

COPD can be a debilitating chronic illness. Patients may develop acute exacerbations, as well as severe activity intolerance and nutritional deficits related to chronic shortness of breath. Those with advanced disease may require supplemental oxygen and can develop depression. Patients are at an increased risk for further respiratory issues, such as pneumonia, chronic respiratory failure, and pulmonary hypertension. Patients are also at an increased risk for cardiac issues, such as right-sided heart failure and cardiomyopathy. Close monitoring and management of symptoms can help decrease the risk of developing these complications and improve quality of life.

Signs and Symptoms

- Accessory muscle use
- Barrel chest
- Cachexia
- Chest tightness
- Chronic, productive cough
- Clubbing of the nails
- Cyanosis
- Distant/diminished lung sounds
- Dyspnea
- Hypoxia ▶

[ ]   **ALERT!**

Patients with COPD may have a baseline SpO_2 value of less than 90% on supplemental oxygen. This makes SpO_2 an unreliable diagnostic tool for assessing respiratory status. ABGs are a more accurate indicator of respiratory status in this population because they accurately provide values for PaO_2, CO_2, and HCO_3^- to indicate acid-base imbalances and hypercapnia. These values are especially important with mechanically ventilated patients and should be frequently monitored.

Signs and Symptoms *(continued)*

- Increased anteroposterior diameter
- Pursed-lip breathing
- Shortness of breath
- Tachypnea
- Weight loss
- Wheezing and/or rhonchi

Diagnosis

Labs

- Usually diagnosed in outpatient setting with pulmonary function testing
- May be ordered in ED for differential diagnosis of COPD exacerbation: ABG—hypercarbia/hypoxia; brain natriuretic peptide (BNP); CBC—elevated white blood cells (WBCs); CMP; sputum cultures—organism growth; troponin

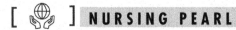

[🌐] NURSING PEARL

The body may attempt to correct for chronic hypoxemia by producing more red blood cells, causing patients with COPD to develop polycythemia.

Diagnostic Testing

- Usually diagnosed in outpatient setting with pulmonary function testing via spirometry
- May be indicated in ED for patients experiencing COPD exacerbation: chest CT scan; chest x-ray.

Treatment

- Additional medications possible in acute exacerbation. Possible antibiotics if underlying infection is discovered (see Table A.1). Advanced COPD and acute exacerbations: possible opioid analgesics (see Table A.2) to reduce air hunger.
- Disease management, often with use of several inhaled medications (see Table 3.1), such as short-acting beta agonists, such as albuterol; muscarinic antagonists, such as ipratropium; inhaled corticosteroids, such as fluticasone.
- More likely to require supplemental oxygen with progression. Patients may require respiratory support with noninvasive measures, such as CPAP or BIPAP. If refractory to initial therapy, patients may require intubation and mechanical ventilation.
- Possible benefit from chest physiotherapy to mobilize secretions and increase sputum expectoration
- Possible lung transplantation for end-stage COPD
- Regular follow-up with pulmonologist for ongoing disease management and pulmonary rehabilitation
- Small, frequent meals; intake of adequate calories; and daily multivitamin supplement

Nursing Interventions

- Apply supplemental oxygen if needed. In acute COPD exacerbations, oxygen should be titrated to an SpO_2 of 88% to 92%. Assist with placement of nasal intermittent positive pressure ventilation (NIPPV), such as CPAP or BIPAP, if needed. Prepare for emergent intubation if patient becomes fatigued and can no longer protect airway.
- Administer medications as prescribed. Medications may be inhaled/nebulized or administered IV. Patients with respiratory distress may be unable to tolerate oral medications. Reassess lung sounds and respiratory effort after medication administration, and deliver additional PRN medications as ordered.
- Assist with patient positioning; patients may feel most comfortable sitting or in the tripod position.
- Closely monitor ABGs.
- Establish IV access and draw lab tests as ordered.

Nursing Interventions *(continued)*

- Manage patient anxiety.
- Monitor airway and use suctioning for secretions as needed.
- Perform head-to-toe assessment with focus on respiratory and cardiovascular evaluation.
- Place patient on continuous pulse oximetry and cardiac monitoring, alerting emergency provider to any changes in vital signs or cardiac rhythm.
- Quickly obtain an EKG for interpretation by the emergency provider.

Patient Education

- Learn reasons to seek care, such as increased shortness of breath, chest tightness, or signs of infection such as fever, chills, and productive cough.
- Learn risk factors for development of COPD and prevention of future COPD exacerbations. Avoid irritants such as smoke and fumes. Obtain appropriate vaccinations, such as flu and pneumonia inoculation, to reduce risk of community-acquired respiratory infections. Maintain a calorie-dense diet to ensure adequate nutrition. Maintain a healthy level of activity, limiting strenuous exercise if it exacerbates symptoms. Obtain support and resources regarding smoking cessation, if needed.
- Recognize the importance of adhering to the treatment plan as prescribed, including maintaining regular follow-up with outpatient pulmonology, if needed. Learn about prescribed medications, medication administration, and cleaning/maintenance of devices, such as nebulizers and oxygen-delivery devices. Rinse mouth after using inhaled steroid medications to prevent infection.

[ ] **POP QUIZ 3.2**

What is the oxygen saturation goal for the patient with COPD?

INFECTIONS

Overview

- Respiratory infections are often classified as upper or lower and may be viral or bacterial.
- Upper respiratory infections (URIs) affect the airway from nostrils to vocal cords in the larynx and the paranasal sinuses, including the middle ear. Some examples of URIs are laryngitis, strep throat, and epiglottitis.
- Lower respiratory infections (LRIs) affect the trachea and bronchi to the bronchioles and alveoli. Some examples of LRIs are bronchitis, pneumonia, and tuberculosis.
- Viruses such as respiratory syncytial virus (RSV), SARS-CoV-2, and influenza can affect both upper and lower airways.

[ ] **COMPLICATIONS**

Infections not treated appropriately may spread to the blood, leading to sepsis or septic shock. This may be indicated by elevated lactate level, tachycardia, hypotension, and altered mental status. Blood cultures should be drawn from two different sites prior to starting antibiotics. Fluid resuscitation must be started urgently.

- Pneumonia is an infection of the alveoli and may be a result of virus, bacteria, fungi, or aspiration, which may lead to impaired gas exchange and ARDS. Common bacteria that cause infection are *Streptococcus pneumoniae* and *Klebsiella pneumoniae*. Bacterial pneumonia may also be classified as community acquired or hospital acquired, which directs treatment decisions. Aspiration pneumonia occurs when oropharyngeal contents enter the lower airways due to impaired swallowing. Aspirated contents may include fluids, food, or foreign bodies, such as small toys/objects (more common in children) or teeth (possible after facial trauma).

Signs and Symptoms

- Patients with URI are more likely to experience symptoms associated with the upper portion of the respiratory tract: cough, nasal congestion/ rhinorrhea, sinus pressure, headache, sore throat, pain with swallowing.

- Patients with LRIs are more likely to experience symptoms associated with the lower respiratory tract: cough (productive or nonproductive), fever/chills, pleuritic chest pain, shortness of breath, tachypneac wheezing.

- Patients with LRIs not treated early or effectively may progress to sepsis and show additional signs: altered mental status, cyanosis, fatigue, fever, hypoxia, hypotension, tachycardia.

Diagnosis

Labs

- ABG/venous blood gas (VBG): indicating hypercarbia/hypoxia
- Blood cultures: two sets from different sites
- CBC: elevated WBCs
- CMP
- Serum lactate: elevated
- Sputum culture and Gram stain
- Viral nasal swab

Diagnostic Testing

- Bronchoscopy with bronchoalveolar lavage
- Chest CT scan
- Chest x-ray
- Thoracentesis

[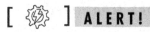] **ALERT!**

Pneumonia is a leading cause of sepsis and septic shock. Patients may progress to respiratory failure, with shock quickly resulting.

[🌐] **NURSING PEARL**

In addition to identifying infections such as pneumonia, imaging also investigates for further complications of respiratory infections, such as pleural effusions and lung abscesses.

Treatment

- Possible chest physiotherapy to mobilize secretions and exudate to promote improved gas exchange.
- For conditions such as asthma and COPD, administration of corticosteroid medications to combat increased inflammation of the respiratory system (see Table 3.1).
- Possible supplemental oxygen to maintain SpO_2 greater than 92%. Patients with severe infection may require NIPPV or placement of endotracheal tube (ETT) and mechanical ventilation. Some conditions, such as *epiglottitis*, an infection of the epiglottis commonly caused by *Haemophilus influenzae* type B, may make intubation increasingly difficult or impossible, and patients may require emergent percutaneous transtracheal ventilation to maintain the airway before a tracheostomy can be surgically placed. Specific strategies for ventilation are recommended for certain conditions, such as low tidal volume ventilation for patients with ARDS.
- Respiratory infections with volume depletion: fluid replacement with IV isotonic crystalloid fluids.
- Self-limiting viral URI management focused on reducing symptoms (see Table A.2 and Table 3.1): analgesics and antipyretics such as acetaminophen and nonsteroidal anti-inflammatory drugs; anticholinergics such as diphenhydramine; bronchodilators such as albuterol; decongestants such as pseudoephedrine; expectorants such as guaifenesin.
- Suspected bacterial infection or aspiration pneumonia: appropriate antibiotics (see Table A.1); initial broad-spectrum coverage possible until sputum culture and sensitivity results available.

Nursing Interventions

- Administer medications as prescribed. Medications may be inhaled/nebulized or administered IV. Patients with respiratory distress may be unable to tolerate oral medications. Reassess lung sounds and respiratory effort after medication administration, and deliver additional medications as ordered. Provide IV fluids and monitor urine output.
- Apply supplemental oxygen if needed to maintain SpO_2 greater than 92%. Assist with placement of NIPPV, such as CPAP or BIPAP, if needed. Prepare for emergent intubation, if needed.
- Assist with patient positioning to improve ventilation. Many patients with respiratory illness are most comfortable in high Fowler's or tripod position to assist with lung expansion. Use specific positioning strategies, such as placing mechanically ventilated patients with ARDS in the prone position to facilitate improved gas exchange.
- Establish IV access and draw blood for lab tests as ordered. Collect samples for additional microbiology studies, such as sputum and blood cultures, before administering antibiotics if clinically indicated.
- Maintain pulmonary hygiene (encourage mobility, coughing and deep-breathing exercises, use of incentive spirometer, mobilizing of secretions, suction as needed, and chest physiotherapy).
- Monitor fever curve and provide cooling interventions if necessary.
- Perform head-to-toe assessment with focus on respiratory and HEENT (head, ears, eyes, nose, throat) systems. Alert provider immediately if respiratory distress or any other emergent concerns are present, such as airway edema/symptoms of epiglottitis. Place patient in appropriate isolation precautions.
- Place patient on continuous pulse oximetry and cardiac monitoring. Alert emergency provider to any changes in vital signs or cardiac rhythm.
- Prevent hospital-acquired pneumonia by providing oral care with chlorhexidine (CHG), especially in ventilated patients.

Patient Education

- If hospital admission is required for treatment of respiratory infections, learn plan of care.
- Learn about risk factors for development of respiratory infections and prevention of future infections. Understand the importance of ongoing treatment for any underlying lung disease in preventing future infections. Follow up with primary care provider to obtain appropriate vaccinations, such as flu and pneumonia inoculation, to reduce risk of community-acquired respiratory infections. Obtain support and resources regarding smoking cessation, if needed.
- Learn reasons to seek care, such as worsening cough, shortness of breath, chest tightness, fever, or chills.
- Learn the importance of adhering to the treatment plan as prescribed, including maintaining regular follow-up with outpatient pulmonology, if needed. Learn about prescribed medications, medication administration, and cleaning/maintenance of devices, such as nebulizers and oxygen-delivery devices. Rinse mouth after using inhaled steroid medications to prevent infection.
- If provided with a prescription for antibiotics and discharged home: Learn about medication ▶

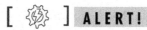 **ALERT!**

Epiglottitis can rapidly lead to obstructed upper airway, requiring intubation. The most frequent cause is a viral or bacterial infection. Encourage calming measures and avoid actions that irritate the tongue and throat.

[📝] **POP QUIZ 3.3**

An older adult patient has a past medical history of a cerebrovascular accident, diabetes mellitus, hypertension, and recent hospitalization. The patient is lethargic, is hypoxic at 87% on 4 L/min supplemental oxygen through nasal cannula (NC), has a weak gag reflex, and is unable to cough up secretions. Recently, the patient was being fed dinner, and the nursing student reported that the patient was coughing profusely after swallowing. Which type of pneumonia is this patient at risk for contracting?

Patient Education *(continued)*

self-administration and the importance of adhering to the treatment plan, including completing the full course of antibiotic therapy as prescribed. Learn about any additional therapies, such as metered-dose inhalers (MDIs) and nebulizer treatments, including the use of these medication delivery devices. If instructed to continue to monitor oxygenation at home using a pulse oximeter, learn proper use of the device, discuss normal parameters, and seek care if SpO_2 falls below defined limits (usually 90%).

INHALATION INJURY

Overview

Three factors need to be considered when treating a patient who has an inhalation injury: exposure to asphyxiants, smoke inhalation, and thermal or heat injury.

- Exposure to asphyxiants, or asphyxiation (CO): due to CO binding to hemoglobin, displacing oxygen, and forming carboxyhemoglobin. CO poisoning: frequently seen in fire-related smoke inhalation. Other sources of CO poisoning: improper heating systems, inadequately vented fuel-burning devices (e.g., gas-powered generators), operation of vehicles in enclosed spaces (e.g., garage), exposure to exhaust behind an operating motorboat.
- Smoke inhalation/injury (or pulmonary irritation): Pulmonary edema can develop after the initial injury, within 24 to 48 hours. It typically affects the lower airways and lung parenchyma.
- Thermal or heat injury (e.g., hot air from a fire): It is important to observe these patients closely for the first 24 to 48 hours after the initial incident and watch for possible increasing edema, especially in the upper airways. Thermal or heat injury may cause direct injury to the respiratory tract.

Signs and Symptoms

- Carbonaceous sputum (smoke inhalation)
- Cherry-red lips and skin (CO poisoning)
- Confusion
- Dyspnea
- Headache (common in CO poisoning)
- Lethargy
- Nausea and vomiting
- Soot around mouth and nose
- Ulcerations of the nasal/oral mucosa (thermal injury)

Diagnosis

Labs

- ABG
- Carboxyhemoglobin level
- CBC
- CMP
- Lactate acid
- Urine pregnancy test or beta-human chorionic gonadotropin hormone level

 COMPLICATIONS

Pregnant patients should exercise caution with activities that may expose the fetus to CO poisoning. CO binds to fetal hemoglobin with a higher affinity and has a longer half-life.

 COMPLICATIONS

Complications with an inhalation injury vary. Some possible complications are asthma, ARDS, and the need for an artificial airway.

 ALERT!

CO is a result of fire and incomplete combustion of fuels. Other potential asphyxiants may also be present in the fire. Consider cyanide poisoning, especially in incidents where polyurethane, plastics, rubber, and textiles are involved. Cyanide poisoning affects multiple body systems, and possible antidotes include amyl nitrate, sodium nitrate, and thiosulfate. Hydroxocobalamin may also be used.

 NURSING PEARL

Cigarette smokers have chronically elevated carboxyhemoglobin levels, so their baseline is always elevated and may affect length of oxygen treatment.

Diagnostic Testing

- Chest x-ray
- Fiberoptic bronchoscopy (standard for determining inhalation injury)
- Pulse oximetry (may give a false value due to CO binding to hemoglobin instead of oxygen)

Treatment

- CO poisoning: removal of CO source and placement of non-rebreather mask with 100% oxygen. Carboxyhemoglobin half-life: 4 to 5 hours in room air, decreases with 100% oxygen. Consideration of hyperbaric chamber.
- Consideration of early intubation, as airway edema makes intubation more difficult
- Hyperbaric oxygenation
- Medications such as albuterol for bronchospasm (see Table 3.1)
- Tracheostomy possibly indicated in cases with airway edema

Nursing Interventions

- Assess the patient for burns and injuries.
- Administer oxygen therapy via non-rebreather mask for nonintubated patients.
- Obtain a detailed history of preceding events, if possible.
- Prepare for ventilatory care.
- Prepare for possible tracheostomy care.

Patient Education

- Do not use a gas oven to heat the home.
- Do not use a kerosene heater or gas-powered generator in enclosed spaces.
- Do not use vehicles in enclosed and poorly ventilated spaces.
- Have CO detectors and smoke detectors installed in the home, and change batteries every 6 months.

OBSTRUCTION

Overview

- Maintaining a patent airway is a top priority and should be assessed immediately in every patient.
- Airway obstructions may be categorized by location (upper versus lower), acuity (acute versus chronic), and severity (partial versus complete).
- Patients with partial airway obstruction may be able to maintain adequate oxygenation, while patients with complete airway obstruction require immediate intervention to prevent respiratory arrest and death.
- *Upper airway obstruction* is blockage of the pharynx and larynx (often as a result of swelling), as noted by the following: Anaphylaxis causes rapid-onset acute upper airway obstruction. *Aspiration pneumonia* is the result of food, fluid, or another foreign body entering the airways, causing airway infection. Beta-blocker medications often cause angioedema. Infections can cause swelling to soft tissues, such as croup, which is characterized by inspiratory stridor and barking cough. Tongue-related obstructions are the most common cause of upper airway

[ ]   **COMPLICATIONS**

Acute airway obstructions require emergent identification and treatment. Patients with partial airway obstructions may progress to complete obstruction as the airway becomes inflamed. Complete airway obstruction will lead to respiratory failure and death. Patients with chronic obstructions, such as those with obstructive sleep apnea, may develop chronic cardiac and respiratory issues secondary to chronically impaired ventilation.

▶

Overview *(continued)*

obstruction in patients with altered mental status or decreased level of consciousness. Foreign body upper airway obstruction is more common in pediatric patients, often between the ages of 6 months and 4 years. Acute upper airway obstructions may also be caused by facial trauma, cancer, enlarged tonsils, edema, chemical and thermal burns, and infection. Obstructive sleep apnea is the most common cause of chronic upper airway obstruction; other causes include masses and malignancy.

- *Lower airway obstructions* are obstructions of the trachea, bronchi, and bronchioles, as noted by the following: Lower airway obstructions are more commonly caused by chronic diseases, such as asthma, tracheomalacia, and cystic fibrosis. *Bronchiolitis* is a common cause of acute lower airway obstruction, often as a result of RSV infection. *Tracheobronchial foreign body aspiration* is a potentially life-threatening, acute lower airway obstruction that requires emergent intervention to restore/ maintain gas exchange.

Signs and Symptoms

Symptoms of airway obstruction vary with severity:

- Partial airway obstruction: changes in voice, coughing, dyspnea, shortness of breath, snoring, stridor, wheezing
- Complete airway obstruction: apnea, cyanosis, death, respiratory distress, retractions, inability to speak, inability to swallow secretions

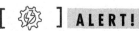 **ALERT!**

Airway is the top priority when assessing and treating a patient. If the airway is not patent, the patient will decompensate rapidly and go into cardiac arrest due to respiratory failure and hypoxia.

Diagnosis

Labs

There are no lab tests specific to diagnosing an airway obstruction. However, the following may be done in preparation for a surgical intervention:

- ABG/VBG: indication of hypercarbia/hypoxia
- CBC: elevated WBCs
- CMP
- Type and screen: preoperative

Diagnostic Testing

- Bronchoscopy
- CT scan: chest, soft tissue, neck
- Laryngoscopy
- X-ray: chest, neck

 NURSING PEARL

Note that the narrowest part of an adult airway is at the glottis, and the narrowest part of a pediatric airway is at the cricoid tissue.

Treatment

- Immediate clearing of complete obstructions to prevent respiratory arrest and death: Emergent endotracheal intubation is indicated. Nasotracheal intubation may be attempted to bypass occlusion in oral cavity. If an endotracheal tube is not able to bypass the obstruction, emergent cricothyrotomy and tracheostomy are indicated. If the obstruction is not cleared urgently and cardiac arrest occurs, proceed with resuscitation per ACLS guidelines. ▶

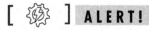 **ALERT!**

The Heimlich maneuver may have been administered before arriving at the hospital in an attempt to clear the airway obstruction. If it was not successful, the nurse should anticipate more aggressive measures, such as direct visualization and retrieval with Magill forceps, intubation, or tracheostomy.

Treatment *(continued)*

- Partial airway obstruction: benefits from supplemental oxygen, possibly humidified to moisten secretions and assist in mobilizing mucus
- Additional medications, such as bronchodilators and corticosteroids (see Table 3.1), to possibly relax bronchial smooth muscle and decrease airway inflammation
- Antibiotics (see Table A.1) indicated for infection prophylaxis after foreign body aspiration
- Bronchoscopy and laryngoscopy: possibly diagnostically to visualize obstruction and possibly therapeutically to remove foreign bodies/aspirated contents, secretions, mucus plugs, and masses
- Immediate administration of intramuscular epinephrine for anaphylaxis
- Possible specialist consultation for continued management of chronic airway obstructions, such as those caused by malignancy

Nursing Interventions

- Apply supplemental oxygen if needed to maintain SpO_2 greater than 94%.
- Administer medications as prescribed.
- Assist in gathering equipment, such as Magill forceps, for extraction of foreign body.
- Assist in opening the airway in an unresponsive patient by using the head tilt or jaw thrust maneuver.
- Be prepared to insert a nasopharyngeal or oral airway if the tongue is obstructing the airway (often evidenced by snoring respirations).
- Establish IV access and draw lab tests as ordered.
- Gather equipment for placement of an advanced airway, including emergency cricothyrotomy if an endotracheal intubation is unsuccessful.
- Perform head-to-toe assessment with focus on HEENT and respiratory systems. Note signs of airway obstruction upon auscultation, such as stridor or rhonchi. Alert provider immediately if signs of respiratory distress are present in the patient with suspected airway obstruction.
- Place patient on continuous pulse oximetry and cardiac monitoring, alerting emergency provider of any changes in vital signs or cardiac rhythm. If respiratory and/or cardiac arrest occurs, proceed with resuscitation per ACLS guidelines.

Patient Education

- Understand prevention of future airway obstructions. Caregivers of young children: Learn choking prevention measures.
- Learn about risk for airway obstruction. Patients with chronic conditions, such as asthma and COPD: Learn about specific underlying disease process to control symptoms and prevent further exacerbations.
- If there is a history of anaphylaxis, know that a prescription for two epinephrine auto-injectors will be provided. Keep auto-injector available at all times. Learn indications and use of auto-injector. Seek emergent care immediately after epinephrine administration.
- Patients with an airway obstruction: Understand that hospitalization may be required for ongoing treatment. Know the plan of care, if applicable.
- Recognize reasons to return for emergent evaluation, such as airway edema, shortness of breath, stridor or wheezing, chest pain, or throat tightness.

[📝] **POP QUIZ 3.4**

A 4-year-old patient presents to the ED by ambulance with a complete airway obstruction after choking on a toy. Back and abdominal thrusts were attempted by the parent on scene but were not successful. Paramedics were unable to clear the foreign body, and intubation was unsuccessful. CPR is now in progress. What intervention does the nurse anticipate will next be attempted to bypass the obstruction?

PLEURAL EFFUSION

Overview

- A *pleural effusion* is a collection of fluid between the membranes surrounding the lungs and the visceral and parietal pleurae.
- Pleural effusions are categorized by composition. A transudative effusion is caused by fluid shifting, which may occur as a result of a variety of conditions such as heart failure, cirrhosis with ascites, and nephrotic syndrome. Exudative effusions occur as a result of inflammation and cellular damage, which may develop secondary to pneumonia, pulmonary embolism, or malignancy. Chylothorax (chylous effusion) occurs when chyle from the lymphatic system leaks into the pleura, which may occur secondary to trauma or malignancy. Hemothorax refers to a collection of blood within the pleura, most often occurring secondary to trauma.
- Patients with preexisting lung disease, sarcoidosis, liver disease, malignancies, and infections such as pneumonia are at increased risk for developing a pleural effusion.

Signs and Symptoms

Patients can be asymptomatic or present with the following symptoms:

- Cough
- Diminished breath sounds on the affected side
- Dullness noted on percussion
- Dyspnea
- Egophony
- Fever
- Hypoxia
- Pleuritic or sharp chest pain
- Pleural rub

Diagnosis

Labs

- ABG
- Blood cultures (if infection is suspected)
- BNP
- CBC
- CMP
- Coagulation panel
- Pleural fluid cultures

Diagnostic Testing

- Chest CT
- Chest x-ray
- Thoracentesis for pleural fluid analysis
- Ultrasound

[ ] **COMPLICATIONS**

Pleural effusions may lead to impaired gas exchange and decreased cardiac output. Patients may also develop infection within the pleural space, leading to empyema and sepsis.

[🌐] **NURSING PEARL**

A pleural friction rub is an adventitious lung sound that may be described as a rasping noise. This occurs as the result of inflamed pleural membranes rubbing against each other upon inspiration and expiration.

Treatment

- Thoracentesis: May be performed for both diagnostic and therapeutic reasons. Thoracentesis indicated if etiology of pleural effusion unclear (even in cases of small effusions) to obtain fluid for analysis. Possible indication for drainage of pleural fluid for symptom relief in patients with larger effusions. May require placement of indwelling pleural catheter for continued drainage of pleural fluid.

- Treatment may be guided by addressing underlying cause. Hemothorax/pneumothorax secondary to therapeutic anticoagulation: may need to pause or reverse anticoagulant. Possible chest tube or needle decompression indication for complications related to hemothorax/pneumothorax. Possible requirement for patients with congestive heart failure of alteration in prescribed therapies to reduce recurrence of effusions; for example, increased diuretic and nitrate medications. Pleural effusions secondary to pneumonia: antibiotics (see Table A.1). Underlying malignancy: oncology consultation for ongoing disease management.

Nursing Interventions

- Administer medications as prescribed.
- Apply supplemental oxygen if needed to maintain SpO_2 greater than 94%.
- Establish IV access and draw blood for lab tests as ordered.
- Perform head-to-toe assessment with focus on respiratory system. Note adventitious sounds upon auscultation, such as pleural friction rub.
- Place patient on continuous pulse oximetry and cardiac monitoring, alerting emergency provider to any changes in vital signs or cardiac rhythm.
- Prepare for and assist with bedside thoracentesis, if needed. Assist with patient positioning (seated, leaning forward, with head and arms resting on a bedside table; if patient is unable to maintain positioning, lay the patient on their side with arm raised over head). Collect fluid for analysis. Assess thoracentesis puncture site. Apply an occlusive dressing post procedure. Continually monitor respiratory status throughout and following procedure.
- Promote pulmonary hygiene. Have patient turn, cough, and deep breathe. Instruct patient on use of incentive spirometer (performed at least 10 times per hour) to improve lung capacity.

Patient Education

- Know risk factors for pleural effusions. Recognize the importance of managing chronic conditions that increase the risk for pleural effusions, such as congestive heart failure and liver disease.
- Follow instructions for administration of any prescribed medications, such as antibiotics.
- If discharged with a pleural drainage catheter, follow instructions regarding care and monitoring of the drain. Keep home-care follow-up appointments for ongoing assessment and management of pleural drainage catheters.
- If thoracentesis was performed, follow instructions regarding wound care and monitoring. Return for evaluation if any signs of infection occur, such as wound drainage or erythema. ▶

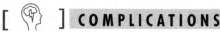 **COMPLICATIONS**

A possible complication of thoracentesis is pneumothorax. Respiratory status should be monitored throughout the procedure. No more than 1500 mL of pleural fluid should be removed in a single procedure to minimize risk of pleural edema. This procedure should be guided by ultrasound.

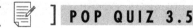 **POP QUIZ 3.5**

During a bedside thoracentesis, the patient suddenly develops increasing pain, cough, and shortness of breath. What complication of thoracentesis should the nurse suspect may have occurred?

Patient Education *(continued)*

- If pleural effusion, know that hospitalization for ongoing treatment may be required. Understand the plan of care, if applicable.
- Recognize reasons to return for emergent evaluation, such as shortness of breath, stridor or wheezing, chest pain, or throat tightness.

PNEUMOTHORAX

Overview

- Pneumothorax occurs when air enters the pleural space between the visceral and parietal pleurae, causing a partially or fully collapsed lung.
- A pneumothorax may be the result of preexisting medical conditions such as COPD, asthma, or lung cancer.
- Iatrogenic pneumothorax may be the result of a medical procedure (e.g., a biopsy).
- A spontaneous pneumothorax is more common in the following patients: cigarette smokers; patients with a history of Marfan's syndrome; tall, thin, male patients.
- A pneumothorax may be classified as the following: *Simple pneumothorax* is generally not severe and does not cause pressure on other organs. *Tension pneumothorax* occurs when the lung is fully collapsed, causing a shift in mediastinal structures. This is a life-threatening emergency.
- A pneumothorax may be the result of trauma: penetrating (e.g., gunshot wounds that are open, allowing air to pass through); nonpenetrating (e.g., as in blunt trauma rupturing the alveoli inside the chest cavity).

[🧠] **COMPLICATIONS**

Increased intrapleural pressure in tension pneumothorax leads to hemodynamic compromise. Cardiac compression leads to decreased cardiac output and JVD. Patients often will become hypotensive and tachycardic. If tension pneumothorax is not emergently decompressed, this condition will lead to rapid decompensation and death.

Signs and Symptoms

- Absent or diminished breath sounds (occurring in affected lung)
- Cyanosis
- Dyspnea
- Hypoxia
- Jugular venous distention (JVD)
- Narrowing pulse pressure
- Sharp chest pain, which may worsen with breathing
- Subcutaneous emphysema
- Tracheal deviation (in tension pneumothorax)

Diagnosis

Labs

There are no lab tests specific to diagnosing pneumothorax. However, the following tests may be indicated:

- ABG/VBG
- CBC
- CMP
- Type and screen

Diagnostic Testing
- Chest CT scan
- Chest x-ray
- Ultrasound

Treatment

- Immediate management of any open pneumothorax. Placement of an occlusive sterile dressing secured on three sides or use of a commercially prepared dressing with a one-way valve placed over the puncture site; prevents outside air from entering the pleural space during inspiration and allows interpleural air to escape during expiration.
- Emergent needle decompression required for any tension pneumothorax. Decompression of a tension pneumothorax: insertion of a 14- to 16-gauge needle into the pleural space to release air and reduce intrapleural pressure prior to placement of a thoracostomy tube. Preferred insertion site for needle decompression: second intercostal space at the midclavicular line.
- All patients with suspected pneumothorax: high-flow supplemental oxygen; positive-pressure ventilation contraindicated prior to thoracostomy tube placement
- Chest tube thoracostomy placement indicated for large or recurrent pneumothorax or any open or tension pneumothorax, and for patients requiring positive-pressure ventilation. Pain management: local anesthesia and medications, such as opiate analgesics (see Table A.2), recommended prior to chest tube placement in patients who are alert and hemodynamically stable. Prophylactic antibiotics (see Table A.1) possible for chest tube placement to prevent infection based on patient presentation.
- Patients with recurrent pneumothorax: may require surgical intervention to reduce risk for developing pneumothorax. Thoracoscopy: may be used to investigate for and resect blebs, if found. Pleurodesis: may be indicated to create inflammation within the pleura, preventing recurrence of pneumothorax.

Nursing Interventions

- Assist in gathering the following equipment for emergent needle decompression: extended-length 14- to 16-gauge IV needle catheter or commercially prepared device; cleaning solution for the site, such as iodine; tape or securing device.
- Perform head-to-toe assessment with focus on respiratory system. Apply a three-sided sterile occlusive dressing or commercially prepared device to any open chest wound. If tracheal deviation is present, alert provider immediately and perform emergent needle decompression. Observe work of breathing and auscultate lung fields, noting any abnormality, such as hyperresonance or diminished/absent breath sounds. Assess head, neck, and chest for subcutaneous emphysema.
- Place patient on continuous pulse oximetry and cardiac monitoring, alerting emergency provider to any changes in vital signs or cardiac rhythm.
- Apply high-flow supplemental oxygen.
- Establish IV access and draw blood for lab tests as ordered.
- Administer medications as prescribed, such as analgesics and antibiotics. ▶

[🌐] **NURSING PEARL**

DOPE is a mnemonic used to troubleshoot causes of potential air leaks in chest tube system:

Displaced tube

Obstruction

Pneumothorax

Equipment failure

Nursing Interventions *(continued)*

- Prepare for and assist with chest tube placement, if needed. Collect necessary equipment, and prepare chest tube drainage system. Don appropriate personal protective equipment. Assist with patient positioning (varies depending on patient condition and location of pneumothorax). Once tube is inserted and secured, attach chest tube to drainage system. Keep drainage system below the level of the patient's chest at all times. Initiate chest tube drainage system suction as ordered. Assess chest tube insertion site, ensuring that no air leak is present and tubing is not kinked, and apply sterile dressing. Continually monitor patient's respiratory status and chest tube output both throughout and after procedure. Use FOCA (**F**luctuation in the water seal chamber, **O**utput, **C**olor of drainage, **A**ir leak assessment) mnemonic to assess chest tube after insertion.
- Endotracheal intubation and mechanical ventilation may be indicated after chest tube placement if respiratory status does not improve.

Patient Education

- Adhere to activity restrictions as prescribed. Avoid high altitudes and flying for up to 6 weeks after recovering from pneumothorax. Ambulate frequently, as tolerated, to promote lung expansion and prevent infection after a pneumothorax.
- Learn about medications, recognizing the importance of completing the full course of antibiotics as prescribed.
- Learn risk factors for development of pneumothorax. Learn about high rate of recurrence of spontaneous pneumothorax. Seek support and resources regarding smoking cessation to reduce risk of future pneumothorax and other respiratory issues.
- Monitor for signs of infection, such as fevers, chills, and cough.
- Know that hospitalization may be required for ongoing treatment of a pneumothorax. Understand plan of care, if applicable.
- If discharged home with a Heimlich valve and portable collection device due to chest tube placement: Know that this one-way valve, often used for smaller, spontaneous pneumothorax, may be safer and more easily managed because the collection device may be held in any position without causing air to enter the pleural space. Follow up with home-care services for continued assessment and management of the chest tube.
- Recognize reasons to return for emergent evaluation, such as worsening chest pain; shortness of breath; or issues with chest tube insertion site and drainage system, such as insertion site erythema, warmth, bleeding, or air leak, or changes in output, such as increased bleeding or purulent drainage.

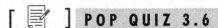 **POP QUIZ 3.6**

The nurse has received a report on an adult patient with single puncture wound to the chest. Emergency medic services (EMS) applied a three-sided occlusive dressing the wound prior to arrival. The nurse assesses the patient a notices that they are now restless and tachypneic and ha developed tracheal deviation. What should the nurse do nex

PULMONARY EDEMA

Overview

- Pulmonary edema refers to an accumulation of fluid within the alveolar spaces and may be categorized as cardiogenic or noncardiogenic.
- *Cardiogenic pulmonary edema* occurs due to increased hydrostatic pressure within pulmonary ▶

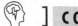 **COMPLICATIONS**

Extra fluid accumulation in the parenchyma leads decreased gas exchange, increasing the risk for respiratc failure.

Overview *(continued)*

capillaries, causing fluid to shift and flood the alveoli. It may occur as a result of heart failure and cardiomyopathy.

- *Noncardiogenic pulmonary edema* occurs as a result of increased capillary permeability caused by an increase in pulmonary vascular pressure, which may occur secondary to a variety of causes such as ARDS, high-altitude pulmonary edema, and pulmonary embolism.

[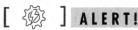] **ALERT!**

Flash pulmonary edema may occur in patients with acute decompensated congestive heart failure, as left-sided filling pressures in the heart suddenly increase. A combination of medications, such as nitrates, diuretics, and opiate analgesics such as morphine, may be used to urgently resolve acute pulmonary edema. Patients may also require inotropic support and positive-pressure ventilation.

Signs and Symptoms

Patients with chronic pulmonary edema may experience more subtle symptoms with gradual onset, such as progressively worsening orthopnea and fluid retention, while more acute presentations may be accompanied by rapid onset of the following symptoms:

- Anxiety
- Crackles
- Cough
- Diaphoresis
- Dyspnea
- Hypertension
- Orthopnea
- Pink or white frothy sputum
- Tachycardia
- Tachypnea
- Wheezing

Diagnosis

Labs

- ABG
- Cardiac enzymes: BNP, creatine kinase–myoglobin binding (CK-MB), troponin
- CBC
- CMP

Diagnostic Testing

- Chest CT scan
- Chest x-ray
- EKG
- Echocardiogram
- Pulmonary artery catheterization
- Ultrasound

Treatment

- Administration of supplemental oxygen to maintain oxygenation. Patients with pulmonary edema likely require positive-pressure ventilation using CPAP or BiPAP to maintain adequate ventilation. Endotracheal intubation may be indicated if NIPPV is unsuccessful or contraindicated (e.g., due to altered mental status, nausea, or vomiting). ▶

Treatment *(continued)*

- Medical management focused on reducing dyspnea, promoting vasodilation, improving cardiac function, and correcting fluid overload. Bronchodilators, such as albuterol, to improve oxygenation (see Table 3.1). Nitrates, such as nitroglycerin, to relax smooth muscle and decrease preload to reduce fluid transudation. Diuretic medications, such as furosemide, to reduce preload and promote elimination of excess fluid. Inotropic agents, such as dopamine, to possibly improve cardiac output. Opiate analgesics, such as morphine, to improve comfort and reduce air hunger (see Table A.2).
- Prevention and treatment of pulmonary edema: management of underlying etiology. Possible prevention of cardiogenic pulmonary edema by optimizing management of chronic cardiac and lung disease. Varied management of noncardiogenic causes, depending on etiology.

Nursing Interventions

- Administer medications as prescribed. Assess pain level and air hunger to assess need for opiate analgesics such as morphine. Reassess vital signs and respiratory pattern after medication administration, and administer additional doses or titrate medications, such as inotropic agents, as needed.
- Apply supplemental oxygen if needed to maintain SpO_2 greater than 94%.
- Assist with patient positioning for comfort and ease of breathing. Patients are often most comfortable in high Fowler's or tripod position to promote lung expansion.
- Establish IV access and draw blood for lab tests as ordered.
- Monitor I/O. Placement of an indwelling urinary catheter may be required for strict output monitoring. Fluid and sodium restrictions may be prescribed to better control fluid balance.
- Perform head-to-toe assessment with focus on respiratory system. Note adventitious sounds that may signify pulmonary edema, such as coarse crackles.
- Place patient on continuous pulse oximetry and cardiac monitoring, alerting emergency provider to any changes in vital signs or cardiac rhythm. Assist to obtain an EKG for prompt interpretation by the emergency provider. Patients may require positive-pressure ventilation to maintain adequate oxygenation; prepare for and assist with placement of CPAP or BIPAP as ordered. If noninvasive ventilation is contraindicated or is not successful, emergent intubation may be required. Specific strategies, such as prone positioning and use of low tidal volume ventilation, may be used to optimize outcomes for certain conditions, such as ARDS. Intubated patients may require frequent suctioning of ETT.
- Provide incentive spirometer for patient to use at least 10 times per hour.

Patient Education

- Learn about prescribed treatment plan. Adhere to any prescribed fluid or sodium restrictions. Monitor weight daily. Recognize normal parameters for weight fluctuation and when to seek care (generally if greater than 3-lb weight gain occurs within 2–3 days). Recognize the importance of taking all medications as prescribed. Recognize the potential effects of medications, such as bleeding risk if anticoagulated and risk for hypokalemia with use of diuretics.
- Learn about risk factors for development of pulmonary edema. If living at or traveling to high altitudes, mitigate risk by slowing rate of ascent and descent. Learn proper management of chronic diseases that may lead to the development of pulmonary edema, such as heart failure, coronary artery disease, hypertension, and obstructive sleep apnea.
- Know that hospitalization may be required for ongoing treatment of a pulmonary edema and its underlying cause. Understand the plan of care, if applicable. ▶

Patient Education *(continued)*

- Recognize reasons to return for emergent evaluation, such as worsening shortness of breath, dyspnea, productive cough, increased fluid retention, and orthopnea, or signs of infection, such as fever and chills.
- Use incentive spirometer 10 times per hour.

PULMONARY EMBOLUS

Overview

- *PE* is a partial or complete blockage of the pulmonary arteries, which may cause life-threatening cardiovascular and respiratory compromise.
- Most PEs are composed of thrombi, which is a portion of a blood clot that has traveled from elsewhere in the body, usually a deep vein thrombosis (DVT).
- Other materials may cause a PE, including the following: Fat embolism occurs when particles of fat enter circulation and travel to the lungs; this may occur as a result of trauma, often secondary to long-bone fracture. Air emboli may occur secondary to medical procedures, such as vascular cannulation. Amniotic fluid embolism may occur if amniotic fluid or fetal materials enter the bloodstream, usually as a result of trauma.
- Septic emboli may occur if infected particles, such as pieces of bacterial vegetation that have formed on an implanted medical device (such as a mechanical valve), travel through the bloodstream and enter pulmonary circulation.

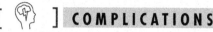 **COMPLICATIONS**

Complications for PE include pulmonary hypertension, obstructive shock, and death.

Signs and Symptoms

- Anxiety
- Apprehension
- Chest pain
- Cough, with or without hemoptysis
- Crackles upon auscultation
- Diaphoresis
- Dyspnea
- Feeling of impending doom
- Mental status changes
- Pain with deep breathing
- Petechial rash
- Pleural friction rub
- Sudden shortness of breath
- Tachycardia
- Tachypnea

[⚡] **ALERT!**

Patients with suspected air embolism should be immediately placed onto their left side in the Trendelenburg position. This may prevent right ventricular outflow obstruction by preventing air from traveling into the pulmonary arteries from the right side of the heart.

Diagnosis

Labs

There are no lab tests specific to diagnosing a pulmonary embolus. However, the following tests may be indicated when caring for the patient with this condition:

- ABG: evaluate for hypercarbia/hypoxia
- CBC

Labs (continued)

- CMP
- Coagulation panel
- D-dimer: may indicate that a clot is in the process of being broken down
- Troponin: elevated levels indicates cardiac ischemia

Diagnostic Testing

- Chest x-ray
- CT chest scan with and without contrast
- CT angiography
- EKG
- Echocardiogram
- Ventilation/perfusion scan
- Venous Doppler ultrasound

Treatment

- Administration of supplemental oxygen to maintain oxygenation. PE: causes impaired perfusion rather than impaired ventilation; intubation and mechanical ventilation may not improve hypoxia. May require advanced supportive measures, such as ECMO, to sustain life.
- Anticoagulants such as heparin, low-molecular-weight heparin, and warfarin for nearly all patients with a PE. Patients with larger PEs: may require fibrinolytic therapies. Monitor for bleeding after any anticoagulant or thrombolytic medications.
- Patients with known risk factors for thrombus formation and embolization: prevention of PE. Placement of an inferior vena cava filter to prevent PE, although the device itself may increase risk of thrombus formation.
- PE may be deadly; perform resuscitation per ACLS guidelines if cardiac arrest occurs.
- Severely compromised patients with a massive PE: embolectomy or thrombectomy possibly indicated.

Nursing Interventions

- Administer medications as prescribed. Assess patient before, during, and after administration of thrombolytic medications, and remain vigilant regarding risk for bleeding. Continually reassess respiratory status to monitor response to prescribed therapies.
- Apply supplemental oxygen if needed to maintain SpO_2 greater than 94%. While high-flow oxygen is beneficial in optimizing oxygenation of functioning lung tissue, impaired perfusion due to PE may lead to marked hypoxia despite interventions. If indicated, prepare for and assist with cannulation for ECMO and expedite transfer to critical care unit for continued management.
- Establish IV access and draw blood for lab tests as ordered, including serial partial thromboplastin times every 6 hours for patients on heparin drip.
- Monitor I/O. Placement of an indwelling urinary catheter may be required for strict output monitoring in the critically ill patient.
- Perform head-to-toe assessment with focus on respiratory and cardiovascular system. Note adventitious sounds that may signify a PE, such as basilar crackles and wheezing. Note any signs of right heart strain, such as JVD.
- Place patient on continuous pulse oximetry and cardiac monitoring, alerting emergency provider to any changes in vital signs or cardiac rhythm. Assist to obtain an EKG for prompt interpretation by the emergency provider.
- Prepare for surgical intervention, if indicated.

Patient Education

- Understand risk factors for thromboembolic disease and consider lifestyle changes, which may reduce risk for thrombosis and embolization. If medications increase risk for venous thromboembolism (VTE), such as oral contraceptives or hormone replacement medications, learn about potential adverse effects and monitor for symptoms of a PE. Seek smoking cessation resources, if applicable. Wear compression stockings daily and ambulate frequently to reduce venous stasis.
- Learn administration of anticoagulants as prescribed. Comply with treatment plan, including taking all medications as prescribed. Depending on anticoagulant prescribed, adhere to any routine intermittent blood sampling schedule to assess coagulation. Discuss risk for bleeding and learn signs of occult bleeding, such as abdominal discomfort, dark/tarry stools, and coffee-ground emesis. Take fall prevention measures to reduce risk for injury and bleeding.
- Seek emergent evaluation of any worsening symptoms such as chest pain, shortness of breath, altered mental status, unilateral weakness or numbness/tingling, changes in speech or vision, or abnormal gait.

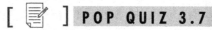

POP QUIZ 3.7

A young adult patient presents to the ED with shortness of breath and chest pain after a recent transatlantic flight. The patient states that their legs were swollen a few days ago, but that it is now resolved. The patient is a current smoker and takes oral contraceptives. The patient has a negative urine pregnancy test. After imaging is performed, the patient is diagnosed with a PE. What risk factors may have contributed to this diagnosis?

TRAUMA

Overview

- Thoracic trauma may be blunt or penetrating in nature and may result in injury to respiratory and cardiac structures.
- Rib fractures are the most common consequence of blunt thoracic injury. Patients may develop a pneumothorax or hemothorax secondary to rib fractures. A flail chest is destabilization of the chest wall, which occurs when fractures are present in two or more contiguous ribs. This causes paradoxical movement in the injured area of the chest, leading to ineffective ventilation.

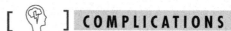

COMPLICATIONS

Complications from trauma to the respiratory system include ARDS, pneumothorax or hemothorax, pneumonia, and pulmonary contusions.

- Blunt thoracic injury may also cause pulmonary contusions (bruising of the lungs). Injury to the lung parenchyma causes edema and bleeding from damaged capillaries; this may cause pulmonary edema. Severe pulmonary injury may lead to the development of ARDS.
- Trauma to the neck and chest may cause tracheobronchial and esophageal injuries. Tracheobronchial injury is usually caused by penetrating trauma or a "clothesline" mechanism of injury. Esophageal injury is rare because the esophagus is well protected; injury is often associated with trauma to the epigastrium secondary to an motor vehicle crash (MVC)
- A ruptured diaphragm can be caused by blunt or penetrating trauma. Diaphragmatic injury may lead to herniation of abdominal organs into the chest cavity.
- In addition to blunt and penetrating trauma, barotrauma may cause damage to thoracic structures, such as pulmonary contusions secondary to blast injuries.

Signs and Symptoms

Table 3.2 shows signs and symptoms of thoracic trauma with interventions.

TABLE 3.2 Signs and Symptoms of Thoracic Trauma With Interventions

TRAUMA	SIGNS AND SYMPTOMS	INTERVENTIONS
Blunt esophageal injury	• Dysphagia • Odynophagia • Subcutaneous emphysema	• Analgesia • Surgery
Flail chest	• Bruising to the chest • Dyspnea • Pain with palpation of the fracture • Paradoxical chest wall movement with breathing • Pneumothorax	• Analgesia • Intubation and mechanical ventilation • See Pneumothorax section for more information regarding treatment of pneumothorax and hemothorax
Pulmonary contusions	• Bruising to the chest • Dyspnea • Hemoptysis (if severe) • Pain • Possible rib fractures	• Analgesia • Intubation and mechanical ventilation, if indicated • Supportive care
Rib fractures	• Dyspnea: Pain with breathing and with palpation of area	• Analgesia • Oxygen therapy: can vary from nasal cannula administration to intubation and mechanical ventilation
Ruptured diaphragm	• Abdominal pain • Bowel sounds present in the lung fields • Dyspnea	• Analgesia • Surgery
Tracheobronchial injury	• Dyspnea • Hoarse voice • Stridor • Subcutaneous emphysema in the upper chest, neck, or face	• Conservative management if patient is stable and without respiratory distress • Possible indication for cricothyrotomy • Possible indication for intubation and mechanical ventilation

Diagnosis

Labs

There are no lab tests specific to diagnosing trauma. However, the following tests may be indicated in the patient presenting with suspected traumatic injury:

- ABG/VBG
- CBC
- CMP
- Coagulation panel
- Lactate
- Type and screen

Diagnostic Testing

- Prioritized focused sonography with assessment in trauma (FAST) examination for any trauma patient, performed after provider completes primary survey to quickly identify internal injuries in any patient presenting with blunt or penetrating trauma. FAST: bedside ultrasound of the heart, right upper quadrant, left upper quadrant, and pelvis. If severe injury/uncontrolled bleeding identified with ▶

Diagnostic Testing (continued)

initial FAST and patient is hemodynamically compromised, further imaging may be deferred to expedite surgical intervention.

■ If patient hemodynamically stable, possible further investigation of injuries. CT scan: chest, neck. Ultrasound: chest, neck. X-ray: chest, neck.

Treatment

■ Provider to conduct primary trauma survey; trauma team to immediately proceed with stabilizing interventions if complications of thoracic trauma, such as tension pneumothorax, flail chest, or life-threatening uncontrolled bleeding, are present.

■ All trauma patients: cardiac monitoring and IV access. Supplemental oxygen to maintain SpO_2 greater than 90%. Patients with chest trauma likely to require ventilatory support.

■ If external hemorrhage noted or if provider notes concern for hemorrhage upon performing FAST examination, the following may be indicated: emergent procedures at the bedside, such as needle decompression and chest tube placement for tension pneumothorax. Surgical intervention: possibly required to investigate and repair injuries.

■ Administration of medications and volume replacement guided by patient condition; the following may be required: blood products; fluid resuscitation with isotonic crystalloid solution; pain medications, such as opiate analgesics (see Table A.2); prophylactic antibiotics for penetrating injuries (see Table A.1).

■ Treatment specific to certain conditions is noted in Table 3.2.

Nursing Interventions

■ Administer medications as prescribed, such as analgesics and antibiotics.

■ Apply supplemental oxygen to maintain SpO_2. Assist with endotracheal intubation and monitoring/management of mechanical ventilation, if needed.

■ Assess and assist with emergent airway, breathing, and circulation interventions.

■ Establish IV access and draw blood for lab tests as ordered.

■ Patients may require expedited transfer to operating room for surgical intervention or critical care unit for continued treatment and monitoring.

■ Perform head-to-toe assessment with focus on cardiovascular and respiratory system. Observe pattern and quality of respirations, noting any penetrating injuries or abnormal chest wall movement. Auscultate lung fields and note any abnormalities such as diminished or absent breath sounds.

■ Place patient on continuous pulse oximetry and cardiac monitoring, alerting emergency provider to any changes in vital signs or cardiac rhythm.

■ Prepare for and assist with any bedside procedures, such as chest tube placement. Report a loss of more than 1,500 mL after chest tube placement.

■ Transfuse blood products if indicated.

Patient Education

■ Learn methods to prevent thoracic trauma. Use seat belts to prevent chest trauma related to motor vehicle crashes. Know strategies to minimize risk for falls.

■ If discharged from the ED after minor thoracic trauma: Adhere to any necessary follow-up and recognize reasons to return for emergent evaluation, such as worsening chest pain or shortness of breath or signs of infection such as fevers, chills, or productive cough. If provided with an incentive spirometer,   ▶

Patient Education *(continued)*

learn use of spirometry and recognize the importance of deep breathing to prevent atelectasis and pneumonia.

▪ With moderate to severe thoracic trauma, know that hospital admission for continued treatment and monitoring will likely be required. Understand the plan of care.

RESOURCES

Agency for Clinical Innovation. (n.d.-a). *Pleural effusion*. Emergency Care Institute. https://www.aci.health.nsw.gov .au/networks/eci/clinical/clinical-resources/clinical-tools/respiratory/pleural-effusion

Agency for Clinical Innovation. (n.d.-b). *Pleural effusion—Classification*. Emergency Care Institute. https:// aci.health.nsw.gov.au/networks/eci/clinical/clinical-resources/clinical-tools/respiratory/pleural-effusion/ pleural-effusion-classification

Agency for Clinical Innovation. (n.d.-c). *Pleural effusion—Management and disposition*. Emergency Care Institute. https://aci.health.nsw.gov.au/networks/eci/clinical/clinical-resources/clinical-tools/respiratory/pleural-effusion/ pleural-effusion-management-and-disposition

American College of Allergy, Asthma and Immunology. (n.d.). *Asthma attack*. https://acaai.org/asthma/symptoms/ asthma-attack

American Lung Association. (n.d.-a). *Emphysema*. https://www.lung.org/lung-health-diseases/lung-disease-lookup/ emphysema

American Lung Association. (n.d.-b). *Pulmonary embolism symptoms and diagnosis*. https://www.lung.org/lung -health-diseases/lung-disease-lookup/pulmonary-embolism/symptoms-diagnosis

American Lung Association. (n.d.-c). *Treating and managing pulmonary embolism*. https://www.lung.org/lung-health -diseases/lung-disease-lookup/pulmonary-embolism/treating-and-managing

The ARDS Definition Task Force. (2012). Acute respiratory distress syndrome: The Berlin definition. *Journal of the American Medical Association, 307*(23), 2526–2533. doi:10.1001/jama.2012.5669

Campo, T. M. (2017). *Medical imaging for the health care provider: Practical radiograph interpretation* (pp. 67–71). Springer Publishing Company.

Casey, R. (2020). Thoracic and neck trauma. In Emergency Nurses Association (Ed.), *Provider manual eighth edition TNCC trauma nursing core course* (8th ed., pp. 130–139). Jones & Bartlett.

Centers for Disease Control and Prevention. (n.d.). *Basics about COPD*. U.S. Department of Health & Human Services. https://www.cdc.gov/copd/basics-about.html

Chakraborty, R. K., & Basnet, S. (2021, March 1). Status asthmaticus. In *StatPearls*. StatPearls Publishing. https:// www.ncbi.nlm.nih.gov/books/NBK526070

Clardy, P., Manaker, S., & Perry, H. (2019). Carbon monoxide poisoning. *UpToDate*. https://www.uptodate.com/ contents/carbon-monoxide-poisoning

Clark, S. B., & Soos, M. P. (2021, January 30). Noncardiogenic pulmonary edema. In *StatPearls*. StatPearls Publishing. https://www.ncbi.nlm.nih.gov/books/NBK542230

Cramer, N., Jabbour, N., Tavarez, M. M., & Taylor, R. S. (2020, August 23). Foreign body aspiration. In *StatPearls*. StatPearls Publishing. https://www.ncbi.nlm.nih.gov/books/NBK531480

Dasaraju, P. V., & Liu, C. (1996). Infections of the respiratory system. In S. Baron (Ed.), *Medical microbiology* (4th ed.). University of Texas Medical Branch at Galveston. https://www.ncbi.nlm.nih.gov/books/NBK8142

Diamond, M., Peniston, H. L., Sanghavi, D., & Mahapatra, S. (2021, November 9). Acute respiratory distress syndrome. In *StatPearls*. StatPearls Publishing. https://www.ncbi.nlm.nih.gov/books/NBK436002/#_NBK436002

Edgecombe, L., Sigmon, D. F., Galuska, M. A., & Angus, L. D. (2020, June 1). Thoracic trauma. In *StatPearls*. StatPearls Publishing. https://www.ncbi.nlm.nih.gov/books/NBK534843

Foley, A., & Sweet, V. (2020). Respiratory emergencies. In V. Sweet & A. Foley (Eds.), *Sheehy's emergency nursing: Principles and practice* (7th ed., pp. 216–226). Elsevier.

Ghaye, B. (2016). Non-thrombotic pulmonary embolism. *Journal of the Belgian Society of Radiology, 100*(1), 96. https://doi.org/10.5334/jbr-btr.1226

Iqbal, M. A., & Gupta, M. (2020, December 16). Cardiogenic pulmonary edema. In *StatPearls*. StatPearls Publishing. https://www.ncbi.nlm.nih.gov/books/NBK544260

Jalota, R., & Sayad, E. (2021, January 23). Tension pneumothorax. In *StatPearls*. StatPearls Publishing. https://www.ncbi.nlm.nih.gov/books/NBK559090

Jany, B., & Welte, T. (2019). Pleural effusion in adults-etiology, diagnosis, and treatment. *Deutsches Arzteblatt International*, *116*(21), 377–386. https://doi.org/10.3238/arztebl.2019.0377

Light, R., & Lee, Y. C. G. (2020). Pneumothorax in adults: Epidemiology and etiology. *UpToDate*. https://www.uptodate.com/contents/pneumothorax-in-adults-epidemiology-and-etiology

McKnight, C. L., & Burns, B. (2020, November 16). Pneumothorax. In *StatPearls*. StatPearls Publishing. https://www.ncbi.nlm.nih.gov/books/NBK441885

Micak, R. (2020). Inhalation injury from heat, smoke, or chemical irritants. *UpToDate*. https://www.uptodate.com/contents/inhalation-injury-from-heat-smoke-or-chemical-irritants

National Heart, Lung, and Blood Institute. (n.d.-a). *Acute respiratory distress syndrome*. U.S. Department of Health and Human Services, National Institutes of Health. https://www.nhlbi.nih.gov/health-topics/acute-respiratory-distress-syndrome

National Heart, Lung, and Blood Institute. (n.d.-b). *Asthma*. U.S. Department of Health and Human Services, National Institutes of Health. https://www.nhlbi.nih.gov/health-topics/asthma

National Heart, Lung, and Blood Institute. (n.d.-c). *COPD*. U.S. Department of Health and Human Services, National Institutes of Health. https://www.nhlbi.nih.gov/health-topics/copd

National Heart, Lung, and Blood Institute. (n.d.-d). *Pleural disorders*. U.S. Department of Health and Human Services, National Institutes of Health. https://www.nhlbi.nih.gov/health-topics/pleural-disorders

National Heart, Lung, and Blood Institute. (n.d.-e). *Pneumonia*. U.S. Department of Health and Human Services, National Institutes of Health. https://www.nhlbi.nih.gov/health-topics/copd. https://www.nhlbi.nih.gov/health-topics/pneumonia

National Heart, Lung, and Blood Institute. (n.d.-f). *Venous thromboembolism*. U.S. Department of Health and Human Services, National Institutes of Health. https://www.nhlbi.nih.gov/health-topics/venous-thromboembolism

Paralikar, S. J. (2012). High altitude pulmonary edema-clinical features, pathophysiology, prevention and treatment. *Indian Journal of Occupational and Environmental Medicine*, *16*(2), 59–62. https://doi.org/10.4103/0019-5278.107066

Pilcher, J., & Beasley, R. (2015). Acute use of oxygen therapy. *Australian Prescriber*, *38*(3), 98–100. https://doi.org/10.18773/austprescr.2015.033

Pinto, D., & Garan, A. (n.d.). Pathophysiology of cardiogenic pulmonary edema. *UpToDate*. https://www.uptodate.com/contents/pathophysiology-of-cardiogenic-pulmonary-edema.

Prescribers' Digital Reference. (n.d.-a). *Acetylcysteine* [Drug information]. https://www.pdr.net/drug-summary/Acetylcysteine-acetylcysteine-668

Prescribers' Digital Reference. (n.d.-b). *Albuterol sulfate* [Drug information]. https://www.pdr.net/drug-summary/Albuterol-Sulfate-Inhalation-Solution-0-083--albuterol-sulfate-1427.4212

Prescribers' Digital Reference. (n.d.-c). *Azithromycin* [Drug information]. https://www.pdr.net/drug-summary/Azithromycin-azithromycin-24249#10

Prescribers' Digital Reference. (n.d.-d). *Digoxin* [Drug information]. https://www.pdr.net/drug-summary/Digoxin-digoxin-724#14

Prescribers' Digital Reference. (n.d.-e). *Dobutamine hydrochloride* [Drug information]. https://www.pdr.net/drug-summary/Dobutamine-dobutamine-hydrochloride-3534#10

Prescribers' Digital Reference. (n.d.-f). *Dopamine hydrochloride* [Drug information]. https://www.pdr.net/drug-summary/Dopamine-Hydrochloride-dopamine-hydrochloride-3710#15

Prescribers' Digital Reference. (n.d.-g). *Guaifenesin* [Drug information]. https://www.pdr.net/drug-summary/Mucinex-guaifenesin-1275#14

Prescribers' Digital Reference. (n.d.-h). *Ipratropium bromide* [Drug information]. https://www.pdr.net/drug-summary/Ipratropium-Bromide-ipratropium-bromide-3270.2526

Prescribers' Digital Reference. (n.d.-i). *Prednisone* [Drug information]. https://www.pdr.net/drug-summary/Prednisone-Tablets-prednisone-3516.6194

Purvey, M., & Allen, G. (2017). Managing acute pulmonary oedema. *Australian Prescriber, 40*(2), 59–63. https://doi
.org/10.18773/austprescr.2017.012

Reed, K. D. (2015). Respiratory tract infections: A clinical approach. *Molecular Medical Microbiology, 3*, 1499–1506.
https://doi.org/10.1016/b978-0-12-397169-2.00084-6

Rose, D., & Dubensky, L. (2020, August 10). Airway foreign bodies. In *StatPearls*. StatPearls Publishing. https://www
.ncbi.nlm.nih.gov/books/NBK539756

Saadeh, C. K. (2020, June 17). What is the role of magnesium sulfate in the treatment of status asthmaticus?
Medscape. https://www.medscape.com/answers/2129484-51987

Sanivarapu, R. R., & Gibson, J. (2020, November 18). Aspiration pneumonia. In *StatPearls*. StatPearls Publishing.
https://www.ncbi.nlm.nih.gov/books/NBK470459

Shubert, J., & Sharma, S. (2020, November 21). Inhalation injury. In *StatPearls*. StatPearls Publishing. https://www
.ncbi.nlm.nih.gov/books/NBK513261

Thompson, B. T., & Kabrhel, C. (2020). Patient education: Pulmonary embolism (beyond the basics). *UpToDate*.
https://www.uptodate.com/contents/pulmonary-embolism-beyond-the-basics

Zanni, J. (n.d.). *Module 4: Understanding mechanical ventilation*. Johns Hopkins Medicine. https://www
.johnshopkinssolutions.com/wp-content/uploads/2017/10/4-Understanding-Mechanical-Ventilation.pdf

ACUTE SPINAL CORD INJURIES

Overview

- *Spinal cord injury* is damage to the spinal nerves that can cause disrupted motor and sensory function below the level of injury; it may occur as a result of direct spinal trauma.
- The neurologic injury may be categorized according to spinal cord level. Cervical spinal cord injuries (C1-C7) cause the most severe deficits, potentially resulting in loss of respiratory function, loss of speech and swallowing ability, loss of bowel and bladder control, and quadriplegia. Thoracic spinal cord injuries (T1-T12) may impact respiratory function and bowel/bladder function and frequently result in paraplegia. Lumbar spinal cord injuries (L1-L5) frequently impact lower extremity function and cause loss of bowel and bladder function. Sacral spinal cord injuries (S1-S5) may impact function and sensation of lower extremities and sexual organs/perineum; patients may also experience loss of bowel and bladder control.
- Injuries may also be classified by severity, with complete spinal cord injuries resulting in total loss of motor and sensory function below the level of injury and incomplete spinal cord injuries allowing some retained motor or sensory function. *Anterior cord syndrome*, typically caused by hyperflexion, is an incomplete spinal cord injury that involves damage to the anterior two thirds of the spinal cord. *Brown-Séquard syndrome*, usually caused by penetrating trauma, is due to a partial transection of the spinal cord. *Central cord syndrome*, typically caused by hyperextension, is compression caused by swelling near the center of the spinal cord. *Posterior cord syndrome*, typically caused by hyperflexion or nontraumatic causes such as demyelinating disease, involves damage and ischemia to the posterior third of the spinal cord.
- Trauma (blunt or penetrating) is the most common cause of spinal cord injury.

Signs and Symptoms

Symptoms related to spinal cord injury vary with level and severity of injury (Table 4.2).

[ ] **COMPLICATIONS**

Patients with spinal cord injuries are at risk for severe complications. Autonomic dysfunction as a result of spinal cord injury may cause autonomic dysreflexia, thermoregulatory issues, and spinal or neurogenic shock, which may be deadly. Patients with paralysis and limited mobility are at increased risk for thromboembolic events, skin breakdown, bowel and bladder issues, and infections such as pneumonia and urinary tract infection (UTI). Patients may also suffer complications related to mental health, such as depression and anxiety.

[ ] **ALERT!**

Patients with spinal cord injuries are at risk for both spinal and neurogenic shock. Neurogenic shock is a subset of distributive shock, which causes cardiovascular/circulatory failure (see Chapter 2 for more information), while spinal shock is a response to a sudden loss of spinal reflexes below the level of injury (Table 4.1).

TABLE 4.1 Types of Shock in Spinal Cord Injury

SPINAL SHOCK	NEUROGENIC SHOCK
• Bowel and bladder dysfunction • Damage anywhere on spinal cord • Lack of ability to regulate temperature • Loss of reflexes below level of injury • Muscle flaccidity • Nervous system response	• Form of distributive shock • Can either be temporary or permanent • Damage at T6 or higher • Normal color and warmth to skin • Temperature instability • Vascular system response • Bradycardia • Hypotension • Loss of vascular resistance • Peripheral vasodilation

TABLE 4.2 Signs and Symptoms of Spinal Cord Injuries

CORD SYNDROME	SYMPTOMS
Anterior cord syndrome	• Complete motor loss below level of injury • Pain and temperature sensation loss below level of injury • Maintained proprioception and vibratory sensation
Posterior cord syndrome	• Preserved motor movement and most sensory functions • Deep touch, vibration, and proprioception loss
Central cord syndrome	• Loss of motor and sensory function, more in upper than in lower extremities
Brown-Séquard syndrome	• Contralateral loss of pain and temperature sensation below level of injury • Ipsilateral loss of proprioception, vibration, and motor function below level of injury
Complete spinal cord lesion	• Absent motor and sensory function below injury • Absent reflexes below level of injury • Loss of bowel or bladder control • Flaccid extremities below level of injury • External rotation of the legs at the hips • Hypotension • Bradycardia • Poikilothermia • Paralytic ileus • Priapism • Respiratory depression

Diagnosis

Labs

There are no lab tests specific to diagnosing acute spinal cord injuries. However, the following are often used to assess patients presenting with suspected spinal injuries or trauma:

▪ Arterial blood gas (ABG)
▪ Complete blood count (CBC)
▪ Comprehensive metabolic panel (CMP)
▪ Coagulation panel
▪ Lactic acid
▪ Type and screen

Diagnostic Testing
- CT scan: head, neck, cervical, and/or total spine
- MRI
- X-ray

Treatment

- For spinal cord injury that is likely the result of significant trauma: Emergency provider must first conduct primary trauma survey. Trauma team immediately proceeds with stabilizing interventions while maintaining spinal immobilization with a cervical collar, logrolling, and use of a backboard. Assess pulse and cardiac rhythm. If pulse is not present, immediately proceed with resuscitation per advanced cardiovascular life support (ACLS) guidelines. Address airway, breathing, and circulatory concerns. Manage the potential for neurologic shock complications (bradycardia and hypotension monitoring). This may require the use of atropine or vasopressors, as needed to maintain a mean arterial pressure (MAP) greater than 65 mmHg.

[ ] **NURSING PEARL**

It is possible for patients to have injuries to the spinal cord that are not visible even with radiographic imaging, and the likelihood of detection increases with use of MRI. Spinal cord injury without radiographic abnormality is a rare diagnosis that is more common in children, in which patients show symptoms of spinal cord injury despite normal radiographic findings.

- Medications and intravenous (IV) fluids guided by patient condition
- Fluid resuscitation with isotonic crystalloid solution
- Vasopressors for cardiovascular complications related to neurogenic shock
- Corticosteroid medications, such as methylprednisolone, to reduce inflammatory response (see Table A.4)
- Pain medications, such as opiate analgesics (see Table A.2)
- Prophylactic antibiotics for penetrating injuries (see Table A.1)
- Possible surgical intervention for treatment of spinal cord injuries. Surgical decompression may be indicated in the acute injury phase and is associated with improved outcomes when compared with decompression delayed for longer than 24 hours. Laminectomy and/or spinal fusion may be indicated.
- Referrals to specialty consultation (e.g., neurology, neurosurgery, orthopedic spine) for recommendations, if applicable

Nursing Interventions

- Administer medications as prescribed. Assess pain quality and severity, and medicate patient as ordered.
- Apply supplemental oxygen to maintain SpO_2. Assist with endotracheal intubation and monitoring/management of mechanical ventilation, if needed.
- Assess for signs of autonomic dysreflexia. Investigate for noxious stimuli, such as bladder fullness, skin breakdown, and infection.
- Conduct psychosocial assessment and provide emotional support as needed.
- Establish IV access and draw laboratories as ordered.
- Insert nasogastric (NG) tube for gastric decompression or continuous tube feedings for nutrition.
- Maintain a warm environment. Patients require warming lights or warm blankets due to thermoregulatory dysfunction.
- Maintain spinal immobilization. Apply cervical collar. Use techniques such as logrolling to minimize vertebral movement. Maintain the patient's bed flat in reverse Trendelenburg until further instructed by the neurosurgery or orthopedic spine team. If able, reposition patient frequently to prevent pressure ulcers.
- Monitor intake/output (I/O). Placement of an indwelling urinary catheter is likely indicated.
- Patients may require expedited transfer to the operating room for surgical intervention or the critical care unit for continued treatment and monitoring. ▶

Nursing Interventions *(continued)*

- Perform head-to-toe assessment with focused neurologic and cardiovascular assessments. Assess level of consciousness and cranial nerves. Assess sensation and motor function in all extremities, noting any deficits. Note skin color and temperature, heart rate, and respirations, alerting emergency provider to any signs or symptoms of shock.
- Place patient on continuous pulse oximetry and cardiac monitoring, alerting emergency provider to any changes in vital signs or cardiac rhythm.

Patient Education

- Learn about complications of spinal cord injury, such as autonomic dysreflexia. Return for emergent evaluation if experiencing fever, shortness of breath, pain, diaphoresis, or dizziness/lightheadedness.
- Understand the plan of care. Hospital admission may be required for continued treatment and monitoring. Depending on severity and level of injury, rehabilitation and possible lifelong care will likely be required. Follow up with case management and social work. Learn expectations regarding impact of injury on long-term sensory and motor function. Follow a bowel and/or bladder program to help manage and regulate urination and bowel movements, which may include self-catheterization.
- Recognize importance of maintaining spinal immobilization as ordered to prevent worsening injury.
- Use assistive devices to help regain functioning based on level of spinal cord injury, which may include wheelchairs, walkers, shoehorns, slide boards, or smart hands-free technology.
- Work with physical therapist/occupational therapist to help regain and/or maximize new level of functioning.

> **[📝] POP QUIZ 4.1**
>
> A patient suffered a spinal cord injury at T5 after a motor vehicle crash a few years ago. The patient presents to the ED appearing anxious and diaphoretic, with facial flushing and cool, clammy lower extremities. The patient's blood pressure is elevated. What should the nurse suspect may be the cause of these symptoms?

CHRONIC NEUROLOGIC DISORDERS

Overview

- Chronic neurologic disorders are associated with significant morbidity and mortality and may be caused by a variety of factors, including genetic disorders, brain injuries, spinal cord injuries, congenital abnormalities, and infection and inflammation.

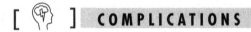

> **[🧠] COMPLICATIONS**
>
> Complications of chronic neurologic disorders include anxiety, bed sores, death, dementia, depression, falls, food aspiration, and pneumonia.

- *Myasthenia gravis* is a chronic autoimmune and neuromuscular disorder that causes painless and varying muscle weakness, especially of the ocular, bulbar, facial, neck, limb, and respiratory muscles. This autoimmune disease disrupts the binding of acetylcholine at the neuromuscular junction, preventing muscle contraction and causing progressively worsening muscle weakness. *Myasthenic crisis* is a medical emergency that causes severe muscle weakness; patients may require intubation and mechanical ventilation due to weakness of respiratory muscles.
- *Multiple sclerosis (MS)* is a demyelinating disorder in which damage to the myelin sheath causes progressive neurologic dysfunction; it is thought to be related to autoimmune dysfunction. Many patients with MS experience acute and chronic neuropathic pain. Patients with MS may present to the ED during an acute exacerbation due to severe weakness and immobility.
- *Amyotrophic lateral sclerosis (ALS)* is a progressive degenerative disorder of the motor neurons; this condition is ultimately fatal, and its cause is unknown. ▶

Overview *(continued)*

■ *Parkinson disease* is caused by the degeneration of dopaminergic neurons and is characterized by progressive muscle rigidity, bradykinesia, and resting tremors.

■ *Huntington disease* is a fatal autosomal dominant genetic disorder that causes degeneration of neurons in the dorsal striatum, leading to chorea (unpredictable and uncontrollable movements). Patients also experience muscle spasms that impair mobility and weakness that may become severe enough to inhibit swallowing.

Signs and Symptoms

Table 4.3 shows signs and symptoms of chronic neurologic disorders.

TABLE 4.3	Signs and Symptoms of Chronic Neurologic Disorders
DISEASE	**SIGNS AND SYMPTOMS**
Myasthenia gravis	• Fluctuating skeletal muscle weakness, most notably bulbar: dysarthria, dysphagia, fatigue with prolonged chewing • Facial muscle weakness: myasthenic sneer • Neck and proximal limb weakness: dropped head syndrome • Ocular: ptosis and/or diplopia • Respiratory muscle weakness • Muscle fatigue • Myasthenic crisis: severe bulbar (oropharyngeal) muscle weakness • Weakness of respiratory muscles
Multiple sclerosis	• Erectile dysfunction • Fatigue • Muscle spasticity/painful contractions • Numbness/tingling • Paralysis • Poor coordination • Slurred speech • Tremors • Urinary incontinence or retention • Visual changes including double vision or loss of vision • Vertigo
Amyotrophic lateral sclerosis	• Cognitive and behavioral changes • Difficulty walking or doing normal daily activities • Inappropriate crying, laughing, or yawning • Muscle cramps and twitching in arms, shoulders, and tongue • Poor coordination: frequent tripping and falling • Slurred speech or trouble swallowing • Weakness/clumsiness to hands, legs, feet, or ankles
Parkinson disease	• Poor balance and coordination • Stiffness of the arms, legs, and trunk • Slowness of movement • Speech difficulty • Symptoms that progressively worsen; typically start on one side of the body and remain more pronounced on that side • Tremors, trembling of hands, arms, legs, jaw, and face

(continued)

TABLE 4.3	Signs and Symptoms of Chronic Neurologic Disorders *(continued)*
DISEASE	SIGNS AND SYMPTOMS
Huntington disease	Movement disorders: • Difficulty with speech and/or swallowing • Impaired gait, posture, and balance • Involuntary jerking or writhing movements • Rigidity or contracture of muscles • Slow or abnormal eye movements • Tremors Cognitive disorders: • Aphasia • Being unaware of one's own behaviors • Difficulty focusing on tasks • Difficulty learning new information • Dysgraphia • Inability to process thoughts • Poor impulse control Psychiatric disorders: • Apathy • Depression and/or mania • Fatigue • Insomnia • Irritability • Social withdrawal • Suicidal thoughts or tendencies

Diagnosis

Labs

While specialized diagnostic tools, such as genetic testing, may be used in the outpatient setting to identify causes of neurologic disorders, the following tests may be performed in the ED for the patient with a chronic neurologic disease:

- CBC
- Cerebrospinal fluid (CSF) sampling
- CMP
- Serum antibody testing
- Urinalysis (if infection is suspected)

Diagnostic Testing

Neurologic examination is the primary diagnostic tool for assessment in the ED; however, the following tests may be indicated to investigate neurologic disease:

- CT scan
- MRI
- Electromyography
- Nerve conduction study
- Lumbar puncture (LP)

Treatment

- Treatment specific to neurologic disorder (see Table 4.4).
- Acute exacerbations or decompensation of chronic neurologic disorders: Patients may present to ED with neurologic deficits, altered mental status, or decreased level of consciousness. Neurologic disease that causes motor dysfunction may impede muscle contraction, impairing movement and limiting mobility. This may progress to cause respiratory compromise; ventilatory support with nasal intermittent positive pressure ventilation or endotracheal intubation may be required.
- Difficulty swallowing for patients with neurologic disorders: Speech pathology consultation and speech therapy may be indicated. Patients may require dietary alterations, such as thickened liquids, to reduce risk of aspiration. Advanced disease with chronic dysphagia may lead to malnutrition; patients may require feeding via NG, gastric, or jejunostomy tube.

[⚡] ALERT!

Treatment of myasthenia gravis includes cholinesterase inhibitors. Overdosing (whether intentionally or accidentally) on these medications can cause a cholinergic crisis. Myasthenia gravis and cholinergic crisis appear similar in presentation, with the exception of diarrhea, increased oral secretions, and diaphoresis, which are present only in a cholinergic crisis. The nurse should be aware of the difference between these diagnoses.

TABLE 4.4 Medications for Neurologic Conditions

INDICATIONS	MECHANISM OF ACTION	CONTRAINDICATIONS, PRECAUTIONS, AND ADVERSE EFFECTS
Anticonvulsant (levetiracetam, phenytoin)		
• Prevent seizures	• Exact mechanism unknown • Limits spread of seizure activity in brain (phenytoin)	• Avoid abrupt disruption in anticonvulsant medications to prevent status epilepticus (except in cases of allergic reactions). • Only reconstitute phenytoin with 0.9 NS for IV route. Check for particulate matter prior to infusing.
Antifungal (amphotericin, fluconazole)		
• Treat fungal meningitis	• Alters fungal cell membrane	• Alert provider right away if patient develops darkening of the skin, diarrhea, and fainting. • Medication is not compatible with many drugs; have pharmacist verify prior to taking.
Anti-Parkinson agents, dopamine precursors (carbidopa-levodopa)		
• Treat PD	• Absorbed by central nervous system and converted into dopamine • Administered concurrently to prevent peripheral conversion of levodopa from being converted into dopamine	• Medication is contraindicated in patients who have malignant melanoma, diabetes, and psychiatric disorders. • Side effects are constipation, trouble sleeping, and loss of muscle coordination.

(continued)

TABLE 4.4 Medications for Neurologic Conditions (continued)

INDICATIONS	MECHANISM OF ACTION	CONTRAINDICATIONS, PRECAUTIONS, AND ADVERSE EFFECTS
Cholinesterase inhibitors (pyridostigmine bromide and donepezil)		
• Treat dementia/ Alzheimer's disease • Myasthenia gravis	• Block destruction of acetylcholine	• Adverse effects are headaches, lightheadedness, weakness, and prolonged muscle contraction. • Use caution in patients who have bradycardia or cardiac conduction problems as medication may increase vagal tone, potentially causing syncope and falls. • IV pyridostigmine may produce uterine contractions; do not give to pregnant patients.
Fibrinolytic therapy (alteplase, streptokinase, tenecteplase, reteplase)		
• Ischemic stroke	• Convert plasminogen to plasmin so plasmin can break down fibrin and fibrinogen to dissolve clot	• Monitor for signs of angioedema, which can occur during and after the infusion (up to 2 hours). • Monitor for signs of worsening mental status, as an intracranial hemorrhage can occur. • tPA is contraindicated with intracranial hemorrhage, blood glucose less than 50 mg/dL, blood pressure greater than 185/110 mmHg despite treatment, endocarditis, INR greater than 1.7, aPTT greater than 40 seconds, PT greater than 15 seconds, intracranial neoplasm, and low platelets (less than 100,000/mm³). • tPA is also contraindicated when the patient has history of intracranial hemorrhage, gastrointestinal bleeding in the past 3 weeks, inhibitors of direct thrombin or direct factor Xa within the last 48 hours (unless laboratory testing shows normal coagulation levels), ischemia stroke in last 3 months, low-molecular-weight heparin in last 24 hours, major surgery in last 2 weeks, severe head trauma in last 3 days, or surgery of head or spine in last 3 days.
Hypertonic (3%) solution		
• Decrease cerebral edema • Decrease ICP	• Increases osmolarity of blood; thus, fluid shifts from extravascular space into intervascular space	• Infusion over long periods of time may cause hyperchloremic metabolic acidosis. • Monitor for hypernatremia.
Immunosuppressants (tacrolimus)		
• Reduce the immune response in MG	• Inhibit first step in T-cell activation	• Patient should not take if current severe infection, cancer, or diabetes.
Monoclonal antibodies (IVIG, rituximab, eculizumab)		
• Treat some autoimmune diseases • MG	• Target specific cells to prevent autoimmune flareup	• Monitor for fever and flu-like symptoms. • Serious but rare infusion reaction in which medication needs to be stopped and possibly restarted at a slower rate.

(continued)

TABLE 4.4 Medications for Neurologic Conditions *(continued)*

INDICATIONS	MECHANISM OF ACTION	CONTRAINDICATIONS, PRECAUTIONS, AND ADVERSE EFFECTS
Muscle relaxer (baclofen)		
• Treat muscle pain, spasms, and stiffness in people with MS or spinal cord injury	• GABA agonist that reduces the release of excitatory neurotransmitters in presynaptic neurons	• Do not use when muscle tone is needed for balance and movement during certain activities. • Do not drive or operate heavy machinery. • Suddenly stopping may cause withdrawal symptoms.
NMDA receptor antagonist		
• Slow progression of Alzheimer disease	• Binds to the excitatory neurotransmitter glutamate to control calcium going into the nerve cells	• Side effects are dizziness, confusion, headache, and constipation. • Watch for misuse of the medication.
Osmotic diuretics (mannitol)		
• To reduce ICP • To reduce cerebral edema	• Stop reabsorption of water and increase osmolarity of extracellular fluid to draw fluid from intracellular system to extracellular system	• Medication is contraindicated in pulmonary edema. • Common adverse reactions are electrolyte abnormalities and dehydration.
Selective serotonin receptor antagonist (sumatriptan)		
• Treat migraine or cluster headaches	• Narrows blood vessels in the head, stopping pain signals	• Common side effects are sleepiness and feeling faint. • Do not take with ergotamine or other triptans. • Use caution in patients with heart disease.

aPTT, activated partial thromboplastin time; GABA, gamma-aminobutyric acid; ICP, intracranial pressure; INR, international normalized ratio; IV, intravenous; IVIG, intravenous immune globulin; MG, myasthenia gravis; NMDA, N-methyl-D-aspartate; NS, normal saline; PD, Parkinson disease, PT, prothrombin time; tPA, tissue plasminogen activator.

Treatment *(continued)*

- Likely benefit from consultation with physical and occupational therapy to develop strategies to maintain mobility and independence
- Pain management for patients with chronic neurologic disorders: Medications for neuropathic pain, such as gabapentin (see Table A.2). Muscle relaxants (e.g., baclofen) for conditions that increase spasticity (see Table 4.4). Opioid analgesia possible for breakthrough pain (see Table A.2).

Nursing Interventions

- Perform head-to-toe assessment with focused neurologic examination. Discuss baseline cognition with patient or caregiver and assess level of consciousness, cranial nerves, and motor function, noting any deficits.
- If indicated, place patient on continuous pulse oximetry and cardiac monitoring, alerting emergency provider to any changes in vital signs or cardiac rhythm.
- Administer medications as prescribed. Assess pain and provide analgesic agents and muscle relaxant medications as indicated.   ▶

Nursing Interventions (continued)

- Apply supplemental oxygen if needed to maintain SpO_2 greater than 94%. Prepare for intubation and mechanical ventilation if needed for patients with advanced neurologic disease.
- Assist with mobility and patient positioning: Patients with chronic neurologic disorders are likely to require mobility aids to safely ambulate; provide assistance, using gait belt to maintain safety if needed. Reposition patient frequently as rigidity and limited mobility may lead to skin breakdown.
- Establish IV access and draw blood for lab tests as ordered. Patients with chronic neurologic disorders may already have an invasive line due to the need for frequent infusions.
- Monitor I/O. Patients with chronic neurologic disease may require placement of an indwelling urethral or suprapubic urinary catheter. Incontinent patients are more likely to experience skin breakdown; provide skin care and perineal cleansing regularly.
- Monitor nutrition and provide feedings as needed. Due to cognitive impairment, limited mobility, and/or swallowing issues, patients are likely to require assistance with feeding; if unable to maintain nutrition, patients may require tube feeding.

Patient Education

- Follow the plan of care and return to the hospital when required, such as when experiencing abnormal breathing, shortness of breath, altered mental status, new onset of weakness, numbness, trouble walking, or changes in speech. Attend outpatient appointments. Collaborate with case management and social work as needed. Continue being monitored by neurology. Continue therapy regimen. Follow the prescribed diet to decrease the risk of choking. Take medications as prescribed. Use fall precautions such as removing trip hazards like cords and throw rugs. Have a family member or caregiver assist with walking.
- Progressive neurologic degeneration requires complex care that may involve routine follow-up with a number of specialists (e.g., urology to manage urinary conditions, physical and occupational therapy to maintain mobility and ability to complete activities of daily living [ADLs]).
- As disease progresses, it may be necessary to discuss palliative and hospice care.

[📝] **POP QUIZ 4.2**

What medications are typically administered to treat Parkinson disease?

DEMENTIA

Overview

- *Dementia* is a general term for progressive and irreversible memory loss and cognitive decline.
- In addition to cognitive issues, patients with dementia often suffer from emotional and behavioral issues, as well as sleep disturbances.
- *Alzheimer disease* is the most common cause of dementia. It causes amyloid plaques and neurofibrillary tangles in the brain, loss of connection between neurons, and shrinking of the brain.
- Vascular dementia causes dementia secondary to cerebrovascular damage, which may occur as a result of vascular disease, ischemia, or hemorrhagic stroke.
- Patients with Parkinson disease are at increased risk for *Lewy body dementia*, a form of dementia in which abnormal protein deposits in the brain cause cognitive impairment, visual hallucinations, and psychosis. Note that Lewy body dementia may be present in patients without Parkinson disease.
- Frontotemporal dementia involves the progressive degeneration of the frontal and temporal lobes, resulting in cognitive dysfunction, personality and behavioral changes, and difficulty with speech and language.
- Other causes of dementia include neurologic disorders such as Huntington disease. ▶

Overview *(continued)*

- Risk for dementia increases with age. Other potential risk factors include history of cardiovascular disease, use of substances such as nicotine and alcohol, head trauma or stroke, and genetic factors/family history of dementia.

Signs and Symptoms

- Cognitive impairments; communication difficulty; difficulty performing tasks; forgetfulness; hallucinations; memory loss.
- Behavioral disturbances; agitation/aggression; mood changes; self-neglect; social withdrawal; personality changes; emotional dysregulation.
- Difficulty performing ADLs
- Difficulty with speech and language
- Failure to thrive

Diagnosis

Labs

While laboratory testing is not used to diagnose dementia in the ED, the following tests may be ordered to assess for illness in patients with dementia:

- CBC
- CMP
- Serum vitamin B_{12}
- Thyroid panel
- Urinalysis and urine culture

[🌐]   NURSING PEARL

Due to impaired cognition, patients with dementia may not exhibit typical complaints when ill. For example, patients with dementia who have a UTI may not complain of dysuria or increased urinary frequency and may instead exhibit more vague signs and symptoms, such as increased weakness or confusion. It is important to assess for possible infection in patients with cognitive decline.

Diagnostic Testing

Neurologic assessment and cognitive function tests are the primary diagnostic tool for dementia; however, radiographic imaging may be used to identify structural changes to the brain that may contribute to cognitive decline:

- Angiography
- CT scan: head
- MRI: brain

Treatment

- For complaints of illness, injury, or behavioral/psychiatric crisis: No cure for dementia; focused treatment on symptom alleviation as disease progression is likely in all patients. Presenting complaint addressed, noting that illness and injury may present differently in patients with dementia.
- Long-term medical management of Alzheimer disease and Lewy body dementia: possible cholinesterase inhibitors (see Table 4.4) to prevent breakdown of acetylcholine and slow progression of symptoms
- *N*-methyl-D-aspartate (NMDA) receptor antagonists (see Table 4.4) possible to slow progression of disease by limiting overactivation of glutamine receptors, which may occur in dementia
- Possible physical therapy and/or occupational therapy to help patients retain existing function
- Complex care planning and ongoing specialist consultation required: Referral to psychiatry for continued management of emotional dysregulation and behavioral issues is needed as disease progresses. Family/caregivers of patients with dementia may require consultation with case management and social work to develop plan of care; as function declines and independence is lost, patients may require placement in a long-term care or skilled nursing facility. Advanced dementia patients may require a consult to hospice and palliative care.

Nursing Interventions

- Administer medications as prescribed.
- Assist with mobility and patient positioning. Patients with dementia may require mobility aids to safely ambulate; provide assistance, using gait belt to maintain safety if needed.
- Conduct psychosocial assessment and provide emotional support to patients and family/caregivers.
- Maintain safety. Assess risk for falls and, if necessary, place patient on continuous observation to prevent injury. Assess risk for elopement and take necessary precautions as needed.
- Monitor I/O. Patients with dementia are at increased risk for dehydration; administer IV fluids as ordered. Most patients with dementia become incontinent, which may lead to skin breakdown; assist with toileting and provide skin care and perineal cleansing regularly.
- Monitor nutrition and provide feedings as needed. Due to cognitive impairment, limited mobility, and/or swallowing issues, patients with dementia are likely to require assistance with feeding.
- Perform head-to-toe assessment with focused neurologic examination. Discuss baseline cognition with patient or caregiver and assess level of consciousness, cranial nerves, and motor function, noting any new deficits.
- Provide support with decision-making and advance care planning.

Patient Education

- Adhere to treatment plans, including taking all medications as prescribed. Follow prescribed dietary restrictions, such as dysphagia diet, to minimize aspiration risk. Learn medication administration and any necessary precautions, such as increased risk for falls with certain psychiatric medications that may be used for agitation/behavioral issues in dementia.
- Discuss plan of care. Follow up as recommended with outpatient care planning, working with case management and social work as needed. Recognize that progressive cognitive decline requires complex care, which may involve routine follow-up with several specialists, such as neurology, psychiatry, and physical and occupational therapy. Know that advanced disease may require palliative and hospice care or placement in a long-term care or skilled nursing facility.
- Recognize reasons to seek emergent evaluation, such as an acute increase in altered mental status or new-onset neurologic deficits, such as weakness, paresthesia, or abnormal gait or speech.
- Reduce risk of falls and injuries. Learn about necessary restrictions on activities that become increasingly unsafe as cognitive decline advances, such as driving and cooking. Learn methods of reducing risk of falls in the home, such as removing throw rugs.
- Caregivers: Learn atypical signs and symptoms of illness for dementia. Monitor for acute increase in altered mental status and increased restlessness, agitation, and lethargy as potential signs of infection. Monitor patients' output, noting changes such as foul-smelling urine, which may indicate UTI.

GUILLAIN–BARRÉ SYNDROME
Overview

- *Guillain–Barré syndrome (GBS)* is a severe and life-threatening form of polyneuritis characterized by ascending paralysis that affects the cranial nerves and peripheral nervous system.
- The exact cause is unknown; however, the syndrome is often preceded by viral infection, viral immunization, HIV infection, trauma, or surgery.

[🧠]   **COMPLICATIONS**

Neuromuscular weakness leading to respiratory failu[re] may occur rapidly. Patients with GBS should have ser[ial] neurologic examinations and be monitored closely for airw[ay] protection. Progressive neurologic weakness may he[lp] identify patients at risk for respiratory failure. Patients w[ith] signs of impending respiratory failure should be intubat[ed] without delay.

Overview *(continued)*

- GBS progresses over 2 to 4 weeks, with peak weakness occurring by the third week.
- One-third of patients with GBS will require mechanical ventilation.

Signs and Symptoms

- Abnormal vagal responses; asystole; bradycardia; heart block
- Absent or depressed deep tendon reflexes
- Difficulty chewing or swallowing
- Difficulty with eye movement
- Loss of bladder control
- Paresthesia
- Pain
- Sensory loss
- Symmetric and progressive weakness; ascending weakness is most common. Descending weakness typically starts in arms or face.
- Vision problems

Diagnosis

Labs

There are no lab tests specific to diagnosing GBS. However, the following tests may be used to rule out underlying causes:

- CBC
- CMP
- CSF analysis
- HIV testing
- Urinalysis

Diagnostic Testing

- Electromyography: may show evidence of an acute polyneuropathy
- LP
- Nerve conduction study
- Spinal MRI

Treatment

- Corticosteroids (see Table A.4), intravenous immunoglobulin, plasmapheresis, or plasma exchange therapy, depending on local availability and patient clinical status (see Table 4.4)
- Monitoring for deterioration of neurologic, respiratory, and cardiovascular status, as well as autonomic dysfunction. Arterial line: may be indicated for hemodynamic monitoring. Mechanical ventilation: may be indicated for respiratory failure.
- Nutritional therapy
- Supportive care to address symptom progression, pain, and deep vein thrombosis (DVT) prophylaxis

Nursing Interventions

- Assist with patient mobility.
- Determine communication method with patient based on patient's ability level.
- Draw serial lab tests as ordered, such as ABGs.
- Ensure a fall-free environment. ▶

Nursing Interventions *(continued)*

- Frequently monitor respiratory assessment, including respiratory rate and oxygen saturation; pulmonary function measurements; incentive spirometry performance; supplemental oxygen therapy, as indicated; tidal volumes, FiO_2, and rate changes or new prolonged periods of apnea if patient is intubated.
- Keep patient NPO (nothing by mouth) until a swallow study has been done.
- Monitor blood pressure and heart rate/rhythm continuously.
- Perform incontinence care, if needed.
- Perform skin assessment and care.
- Provide analgesia for pain relief.
- Perform serial neurologic examinations and peripheral vascular assessments: Cough, gag, and corneal reflex; serial neurologic examinations during acute phase or more frequently for patients at high risk of deterioration or who are rapidly worsening; strength and motor responses in all extremities.

Patient Education

- Discuss future vaccinations with healthcare provider before receiving them.
- Do not eat or drink until a swallow study is completed.
- Engage in exercise slowly.
- Follow up with outpatient resources.
- Know that long-term effects can include fatigue, pain, and weakness.
- Understand that physical therapy may be indicated. Use assistive devices as directed.
- Be aware that the effects of GBS can last weeks or months, with potential for some side effects to last for years.

HEADACHE

Overview

- *Headaches* may be classified as either primary, with no known cause, or secondary, with an identifiable cause. Headache may also be neuropathic in nature, as with chronic conditions such as trigeminal neuralgia. Primary headaches may be further classified as cluster, migraine, and tension headaches (Table 4.5). Secondary headaches may be a sign of an emergent condition, such as cerebrovascular accident, intracranial hemorrhage, temporal arteritis, and hypertensive emergencies. Secondary headache is more commonly attributed to more benign causes, such as sinus inflammation.
- "Thunderclap headache" strikes suddenly and peaks within 60 seconds. It is uncommon but may be a sign of bleeding in and around the brain.

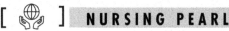

[🌐]   **NURSING PEARL**

A "thunderclap headache" is the abrupt onset of an extremely severe headache, commonly associated with an acute subarachnoid hemorrhage. Patients may describe this pain as the "worst headache of their life."

Signs and Symptoms

A secondary headache is a symptom of a medical condition such as sinusitis, subarachnoid hemorrhage, meningitis, or tumor. Patients with secondary headache often show additional signs and symptoms indicative of an underlying pathology:

- Fever
- Hypertension

[🧠]   **COMPLICATIONS**

Complications from primary headaches include impaired ability to carry out ADLs, chronic pain, and psychosocial complications such as depression and anxiety.

TABLE 4.5	Classifications of Primary Headaches
TYPE	**SIGNS AND SYMPTOMS**
Cluster	• Severe unilateral headache, usually felt behind one eye • Usually occurring at night, often lasting for less than 2 hours • May cause unilateral tearing of the eye or rhinorrhea • Episodes of headache occurring in cycles that may last days to weeks
Migraines	• May be preceded by an aura • Visual disturbances common: field deficits and visual hallucination/distortion • May have identifiable triggers, such as changes in sleep or diet • Chronic, severe episodes often debilitating • Symptoms often lasting 4–72 hours • Pain often unilateral and described as "pulsing" or "stabbing" • Nausea and vomiting • Photophobia and phonophobia
Tension	• Most common type of headaches • "Vise-like" or tight feeling • May also be described as a "muscle-contraction headache" • Usually generalized and last for several hours

Signs and Symptoms *(continued)*

- Nausea
- Neurologic deficits
- Phonophobia
- Photophobia
- Visual disturbance

Temporal arteritis has the following signs and symptoms:

- Headache
- Fatigue
- Fever
- Vision loss

Diagnosis
Labs

Many patients presenting to the ED with headache may not require laboratory testing if pain is mild to moderate and additional signs and symptoms, such as neurologic deficit or fever, are not present. If further testing is indicated, the following laboratory studies may be ordered:

- CBC
- CMP
- Coagulation panel
- Erythrocyte sedimentation rate (ESR) and C-reactive protein (CRP)
- Venereal disease research laboratory test

[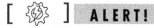]   **ALERT!**

Temporal arteritis is an emergent condition that may be incorrectly identified as a migraine or tension headache in the ED. Assessment of ESR and CRP levels is helpful in ruling out this condition, as serum levels will be elevated in patients with vasculitis.

Diagnostic Testing

- CT/CT angiography scan: head, neck
- MRI/MR angiography: brain
- Temporal artery biopsy (temporal arteritis)
- Visual acuity

Treatment

- Treatment specific to subtype: High-flow supplemental oxygen is the primary therapy for cluster headache. Patients with a migraine headache may benefit from resting in a dark, quiet room to minimize worsening symptoms related to photophobia and phonophobia. Selective serotonin receptor agonists (see Table 4.4) may be prescribed to treat more severe headaches as needed. Tension headaches are often treated with relaxation and over-the-counter pain relievers, such as acetaminophen and nonsteroidal anti-inflammatory drugs (see Table A.2). Patients may require additional medications, such as antiemetics and IV fluids, to manage headache side effects.
- Underlying cause treated for secondary headaches: Some patients may require immediate surgical intervention, such as emergent craniotomy for severe intracranial hemorrhage. Hypertensive patients may require antihypertensive medication, such as beta-blockers, to lower blood pressure and reduce headache. Patients with temporal arteritis must be medicated with corticosteroids, such as prednisone (see Table A.4.), to control inflammation.
- Patients may require consult to neurology for ongoing monitoring and management of headaches.

Nursing Interventions

- Perform head-to-toe assessment with focused neurologic examination. Assess for signs of illness or head trauma and any other potential signs of secondary headache. Alert emergency provider to any concerning symptoms, such as complaint of thunderclap headache. Assess visual acuity, if needed. Collect history regarding headache onset, location, quality, and severity, and assess level of consciousness, cranial nerves, and motor function, noting any neurologic deficits.
- Administer medications as prescribed, such as analgesics and antiemetics.
- Administer supplemental oxygen as needed to maintain SpO_2 greater than 94%; some conditions, such as cluster headache, may require administration of high-flow oxygen.
- Control environment to minimize exposure to harsh light and sound. Provide eye covering if dark environment is not available.
- Establish IV access and draw blood for lab tests as ordered.
- Provide care specific to any identified intracranial cause of headache, such as ischemic stroke or hemorrhage. Expedite transfer for emergent surgical intervention, if indicated.

Patient Education

- Adhere to treatment plans, including taking all medications as prescribed. Learn proper administration of medication taken as needed (PRN) for prescribed migraine therapies. If using anticoagulant therapy, learn about increased risk for bleeding and symptoms of intracranial bleeding. Discuss any necessary follow-up, such as referral to neurology.
- Learn about potential headache triggers. If chronic/recurrent headache, keep a record of headaches as well as daily diet and activities to assist in identifying possible headache causes. If at risk for neurologic emergencies, such as intracerebral hemorrhage or ▶

[📝]   POP QUIZ 4.3

A patient with a history of hypertension presents to the E with complaint of a headache. The patient is writhing in pa and screaming, "This is the worst headache I've ever had What condition should the nurse suspect may be the cau of this headache?

Patient Education *(continued)*

ischemic stroke, learn ways to reduce risk of such catastrophic events, such as smoking cessation and lifestyle modification to reduce blood pressure and manage other chronic cardiovascular disease.

■ Recognize reasons to seek emergent evaluation, such as an altered mental status or new-onset neurologic deficits, such as weakness, paresthesia, or abnormal gait or speech.

INCREASED INTRACRANIAL PRESSURE

Overview

■ *Intracranial pressure (ICP)* is the pressure exerted by neural tissue, blood, and spinal fluid within the skull. It occurs when there is an accumulation of fluid or a foreign body increasing the pressure within the skull onto the brain. ICP is normally less than or equal to 15 mmHg in adults; pathologic intracranial hypertension is present at pressures greater than or equal to 20 mmHg.

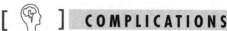

[🧠]   **COMPLICATIONS**

Increased ICP can displace cerebral contents downward, resulting in brainstem herniation and death. All effort should be made to lower and maintain ICP within a manageable value to prevent this severe complication.

■ A normal ICP is crucial in maintaining an adequate cerebral perfusion pressure (CPP). CPP is calculated by measuring the difference in MAP and ICP (MAP − ICP = CPP). Consequently, CPP may be dangerously reduced by increased ICP and decreased blood pressure.

■ Increases in ICP are caused by anything that may increase blood, CSF, or neural tissue volume, such as intracranial hemorrhage, hydrocephalus, and cerebral edema, which may occur secondary to trauma, seizures, or spinal and brain masses. Etiology of increased ICP may be classified as primary factors (intracranial causes, such as a mass) or secondary factors (extracranial causes, such as hypoventilation causing cerebral vasodilation).

Signs and Symptoms

■ Altered or decreased level of consciousness (early sign)
■ Bulging fontanelle (infants)
■ Coma
■ Cushing's triad (late sign indicating possible herniation): bradycardia, irregular respirations (Cheyne-Stokes), hypertension, widened pulse pressure
■ Dilated, nonreactive pupils
■ Headache
■ Nausea and vomiting
■ Posturing (decerebrate or decorticate)
■ Pupillary changes
■ Shrill cry (infants)
■ Visual changes

Diagnosis

Labs

There are no lab tests specific to diagnosing increased ICP. However, the following tests may be indicated if increased ICP is suspected and differential diagnosis of neurologic symptoms is required:

■ ABG
■ CBC
■ CMP   ▶

Labs (continued)
- Coagulation panel
- Ethyl alcohol (ETOH)
- Lactic acid
- Point-of-care glucose
- Serum osmolality
- Type and screen
- Urinary toxicology screen

Diagnostic Testing

Radiographic imaging of the head and neck may help uncover the cause of increased ICP by identifying hemorrhage or mass and may also be used to investigate for complications such as brain herniation.
- CT scan
- MRI
- LP

Treatment

- Treatment focused on resolution of increased ICP cause, such as evacuation of a blood clot, resection of a tumor, CSF diversion in the setting of hydrocephalus, or treatment of a trauma or an underlying metabolic disorder
- LP for measurement of ICP and CSF sampling: Opening pressure of CSF may be obtained via manometry after inserting the needle into the subarachnoid space, prior to any CSF drainage.
- Placement of an intraventricular monitor possible for invasive ICP monitoring: Intraventricular monitors are considered the gold standard of ICP monitoring devices. They are surgically placed into the ventricular system and affixed to a drainage bag and pressure transducer. This allows for the removal of CSF. Intraparenchymal devices use an electronic or fiberoptic transducer at the tip and are inserted directly into the brain parenchyma via a small hole drilled in the skull. Subarachnoid bolts are fluid-coupled systems with a hollow screw that can be placed through the skull adjacent to the dura. After the dura is punctured, the CSF can communicate with the fluid column and transducer. Epidural monitors contain optical transducers that rest against the dura after passing through the skull.
- Possible dangerous bradycardia, hypertension, and abnormal respirations, which may progress to cause cardiac arrest: immediate resuscitation per ACLS guidelines if cardiac arrest occurs.
- Possible rapid decompensation and death with hemorrhage: emergent evacuation of intracranial bleeding. Cranial burr holes may be placed for emergent decompression. Surgical intervention for craniotomy may be required to evacuate hematoma. A decompressive craniectomy may also be indicated to relieve extra pressure.
- Varied management of patients with increased ICP: Administration of antiepileptic medications, such as levetiracetam (see Table 4.4), is often indicated for seizure treatment/prophylaxis because an increase in ICP may lead to seizure activity, which further increases ICP. Administration of antipyretics (see Table A.2) may decrease cerebral edema, which occurs with fever. Administration of pain medications, such as opiate analgesics (see Table A.2), may be indicated to reduce metabolic demand, ventilator dyssynchrony, venous congestion, and sympathetic responses of hypertension and tachycardia. Blood pressure monitoring should be done to maintain a CPP greater than 60 mmHg with pressor support as needed. Conversely, medications for management of hypertension, such as beta-blockers, may be indicated. Fluid management will keep euvolemic and normo- to hyperosmolar. Administer only isotonic fluids (normal saline) and avoid free water. Patient positioning may contribute to increases in ICP; elevating the head of bed (HOB) greater than 30 degrees and maintaining the head midline will ▶

Treatment *(continued)*

maximize venous outflow. Patients with hydrocephalus may be treated with surgical placement of a ventriculoperitoneal shunt to normalize ICP.

- Additional interventions for persistent increase in ICP that is not responsive to the foregoing therapies: Patients may require mechanical ventilation, sedation, and paralysis with neuromuscular blocking agents (see Table A.2) to control airway and intrathoracic pressures and prevent reactions that may contribute to elevated ICP, such as shivering. Hyperventilation may be used to reduce ICP by promoting cerebral vasoconstriction. Osmotic agents, such as mannitol, and hypertonic (3%) saline (see Table 4.4) may be indicated to decrease fluid from the injured brain, thereby reducing ICP and preventing further injury.

Nursing Interventions

- Perform head-to-toe assessment with focused neurologic, cardiovascular, and respiratory examination. Assess level of consciousness using Glasgow Coma Scale (GCS; Table 4.6), and assess cranial nerve function and motor function, noting any deficits. Assess pain, noting onset, severity, location, and quality of any headache. Investigate for signs of head or neck injury. Apply cervical collar and maintain spinal immobilization, if indicated. Ensure collar is not too tight, which could cause increased ICP. Readjust with a second nurse if needed. Assess for symptoms associated with increased ICP, such as nausea, vomiting, and irregular respirations. Immediately alert emergency provider if there is suspicion for increased ICP.
- Place patient on continuous pulse oximetry and cardiac monitoring, alerting emergency provider to any changes in vital signs or cardiac rhythm. Assist with placement and monitoring of any invasive monitoring devices, such as an arterial line. Maintenance of systolic blood pressure greater than 100 mmHg is vital in maintaining CPP. Apply supplemental oxygen to maintain SpO_2 greater than 94%.
- Administer medications as prescribed. Assess pain and administer analgesia as ordered to reduce elevated pain. Administer additional medications, such as antiemetics, antiepileptics, antihypertensives, and osmotic agents per patient status.
- Assist emergency provider with any necessary bedside procedures, such as LP or emergent trephination with burr hole(s).
- Assist with patient positioning, maintaining elevation of the head of the bed unless contraindicated (as with spinal injury).
- If the patient has increased ICP, start with nonpharmacologic interventions to reduce ICP. Attend to pump and/or equipment alarms promptly. Decrease stimulation as much as possible by lowering the lights, stimulations, noise, and distractions in the room. Educate family to minimize patient stimulation. Minimize deep suctioning if possible. Position patient appropriately with head midline and HOB greater than 30 degrees.
- Progress to pharmacologic interventions if ICP remains elevated despite initial interventions. Administer hypertonic saline or mannitol per provider orders. Administer PRN pain medication bolus. Titrate to increase continuous pain/sedation medication.
- Monitor and draw serial lab tests (basic metabolic panel, serum osmolality) as ordered or per protocol.
- Monitor I/O; placement of an indwelling urinary catheter is often ordered for strict output monitoring.
- Notify provider and/or neurosurgery if ICP is greater than 20 mmHg for more than 5 minutes despite initial interventions.
- Perform a detailed serial neurologic assessment every hour or per neurosurgery's recommendations.
- Patients with increased ICP are at increased risk for seizure; pad bed rails and monitor for seizure activity.
- Prepare for a head CT scan if any neurologic changes are noted.
- Expedite transfer to critical care unit for continued care and monitoring, or transfer to operating room for surgical intervention if needed.

TABLE 4.6 Glasgow Coma Scale	
AGE 2 YEARS AND YOUNGER	**AGE 5 YEARS AND OLDER**
Eye Opening Response	**Eye Opening Response**
4: Spontaneous	4: Spontaneous
3: To speech	3: To speech (to sound*)
2: To pain	2: To pain (to pressure*)
1: None	1: None
Best Verbal Response	**Best Verbal Response**
5: Babbles and coos	5: Oriented
4: Irritable/cries	4: Confused
3: Cries in response to pain	3: Inappropriate words
2: Moans in response to pain	2: Incomprehensible words (sounds*)
1: None	1: None
Best Motor Response	**Best Motor Response**
6: Moves spontaneously and purposefully	6: Obeys commands
5: Withdraws from touch	5: Localizes to pain
4: Withdraws from pain (normal flexion)	4: Withdraws from pain (normal flexion)
3: Abnormal flexion (decorticate)	3: Abnormal flexion (decorticate)
2: Extension (decerebrate)	2: Extension (decerebrate)
1: None	1: None

*Updated changes to Glasgow Coma Scale (GCS), now known as GCS-40, but not exclusively adopted into practice to date.

Patient Education

- Be aware of risk factors for increased ICP. Know ways to minimize risk for head trauma, such as helmet use where appropriate. If prescribed anticoagulants, learn about increased risk for spontaneous and traumatic intracerebral bleeding. Learn about any risk for cardiovascular disease and stroke, and seek support and resources to promote lifestyle changes, such as smoking cessation, as needed. For patients with conditions that contribute to increased ICP, such as hydrocephalus or malignancy of the brain or spinal cord, learn necessary therapies for the underlying disease.
- Recognize reasons to return to the ED, such as severe headache, nausea and vomiting, or visual disturbance.
- Understand that symptomatic increases in ICP require hospital admission for continued treatment and monitoring. Discuss plan for admission and ongoing treatment with provider and nurse.

MENINGITIS
Overview

- *Meningitis* is a potentially deadly condition in which the meninges of the brain and spinal cord become inflamed. Bacterial meningitis is a result of bacteria traveling to the brain via the bloodstream. Viral meningitis can be caused by a virus, such as HIV,

[🧠]   COMPLICATIONS

Complications of meningitis include hearing and/or visio loss, cognitive changes, seizures, coordination and/o balance difficulties, behavioral or cognitive difficulties, and in severe cases, increased ICP, herniation, and death.

Overview *(continued)*

mumps, or varicella. It is typically self-limiting and rarely life-threatening; Other causes of meningitis include parasites, fungal infection, brain masses, and trauma.

- Risk for meningitis is increased in infancy and adolescence.

Signs and Symptoms

- Altered mental status
- Decreased level of consciousness
- Headache
- Fatigue
- Fever
- Nausea
- Neck pain/nuchal rigidity
- Petechial rash (meningococcal meningitis)
- Photophobia
- Vomiting

[ ]   **ALERT!**

Patients with meningitis may develop *nuchal rigidity*, or neck stiffness that impairs the ability to flex the neck forward (bring chin to chest).

Diagnosis

Labs

- Blood cultures
- CBC
- CMP
- Coagulation panel
- CSF analysis
- Point-of-care glucose

[ ]   **NURSING PEARL**

Analysis of CSF assists in differentiating between bacterial and viral meningitis. In patients with meningitis, CSF often shows a decreased glucose level and an increased protein and WBC count. Patients with bacterial meningitis typically have purulent CSF, whereas CSF of patients with viral meningitis remains clear.

Diagnostic Testing

LP and CSF sampling is the primary means of diagnosis for meningitis; however, radiographic imaging may be used to further assess patients with meningitis.

- Chest x-ray
- CT scan: head, neck
- LP
- MRI: brain

Treatment

- Intractable seizures, brain herniation, and cardiac arrest: Begin immediate resuscitation per ACLS guidelines if cardiac arrest occurs. See Intracranial Pressure section for more information regarding treatment of increased ICP and risk for brain herniation. See Seizures section for more information regarding treatment of seizures and status epilepticus.
- Meningococcal meningitis: Highly contagious and spreads via droplets. Droplet isolation precautions if meningitis suspected. Prophylactic antibiotics for those who have been in close contact with a patient diagnosed with bacterial meningitis.
- Supportive care for most patients: antipyretics (see Table A.2) for fever; electrolyte correction; nutritional support and hydration; possible fluid resuscitation with isotonic crystalloid; rest and decreased stimulation; supplemental oxygen as needed to maintain SpO_2 greater than 94%.
- Suspected bacterial meningitis priority: prompt broad-spectrum antibiotic administration (see Table A.1). Antibiotic administration should not be delayed while awaiting an LP; a CT should be ▶

Treatment (continued)

performed prior to LP for patients at high risk of herniation. Blood cultures should be drawn prior to antibiotics, but administration of antibiotics should not be delayed if unable to draw cultures prior. Adjunctive dexamethasone should be given shortly before or at the same time as the first dose of antimicrobials.

- No specific treatment for viral meningitis or eosinophilic meningitis caused by parasites. Most cases of viral meningitis are less severe and self-limiting; however, treatment with antiviral medications may be indicated for some, such as immunocompromised patients. Most patients who develop mild viral meningitis usually recover in 7 to 10 days without treatment. For parasitic meningitis, medications can be used to reduce the body's reaction to the parasite rather than for the infection itself. However, treatment of the infection may help some patients.
- Fungal meningitis: long courses of high-dose antifungal medications. Duration is dependent on clinical status and type of fungus causing infection.
- Administration of anticonvulsant medications (see Table 4.4) possible
- Corticosteroids (see Table A.4) possible to reduce inflammation
- Meningococcal vaccine recommended for all children beginning at age 11 years with a booster at age 16 years

Nursing Interventions

- Perform head-to-toe assessment with focused neurologic examination. Assess level of consciousness, cranial nerves, and motor function, noting any deficits. Assess for pain with chin-to-chest movement. Inspect skin for rashes.
- Place patient on continuous pulse oximetry and cardiac monitoring, alerting emergency provider to any changes in vital signs or cardiac rhythm. Critically ill patients may require placement and monitoring of invasive monitoring devices, such as an arterial line. Apply supplemental oxygen to maintain SpO_2 greater than 94%.
- Establish IV access and draw blood for lab tests as ordered.
- Administer medications as prescribed. Antibiotics should not be delayed while awaiting an LP; attempt to draw cultures before starting antibiotics. Administer IV fluids as ordered. Assess pain and administer analgesics as ordered.
- Assist with bedside procedures, such as LP, if needed.
- Assess and manage risk for falls and seizures; pad bedrails to prevent injury.
- Maintain elevation of HOB unless contraindicated.
- Monitor and draw serial lab tests as ordered/per protocol.
- Monitor I/O.
- Position patient appropriately with HOB higher than 30 degrees with head midline.

Patient Education

- Adhere to treatment plans, including taking all medications as prescribed.
- Be aware that bacterial meningitis is likely to require hospital admission for continued treatment and monitoring. Discuss plan of care with nurse.
- Recognize reasons to seek emergent evaluation, such as altered mental status, fever, or new-onset neurologic deficits, such as weakness, paresthesia, or abnormal gait or speech. ▶

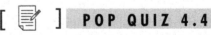 **POP QUIZ 4.4**

A 7-month-old patient is suspected of having meningococcal meningitis. The patient's parents and teenage sibling are present. What education should the nurse provide to the family about this diagnosis?

Patient Education *(continued)*

- Take precautions to reduce risk of meningitis. If in communal living, such as dormitories, shelters, and jails, recognize increased risk for contracting meningitis. If older than 11 years, follow up with primary care physician to receive the meningococcal vaccine. Practice good hand hygiene. Understand that all close contacts must take prophylactic antibiotics.

SEIZURE

Overview

- A *seizure* is a sudden change in behavior, change in awareness, and/or abnormal movements caused by the uncontrolled, excessive electrical activity between the neurons of the brain.
- Seizures may be categorized as provoked, acute symptomatic seizures occurring secondary to a known cause, such as with alcohol withdrawal and electrolyte imbalance. They can also be unprovoked, occurring without an identifiable trigger. *Epilepsy* is characterized by recurrent, unprovoked seizures.
- Seizures are further categorized as either focal or generalized according to whether the onset of electrical activity involves a focal region of the brain or the entire cortex simultaneously. Generalized seizures occur in both hemispheres, while focal onset seizures are noted to have abnormal electrical activity localized to a portion of the brain. Seizures of unknown onset may not be differentiated in this manner. Patients with focal seizures may or may not experience motor symptoms and may or may not retain awareness of their surroundings.
- Seizures can progress to *status epilepticus*, which is a seizure lasting 5 minutes or longer or multiple seizures without a return to consciousness. Patients with status epilepticus require immediate intervention to stop seizures, as well as supportive measures (e.g., mechanical ventilation). Status epilepticus is associated with significant morbidity and mortality because continued damage from repeated seizures may cause severe neurologic damage.
- Largely a clinical diagnosis, seizures can occur due to an underlying medical condition or independently. A thorough history, physical and neurologic examinations, and additional tests are needed to identity an underlying cause.

Signs and Symptoms

Symptoms vary with different types of seizures.

- Focal seizures: sensory distortion, such as visual changes and auditory or olfactory distortion; eye movements such as gaze deviation or epileptic nystagmus; possible motor function involvement, such as jerking motion of a limb; possible retained awareness or disorientation of the patient
- Generalized absence seizures: impaired awareness; "blank stare" or gaze deviation; possible motor function involvement, such as lip smacking or eyelid fluttering/epileptic nystagmus
- Generalized atonic seizure: sudden loss of muscle tone; impaired awareness
- Generalized tonic-clonic seizure: muscle stiffness/rigidity and loss of consciousness (tonic stage); rhythmic involuntary muscle contraction (clonic stage); possible loss of bladder or bowel control ▶

[🧠] **COMPLICATIONS**

Complications from prolonged seizures include acidosis, aspiration, arrhythmias, fever, hypoxia, increased ICP, renal failure, and rhabdomyolysis. Neurologic, respiratory, and cardiac compromise may lead to cardiac arrest. It is important to assess for any injuries sustained from the tonic-clonic seizure itself.

[⚡] **ALERT!**

Patients with generalized seizures often experience symptoms of confusion, decreased level of consciousness, headache, nausea and vomiting, and muscle pain during the postictal period, which usually lasts for up to 30 minutes. There may be additional concerns if disorientation persists for a longer period of time.

Signs and Symptoms *(continued)*

- Myoclonic seizure: brief twitching/jerking motion without loss of awareness
- Febrile seizure: fever over 100.4°F (38°C); shaking or jerking of the arms. Simple seizure: lasts a few seconds to 15 minutes, occurs only once in 24 hours, and is not specific to one part of the body. Complex seizure: lasts longer than 15 minutes, occurs more than once in 24 hours, or is confined to one side of the body.

Diagnosis

Labs

There are no lab tests specific to diagnosing seizures; however, the following may be helpful to rule out a metabolic or infectious cause of the seizure:

- CBC
- CMP
- Lactic acid
- Liver function tests
- Medication levels (e.g., levetiracetam, phenytoin)
- Urinalysis
- Urinary toxicology screen

Diagnostic Testing

- CT scan
- EKG
- EEG
- MRI
- LP

Treatment

- Blood sugar check for all seizure patients.
- Seizures that do not resolve within a couple of minutes: possible benzodiazepine such as lorazepam (see Table A.2.).
- Prolonged seizures and/or status epilepticus: may require rapid loading of IV anticonvulsant medication (e.g., phenytoin, levetiracetam; see Table 4.4).
- Antiseizure medication therapy dependent on multiple factors: estimated risk of recurrent seizure; probability that event represented a true seizure; stability of the patient; suspected or confirmed cause of seizure based on initial evaluation.

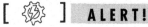

[⚡]   ALERT!

For patients presenting with convulsive status epilepticus, initial treatment with a benzodiazepine is recommended. An IV loading dose of a longer-acting antiseizure medication is also recommended to maintain seizure control. In patients who are actively seizing despite two initial doses of a benzodiazepine, preparation for a continuous midazolam or propofol infusion should occur simultaneously with administration of fosphenytoin, valproate, or levetiracetam. A continuous EEG may be ordered once the patient is stabilized, as well as serial neurologic examinations to monitor neurologic status in the patient post seizure.

- Persistent seizure despite therapies: possible sedation with barbiturate medications (see Table A.2) for their anticonvulsant and neuroprotective qualities.
- Priority treatment: protecting patient from injury and maintaining airway and ventilation; ensure airway is patent and have suction available; seizure patients are at high risk for aspiration. Patients may require intubation and mechanical ventilation. Provide protection against injury, such as padding bedrails and loosening any restrictive clothing, if needed. Patients presenting to the ED after a seizure may have injured the head/neck; spinal immobilization with application of a cervical collar may be indicated.   ▶

Treatment *(continued)*

- Provoked seizures: treatment of underlying cause. Patients require correction of any electrolyte abnormalities that may contribute to risk for seizure, such as hypoglycemia. Patients with known epilepsy with subtherapeutic serum anticonvulsant levels require additional anticonvulsant medications, such as levetiracetam (see Table 4.4), acutely in the ED and may require adjustment to prescribed therapy. Alcohol withdrawal requires close monitoring and evaluation to determine risk for seizure; medications such as benzodiazepines (see Table A.2) should be administered as needed to reduce risk for seizure and control withdrawal symptoms such as tremor and agitation. Patients with seizures of unknown cause require consultation with neurology and further testing and observation to investigate for possible triggers and avoid seizure recurrence.
- Hospital admission: Patients who have a first seizure associated with a prolonged postictal state, incomplete recovery, or serious seizure-related injury. Patients with status epilepticus, neurologic or systemic illness or insult requiring additional evaluation and treatment, or questions regarding compliance.

Nursing Interventions

- Perform head-to-toe assessment with focused neurologic examination. Assess eye movements, noting any gaze deviation or nystagmus. Assess level of consciousness, cranial nerves, and motor function, noting any deficits. Assess risk for seizure and institute seizure precautions if needed, taking appropriate actions such as padding bed rails, using floor mats, and limiting stimuli. Note any abnormal/involuntary jerking movements.

[ ]   **NURSING PEARL**

The Clinical Institute Withdrawal Assessment (CIWA) scale scores patients' symptoms related to alcohol withdrawal, such as tremor, agitation, nausea, headache, and hallucinations, to guide treatment with medications such as benzodiazepines and to reduce risk of seizure.

- Place patient on continuous pulse oximetry and cardiac monitoring, alerting emergency provider to any changes in vital signs or cardiac rhythm. Assist to quickly obtain an EKG for interpretation by the emergency provider. Apply supplemental oxygen to maintain SpO_2 greater than 94%. Ensure suction is available. Capnography may also be indicated.
- If the patient seizes, protect from injury while observing seizure onset, activity, and duration. Do not insert anything in the mouth of a seizing patient. Immediately remove any harmful objects near the patient. Turn the patient on the side, if able. Ensure patient's head is free from injury. Observe motor activity, noting tonic-clonic movements, gaze deviation, or nystagmus. Administer anticonvulsant medications as ordered (IV or intramuscular). Prepare for emergent interventions, such as intubation, if seizure activity persists.
- If the seizure occurred prior to admission to the ED, ask the patient or family member for a detailed description of the event, length of the postictal period, any triggers, family history of seizures, and any prior seizures.
- Establish IV access and draw blood for lab tests as ordered.
- Administer medications as prescribed.
- Patients at risk for ETOH withdrawal–related seizures require frequent assessment of withdrawal symptoms to guide medication administration and reduce risk for seizures.
- Monitor patient during postictal period. Place patient in recovery position (roll onto side, cushioning head). Monitor respirations and provide supplemental oxygen, support/ventilation if needed. Patients may require suctioning of secretions to maintain airway patency. Assess level of consciousness and reorient patient as needed. Assess and treat any injuries sustained as a result of seizure. Assess for incontinence and provide perineal care, if needed.

Patient Education

- Avoid possible seizure triggers. Environmental factors, such as bright, flashing lights and loud music, may increase risk for seizures. Physiologic stressors, such as illness or lack of sleep, may also contribute to seizure risk. Assess substance use history, such as alcohol dependence and misuse of substances such as benzodiazepines, and learn risk for withdrawal-related seizures.
- Learn about prescribed therapies. Take all medications as prescribed to maintain therapeutic levels of any prescribed anticonvulsants. Do not skip a dose. Take a forgotten dose as soon as you remember.
- Recognize and respond to seizure activity. Avoid potentially unsafe activities, such as working at high elevations or swimming/bathing unsupervised, until cleared by neurology. Avoid operating heavy machinery or driving until seizures are considered controlled as determined by a physician, per state guidelines. Modify lifestyle to ensure safety in the event of a seizure. This includes keeping bathrooms unlocked, avoiding taking baths, and considering replacing glass shower doors with safety glass. Caregivers: Monitor onset and duration of any seizure activity, noting presence of any involuntary movements or gaze deviation. Set parameters for seeking emergent care, such as calling 911 when seizures last longer than 5 minutes or when patient does not regain consciousness. Keep a seizure calendar to record seizure events and symptoms. Learn care of the postictal patient, such as placing patient in the recovery position, assisting with reorientation, and seeking emergent care for any respiratory compromise or persistent confusion.

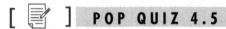

POP QUIZ 4.5

An adult patient presents to the ED with symptoms related to alcohol withdrawal, stating that their last drink was 14 hours ago. What clinical tool would the nurse use to assess the patient's symptoms, and what precautions should be taken to protect this patient?

SHUNT MALFUNCTION

Overview

- Shunts are placed in the brain to reduce hydrocephalus by eliminating fluid collection in the ventricles of the brain and draining it to the chest or abdominal cavity.
- Shunt malfunctions include abdominal complications, blockage, disconnection, infections, overdrainage, and underdrainage.
- Shunts require frequent monitoring

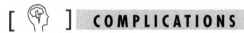

COMPLICATIONS

Complications of shunt dysfunction include increased IC and recurrence of hydrocephalus.

Signs and Symptoms

- Fever
- Headache
- Lethargy
- Nausea and vomiting
- Seizures

Diagnosis

Labs

- CBC
- CSF

Diagnostic Testing
- CT
- Head x-ray

Treatment
- Medications (see Table 4.4); antibiotics for infection (see Table A.1)
- Surgery to either repair or replace the shunt

Nursing Interventions
- Monitor for signs of increasing ICP.
- Be aware of pediatric signs of increasing ICP.
- Monitor for signs of sepsis.

Patient Education
- Seek medical attention immediately if shunt dysfunction is realized.

STROKE

Overview
- A *stroke* (also referred to as a CVA) is a disruption of blood flow to the brain caused by narrowing, occlusion, or hemorrhage of a blood vessel.
- Strokes may be categorized as hemorrhagic or ischemic. Hemorrhagic strokes are caused by arterial bleeding within the brain, which may occur as a result of an arteriovenous malformation, cerebral aneurysm, or intracerebral hemorrhage. Ischemic strokes are the most common types and are the result of total occlusion of a cerebral blood vessel, typically from an embolism or thrombus. *Transient ischemic attack (TIA)* is a temporary disruption of blood flow to the brain that causes temporary, reversible neurologic deficits. A TIA is a warning sign that the patient is at risk for stroke.

 COMPLICATIONS

Complications from a stroke differ depending on the location of the stroke, but include aphasia, contractures, depression, dysarthria, dysphagia, emotional disturbance, personality changes, memory issues, hemineglect, hemianopia, numbness, pain, paralysis, vascular cognitive impairment, vascular dementia, and weakness. In addition to neurologic deficits, strokes may lead to cardiovascular compromise, brain herniation, and death.

Signs and Symptoms
Symptoms are variable depending on affected areas of the brain. The following symptoms may be present.
- Aphagia
- Ataxia
- Altered mental status
- Confusion
- Difficulty walking
- Dysarthria
- Expressive aphasia
- Facial droop
- Headache
- Hypertension (systolic blood pressure greater than 220 mmHg)
- Loss of coordination ▶

 NURSING PEARL

"FAST" is an acronym used to promptly identify signs of a stroke:

F: Facial droop

A: Arm weakness and drift

S: Speech difficulties

T: Time: Onset of symptoms

Signs and Symptoms (continued)

- Nausea
- Numbness or tingling of the face or an extremity
- Ocular abnormalities; blurred vision or visual field deficits; monocular or binocular blindness; nystagmus; unequal pupils
- Rapid change in level of consciousness
- Receptive aphasia
- Vision changes
- Vomiting
- Weakness or paralysis that may affect a single extremity, half of the body, or all four extremities

Diagnosis

Labs

- ABG
- CBC
- CMP
- Coagulation panel
- Point-of-care glucose
- Troponin
- Type and screen
- Toxicology screen

Diagnostic Testing

- CT scan: emergent noncontrast head CT possible initially to assess for hemorrhagic stroke, followed by additional studies to assess for ischemia, such as CT angiography; CT perfusion study.
- Carotid duplex scanning
- EEG
- LP
- MRI/MR angiography

Treatment

- Vital to guide treatment: prompt identification of stroke symptoms and emergent radiographic imaging to determine presence and type of stroke (ischemic vs. hemorrhagic)
- Ischemic stroke management: Tissue plasminogen activator (tPA) (see Table 4.7) is the first-line therapy if initiated within 4.5 hours of symptom onset or "last known normal." This clot-busting medication may restore blood flow to the affected portion of the brain, potentially reversing associated neurologic deficits. Antithrombotic therapy (see Table A.1) with aspirin is initiated within 48 hours of stroke onset (and is often continued at discharge). Additional considerations include blood pressure reduction (after the acute phase of ischemic stroke has passed), lipid-lowering therapy with a high-intensity statin, and prophylaxis for DVT and pulmonary embolus. Patients may require surgical intervention with a mechanical thrombectomy.
- Hemorrhagic stroke management: For patients who present with systolic blood pressure between 150 and 220 mmHg, allow for rapid lowering of systolic blood pressure to a target of 140 mmHg, provided the patient remains clinically stable. Lowering blood pressure beyond this may contribute to cerebral ischemia. For patients who present with systolic blood pressure greater than 220 mmHg, allow for rapid lowering of systolic blood pressure to less than 220 mmHg. Blood pressure is then gradually ▶

Treatment *(continued)*

reduced (over a period of hours) to a target range of 140 to 160 mmHg, provided the patient remains clinically stable. Discontinue all anticoagulant and antiplatelet drugs. Hemorrhagic stroke may be related to anticoagulant and fibrinolytic therapies. Reversal agents may be indicated, such as vitamin K, prothrombin complex concentrate, or fresh frozen plasma for warfarin reversal and protamine sulfate for heparin reversal. Provide management of elevated ICP, if applicable, as well as seizure management and prophylaxis. Patients may require emergent surgical intervention, such as decompressive craniotomy for hemorrhagic stroke or endovascular embolization or clipping/coiling of aneurysm.

- Possible carotid endarterectomy to reduce risk of ischemic stroke (although TIA causes transient symptoms that reverse without intervention)
- Likely supportive care: Patients may require intubation and mechanical ventilation. Blood pressure management is vital in maintaining cerebral perfusion. Dependent on patient condition, permissive hypertension may be used for patients with ischemic stroke to maintain cerebral perfusion. Provide patients with IV resuscitation: isotonic saline without dextrose is preferred for intravascular repletion and maintenance fluid therapy.
- Likely rehabilitation and long-term care planning to manage deficits associated with stroke: Consultation to physical and occupational therapy, speech pathology, neurology, and psychiatry may be required in the post-acute phase of stroke management to optimize function and prevent stroke complications, such as limited mobility and contractures, speech and swallow impairment, emotional dysregulation, and cognitive impairment.

TABLE 4.7 Criteria for tPA Inclusion and Contraindications	
INCLUSION CRITERIA	**CONTRAINDICATIONS**
18 years and older: • Onset of abnormal symptoms less than 4.5 hours ago for patients younger than 80 years • Onset of abnormal symptoms 3 hours ago or less in patients older than 80 years Over 80 years old: • 3 hours or less since "last known normal" if there is a prior history of diabetes or stroke • NIHSS score greater than 25, taking anticoagulants • 4.5 hours since "last known normal" if nothing above is present	Any of the following currently present: • Intracranial hemorrhage • Blood glucose less than 50 mg/dL • Blood pressure greater than 185/110 mmHg despite treatment • Endocarditis • INR greater than 1.7, aPTT greater than 40 seconds, PT greater than 15 seconds • Intracranial neoplasm • Low platelets less than 100,000/mm³ History of • Intracranial hemorrhage • Gastrointestinal bleeding within the past 3 weeks • Inhibitors of direct thrombin or direct factor Xa within the last 48 hours, unless laboratory testing shows coagulation levels within normal limits • Ischemia stroke within the last 3 months • Low-molecular-weight heparin within the last 24 hours • Major surgery within the last 2 weeks • Severe head trauma within the last 3 days • Surgery within the head or spine in the last 3 days

aPTT, activated partial thromboplastin time; INR, international normalization ratio; NIHSS, National Institutes of Health Stroke Scale; PT, prothrombin time.

Nursing Interventions

- Perform head-to-toe assessment with focused neurologic assessment. Immediately alert emergency provider to expedite treatment for stroke patients. Discuss onset of symptoms and establish the time at which the patient was last seen well. Use National Institutes of Health stroke scale to assess stroke symptoms.
- Place patient on continuous pulse oximetry and cardiac monitoring, alerting emergency provider to any changes in vital signs or cardiac rhythm. Assist to obtain an EKG for prompt interpretation by the emergency provider. Invasive blood pressure monitoring with placement of an arterial line may be indicated.
- Obtain point-of-care blood glucose level and treat hypoglycemia, if needed.
- Apply supplemental oxygen to maintain SpO_2. Assist with endotracheal intubation and monitoring/management of mechanical ventilation, if needed.
- Establish IV access and draw blood for lab tests as ordered.
- Expedite transport to radiology for stat head CT. Target door-to-CT time is less than 25 minutes per American Stroke Association guidelines.
- Administer medications as prescribed. Target door-to-tPA administration time is less than 60 minutes per American Stroke Association guidelines. If tPA is indicated, provide bolus dose and begin infusion as ordered, conducting frequent neurologic assessments and vital sign monitoring throughout and following the infusion. Administration of any oral medications may be contraindicated until swallow evaluation is performed. Complete bedside swallow study if patient meets criteria. If there is concern for dysphagia, consult speech language pathology and place patient on aspiration precautions.
- Monitor for signs of increased ICP and neurogenic shock. Maintain elevation of HOB to decrease ICP, if indicated.
- Patients and family are likely to experience emotional distress related to prognosis and neurologic deficits. Provide emotional support as needed.
- Patients may require expedited transfer to the operating room for surgical intervention or the critical care unit for continued treatment and monitoring.

Patient Education

- Know that for ischemic or hemorrhagic stroke, hospital admission will be required for continued treatment and monitoring. Discuss plan of care with nurse and family.
- Learn about health management to prevent ischemic and hemorrhagic stroke. Seek support and resources regarding smoking cessation, if needed. Discuss ways to reduce risk of cardiovascular disease, such as implementing a regular exercise regimen and eating a nutritious diet (e.g., the Mediterranean diet). Promote disease management of conditions that increase stroke risk, such as hypertension and hyperlipidemia. Take all medications as prescribed, such as anticoagulation for atrial fibrillation. If prescribed anticoagulant therapy, learn about risk for bleeding/increased risk for intracranial hemorrhage.
- Know that if diagnosed with TIA, return for emergent evaluation of symptom recurrence is necessary. Learn about any increased risk for stroke following TIA. Attend follow-up visits, such as with neurology and cardiology, for ongoing management and monitoring. ▶

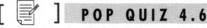 **POP QUIZ 4.6**

A patient presents with altered mental status and discovered to have experienced a hemorrhagic stroke. The patient's family states that the patient is prescribed warfarin for atrial fibrillation. A coagulation panel is drawn, and the patient's INR is found to be supratherapeutic at 13. What reversal medication would the nurse expect to administer?

Patient Education *(continued)*

■ Recognize stroke symptoms and reasons to seek emergent care. Learn FAST acronym for identifying stroke symptoms. Seek emergent evaluation of any severe headache, altered mental status, sudden-onset facial weakness or weakness of extremities, abnormal speech, or gait.

TRAUMA

Overview

■ Head injuries are one of the most common complaints in the ED, with injuries ranging in severity from mild to life-threatening.

■ A *traumatic brain injury* is an alteration in brain function caused by an external force. It includes a broad range of pathologic injuries to the brain of varying clinical severity.

■ Severity of brain injury is largely based on clinical examination using GCS, with mild injuries often defined by a GCS score of 13 to 15, moderate injury within a range of 9 to 12, and severe brain injuries presenting with a GCS score below 8.

■ Table 4.8 describes different types of head trauma.

Signs and Symptoms

See Table 4.8.

[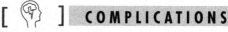]   COMPLICATIONS

Complications of head trauma vary in severity. Some examples include confusion, dizziness, fatigue, hemiparesis, hemiplegia, herniation, insomnia, irritability, memory loss, nausea, persistent headaches, posturing, and death.

TABLE 4.8	Types of Head Trauma	
TYPE	**OVERVIEW**	**SYMPTOMS**
Anoxic brain injury	• Caused by a complete lack of oxygen to the brain; can start in as little as 4 minutes • Common causes: cardiac arrest, stroke, near drowning, and overdose	• Headache • Poor coordination • Vision changes • Seizures • Trouble speaking
Basilar skull fractures	• Usually caused by blunt trauma to the base of the skull	• Causes characteristic ecchymosis to mastoid process (Battle sign) and periorbital region ("raccoon eyes") as well as hemotympanum • May cause CSF rhinorrhea or otorrhea
Concussion	• Mild TBI caused by mild-moderate blunt head trauma • Diagnosis based on clinical assessment; no radiographic evidence of injury • Patients at risk for second-impact syndrome, a condition in which a second concussion occurs while healing from the initial head injury, leading to sudden-onset cerebral edema, increased ICP, and possible death	• Presentation may be mild to severe, with symptoms such as headache, memory loss, dizziness, photophobia, nausea, and vomiting. • Symptoms may last from 10 days to longer than 3 months (postconcussive syndrome).
Coup/contrecoup	• A lesion at the site of impact (coup) and opposite the site of impact (contrecoup) as a result of rapid acceleration and deceleration forces	• May cause mild to severe TBI symptoms such as headache, dizziness, and photophobia • More severe symptoms such as altered mental status, abnormal speech, or uncoordinated gait

(continued)

TABLE 4.8 Types of Head Trauma *(continued)*

TYPE	OVERVIEW	SYMPTOMS
Cerebral contusion	• Bleeding and swelling caused by damage to parenchymal vessels, often as the result of blunt head trauma • Often worsening cerebral edema develops 2–3 days after injury • Lesion may cause focal infarction and necrosis, leading to permanent neurologic damage	• Altered mental status • Loss of memory • Difficulty focusing • Trouble speaking
Diffuse axonal injury	• Brain injury caused by axonal shearing as a result of shaking or rotational forces • Causes lesions to white matter and damage to deep brain structures • Prognosis: poor	• Profound neurologic deficits • Persistent vegetative state
Epidural hematoma	• A collection of blood between the skull and dura mater, often caused by laceration of the middle meningeal artery • Large hematomas may require emergent surgical intervention for craniotomy and hematoma evacuation	• Characteristic loss of consciousness after injury followed by a period of lucidity before neurologic decline
Herniation syndrome	• Increased ICP causes brain tissue to herniate through foramen within the skull; as herniation syndrome progresses, rapid neurologic decline leads to impaired cardiovascular and respiratory function, resulting in death • Herniation may occur as a result of increased pressure secondary to trauma, intracranial hemorrhage, or malignancy	• Rapid neurologic decline • Decreased heart and respiratory function
Penetrating injury	• Occurs when an object breaches the skull, which may be the result of an accident or of intentional acts of violence (for example, gunshot injuries) • Frequently requires surgical intervention for emergent craniotomy and removal of foreign body • Often associated with poor prognosis	• Heavy bleeding from the head • Bleeding from the ears • Difficulty breathing • Seizures • Loss of bowel or bladder control • Changes in pupils
Subarachnoid hemorrhage	• Bleeding between the arachnoid membrane and the pia membrane	• Severe headache • Double vision • Photosensitivity • Nausea and vomiting
Subdural hematoma	• A collection of blood between dura mater and arachnoid layers • Usually caused by tearing of the bridging veins in an acute SDH • Increased risk with anticoagulation and alcohol misuse	• Appearing normal for a few days and then slowly becoming confused and potentially losing consciousness • Headache • Changes in behavior • Lethargy • Nausea and vomiting

(continued)

TABLE 4.8	Types of Head Trauma *(continued)*	
TYPE	**OVERVIEW**	**SYMPTOMS**
TBI (moderate/ severe)	• Usually the result of a significant blow to the head resulting in tissue injury such as bruising, tearing, and bleeding	• Loss of consciousness for minutes to hours • Nausea and vomiting • Seizures • Dilation of one or both pupils • CSF leaking • Agitation • Slurred speech

CSF, cerebrospinal fluid; ICP, intracranial pressure; SDH, subdural hematoma; TBI, traumatic brain injury.

Diagnosis
Labs
There are no lab tests specific to diagnosing trauma. However, the following tests are indicated for patients presenting with head trauma:

- ABG
- CBC
- CMP
- Coagulation panel
- Lactic acid
- Type and screen

Diagnostic Testing
- CT scan
- MRI
- LP

Treatment
- Varied treatment based on severity of injury: Mild head trauma may require observation and pain management, while more severe head trauma may require emergent interventions to sustain life. Brain injury may lead to irreversible neurologic damage, bradycardia, hypertension, and respiratory dysfunction, which may progress to cause cardiac arrest. Begin immediate resuscitation per ACLS guidelines if cardiac arrest occurs. Patients may require intubation and mechanical ventilation if unable to maintain respiratory function.
- Treatment largely focused on maintaining normal ICP and cerebral perfusion; Hyperventilation may be used to reduce ICP by promoting cerebral vasoconstriction. Osmotic agents, such as hypertonic fluid and mannitol (see Table 4.4), may be indicated. Strict monitoring of I/O and neurologic status is required. Patient positioning may contribute to increases in ICP; elevate the HOB to decrease pressure. Administration of antiepileptic medications, such as levetiracetam (see Table 4.4), is often indicated for seizure treatment/prophylaxis, as head injuries and increased ICP may lead to seizures. Medications for management of hypertension, such as beta-blockers, may be indicated.
- Possible emergent evacuation of intracranial bleeding for intracranial hemorrhage with potential rapid decompensation and death: Cranial burr holes may be placed in the ED for emergent decompression. Surgical intervention for craniotomy may be required to evacuate hematoma. ▶

[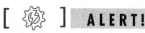]   **ALERT!**

Patients may experience CSF rhinorrhea or otorrhea after skull fracture. Fluid is often mixed with blood, and it may be difficult to differentiate CSF from normal discharge. A halo test may be used to quickly identify CSF. A positive halo test is indicative of CSF drainage, in which a drop of fluid on an absorbent surface will show the drop surrounded by a lighter ring, or "halo."

Treatment *(continued)*

- Likely to require consultation to specialty services for ongoing management of brain injury and associated deficits; may require physical and occupational therapy, speech therapy, and follow-up with neurology, psychiatry, and other specialists to provide comprehensive treatment of brain injuries and neurologic deficits.

Nursing Interventions

- Perform head-to-toe assessment with focused neurologic examination. Assess for symptoms associated with increased ICP, such as nausea and vomiting and irregular respirations. Immediately alert emergency provider if there is suspicion for

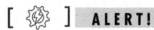

ALERT!

Insertion of anything into the nares, such as NG tube or nasopharyngeal airway, is contraindicated in patients with facial/frontal head trauma until imaging is obtained.

intracranial hemorrhage/increased ICP. Assess level of consciousness using GCS (see Table 4.6), and assess cranial nerve function and motor function, noting any deficits. Assess pain, noting onset, severity, location, and quality of any headache. Inspect for penetrating injuries and external hemorrhage. Investigate for signs of head or neck injury. Apply cervical collar and maintain spinal immobilization, if indicated.
- Place patient on continuous pulse oximetry and cardiac monitoring, alerting emergency provider to any changes in vital signs or cardiac rhythm. Invasive blood pressure monitoring may be indicated. Assist with placement of arterial line, if needed; Apply supplemental oxygen to maintain SpO_2 greater than 94%. Prepare for and assist with intubation and mechanical ventilation, if needed. Proceed with resuscitation per ACLS guidelines if cardiac arrest occurs.
- Assist emergency provider with any necessary bedside procedures, such as emergent trephination with burr hole(s).
- Administer medications as prescribed. Administer additional medications, such as antiemetics, antiepileptics, antihypertensives, and osmotic agents, and titrate as ordered. Assess pain and administer analgesics, such as opiate medications, as ordered.
- Assist with patient positioning, maintaining elevation of HOB unless contraindicated (as with spinal injury).
- Monitor I/O. Placement of an indwelling urinary catheter may be indicated for strict output monitoring for patients with severe injuries.
- Institute seizure precautions, if appropriate, padding bed rails and limiting environmental stimuli such as bright lights and loud noises.
- Expedite transfer to the critical care unit for continued care and monitoring or transfer to the operating room for surgical intervention, if needed.

Patient Education

- Know that moderate to severe head trauma often requires hospital admission for continued treatment and monitoring. Discuss plan for admission and ongoing treatment; Prepare for possible consultation with case management and social work to begin long-term care planning if there are neurologic deficits as a result of traumatic brain injury.
- If discharged after minor head trauma, such as concussion, monitor symptoms. Learn expected symptoms after head injury, such as headache and cognitive issues like impaired memory and concentration.
- Do not lift heavy items or strain. ▶

Patient Education *(continued)*

- Be aware that headaches, difficulty concentrating, and dizziness may persist for days or weeks after the injury. Do not drive or operate heavy machinery until cleared by provider. Call provider or 911 for any changes in vision, clear fluid coming from nose or ears, new or worsening confusion or changes in level of consciousness, persistent nausea or vomiting, seizures, or worsening headache. Learn about second-impact syndrome and prescribed activity restrictions, such as limitations on sports and recreational activities, to reduce risk of repeated head injury. Learn about risk for rapid decompensation and death with repeated head injury. Seek emergent evaluation of any worsening neurologic deficits such as abnormal speech or gait, loss of coordination, weakness, altered mental status, or severe headache.
- Practice fall and injury prevention if at risk for head injuries. If anticoagulated, learn about increased risk for intracranial hemorrhage if head injury occurs. Seek support and resources for management of alcohol dependence and substance use, if needed. Take measures to increase home safety, such as installation of hand rails and removal of throw rugs.

RESOURCES

Campbell, M. (2020). Head trauma. In Emergency Nurses Association (Ed.), *Provider manual eighth edition TNCC trauma nursing core course* (8th ed., pp. 95–116). Jones & Bartlett.

Campo, T. M. (2017). *Medical imaging for the health care provider: Practical radiograph interpretation* (pp. 171–182). Springer Publishing Company.

Centers for Disease Control and Prevention. (n.d.-a). *Signs and symptoms of meningococcal disease*. U.S. Department of Health and Human Services. https://www.cdc.gov/meningococcal/about/symptoms.html

Centers for Disease Control and Prevention. (n.d.-b). *What to expect after a concussion* [Patient Fact Sheet]. U.S. Department of Health and Human Services.

Clarkson, A. (2020). Spinal trauma. In Emergency Nurses Association (Ed.), *Provider manual eighth edition TNCC trauma nursing core course* (8th ed., pp. 172–180). Jones & Bartlett.

Eaton, J., Hanif, A. B., Mulima, G., Kajombo, C., & Charles, A. (2017). Outcomes following exploratory burr holes for traumatic brain injury in a resource poor setting. *World Neurosurgery, 105*, 257–264. https://doi.org/10.1016/j.wneu.2017.05.153

GBS/CIDP Foundation International. (2012). *Guillain-Barré syndrome: An acute care guide for medical professionals*. https://www.gbs-cidp.org/wp-content/uploads/2013/02/AcuteCareICU13.pdf

Jain, S., & Iverson, LM. (2020, June 23). Glasgow coma scale. In *StatPearls*. StatPearls Publishing. https://www.ncbi.nlm.nih.gov/books/NBK513298

Ledford, L. (2020). Neurologic emergencies. In V. Sweet & A. Foley (Eds.), *Sheehy's emergency nursing: Principles and practice* (7th ed., pp. 249–258). Elsevier.

Mayo Foundation for Medical Education and Research. (2020, October 1). *Meningitis*. Mayo Clinic. https://www.mayoclinic.org/diseases-conditions/meningitis/diagnosis-treatment/drc-20350514

MedlinePlus. (2021, May 4). *Increased intracranial pressure*. National Library of Medicine. https://medlineplus.gov/ency/article/000793.htm

National Institute of Neurological Disorders and Stroke. (n.d.-a). *Dementia*. U.S. Department of Health and Human Services, National Institutes of Health. https://www.ninds.nih.gov/Disorders/All-Disorders/Dementia-Information-Page

National Institute of Neurological Disorders and Stroke. (n.d.-b). *Headache: Hope through research*. U.S. Department of Health and Human Services, National Institutes of Health. https://www.ninds.nih.gov/disorders/patient-caregiver-education/hope-through-research/headache-hope-through-research#3138_10

National Institute of Neurological Disorders and Stroke. (n.d.-c). *Headache*. U.S. Department of Health and Human Services, National Institutes of Health. https://www.ninds.nih.gov/Disorders/All-Disorders/Headache-Information-Page

National Institute of Neurological Disorders and Stroke. (n.d.-d). *Huntington's disease*. U.S. Department of Health and Human Services, National Institutes of Health. https://www.ninds.nih.gov/Disorders/All-Disorders/ Huntingtons-Disease-Information-Page

National Institute of Neurological Disorders and Stroke. (n.d.-e). *Multiple sclerosis*. U.S. Department of Health and Human Services, National Institutes of Health. https://www.ninds.nih.gov/disorders/all-disorders/ multiple-sclerosis-information-page

National Institute of Neurological Disorders and Stroke. (n.d.-f). *Parkinson's disease*. U.S. Department of Health and Human Services, National Institutes of Health. https://www.ninds.nih.gov/Disorders/All-Disorders/ Parkinsons-Disease-Information-Page

National Institute of Neurological Disorders and Stroke. (2013, July). *Spinal cord injury: Hope through research*. U.S. Department of Health and Human Services, National Institutes of Health. https://www.ninds.nih.gov/Disorders/ Patient-Caregiver-Education/Hope-Through-Research/spinal-cord-injury-Hope-Through-Research

National Institute of Neurological Disorders and Stroke. (2015, April). *The epilepsies and seizures: Hope through research*. U.S. Department of Health and Human Services, National Institutes of Health. https://www.ninds.nih .gov/Disorders/Patient-Caregiver-Education/Hope-Through-Research/Epilepsies-and-Seizures-Hope -Through#3109_22

National Institute of Neurological Disorders and Stroke. (2018a, June). *Guillain-Barré syndrome fact sheet*. U.S. Department of Health and Human Services, National Institutes of Health. https://www.ninds.nih.gov/Disorders/ Patient-Caregiver-Education/Fact-Sheets/Guillain-Barr%C3%A9-Syndrome-Fact-Sheet

National Institute of Neurological Disorders and Stroke. (2018b, June). *Meningitis and encephalitis fact sheet*. U.S. Department of Health and Human Services, National Institutes of Health. https://www.ninds.nih.gov/Disorders/ Patient-Caregiver-Education/Fact-Sheets/Meningitis-and-Encephalitis-Fact-Sheet

National Institute of Neurological Disorders and Stroke. (2020a, February). *Stroke: Hope through research*. U.S. Department of Health and Human Services, National Institutes of Health. https://www.ninds.nih.gov/Disorders/ Patient-Caregiver-Education/Hope-Through-Research/Stroke-Hope-Through-Research#warningsigns

National Institute of Neurological Disorders and Stroke. (2020b, February). *Traumatic brain injury: Hope through research*. U.S. Department of Health and Human Services, National Institutes of Health. https://www.ninds. nih.gov/health-information/patient-caregiver-education/hope-through-research/traumatic-brain-injury-hop e-through-research.

National Institute of Neurological Disorders and Stroke. (2020c, March). *Myasthenia gravis fact sheet*. U.S. Department of Health and Human Services, National Institutes of Health. https://www.ninds.nih.gov/Disorders/ Patient-Caregiver-Education/Fact-Sheets/Myasthenia-Gravis-Fact-Sheet#1

National Institute of Neurological Disorders and Stroke. (2020d, April). *Hydrocephalus fact sheet*. U.S. Department of Health and Human Services, National Institutes of Health. https://www.ninds.nih.gov/Disorders/ Patient-Caregiver-Education/Fact-Sheets/Hydrocephalus-Fact-Sheet#3125_1

National Institute of Neurological Disorders and Stroke. (2021, May 26). *Amyotrophic lateral sclerosis (ALS) fact sheet*. U.S. Department of Health and Human Services, National Institutes of Health. https://www.ninds.nih.gov/ Disorders/Patient-Caregiver-Education/Fact-Sheets/Amyotrophic-Lateral-Sclerosis-ALS-Fact-Sheet

National Institute on Aging. (n.d.-a). *What is Alzheimer's disease?* U.S. Department of Health and Human Services, National Institutes of Health. https://www.nia.nih.gov/health/what-alzheimers-disease

National Institute on Aging. (n.d-b). *What is dementia? Symptoms, types, and diagnosis*. U.S. Department of Health and Human Services, National Institutes of Health. https://www.nia.nih.gov/health/what-dementia symptoms-types-and-diagnosis

OHSU Stroke Advisory Committee. (2018, June). *Acute stroke practice guidelines for inpatient management of ischemic stroke and transient ischemic attack (TIA) for the administration of tPA*. https://www.ohsu.edu/sites/ default/files/2019-06/OHSU%20Acute%20Stroke%20Practice%20Guidelines%20for%20Administration%20 of%20tPA%202018.pdf

Powers-Jarvis, R. S. (2020). Initial assessment. In *Provider manual eighth edition TNCC trauma nursing core course*. (8th ed., pp. 29–30). Jones & Bartlett.

Prescribers' Digital Reference. (n.d.-a). *Acetaminophen* [Drug information]. https://www.pdr.net/drug-summary/ Ofirmev-acetaminophen-1346.3520

Prescribers' Digital Reference. (n.d.-b). *Alteplase* [Drug information]. https://www.pdr.net/drug-summary/Activase
-alteplase-1332.3358

Prescribers' Digital Reference. (n.d.-c). *Carbidopa/levodopa* [Drug information]. https://www.pdr.net/drug-summary/
Duopa-carbidopa-levodopa-3668.8411

Prescribers' Digital Reference. (n.d.-d). *Donepezil hydrochloride* [Drug information]. https://www.pdr.net/drug
-summary/Aricept-donepezil-hydrochloride-138.4002

Prescribers' Digital Reference. (n.d.-e). *Hydrocortisone sodium succinate* [Drug information]. https://www.pdr.net/
drug-summary/Solu-Cortef-hydrocortisone-sodium-succinate-1880.141

Prescribers' Digital Reference. (n.d.-f). *Ketorolac tromethamine* [Drug information]. https://www.pdr.net/drug
-summary/Acular-ketorolac-tromethamine-1107

Prescribers' Digital Reference. (n.d.-g). *Levetiracetam* [Drug information]. https://www.pdr.net/drug-summary/
Keppra-Injection-levetiracetam-1055.6058

Prescribers' Digital Reference. (n.d.-h). *Mannitol* [Drug information]. https://www.pdr.net/drug-summary/Osmitrol
-mannitol-1149

Prescribers' Digital Reference. (n.d.-i). *Metoclopramide* [Drug information]. https://www.pdr.net/drug-summary/
Metoclopramide-Injection-metoclopramide-3898.5843

Prescribers' Digital Reference. (n.d.-j). *Penicillin G potassium* [Drug information]. https://www.pdr.net/
drug-summary/Penicillin-G-Potassium-penicillin-G-potassium-1150

Prescribers' Digital Reference. (n.d.-k). *Pyridostigmine bromide* [Drug information]. https://www.pdr.net/drug
-summary/Mestinon-pyridostigmine-bromide-761.1037

Prescribers' Digital Reference. (n.d.-l). *Tacrolimus* [Drug information]. https://www.pdr.net/drug-summary/Astagraf
-XL-tacrolimus-3266.4495

Royal College of Physicians and Surgeons of Glasgow. (n.d.). *The Glasgow structured approach to assessment of the
Glasgow coma scale*. https://www.glasgowcomascale.org

5 GASTROINTESTINAL EMERGENCIES

APPENDICITIS

Overview

- *Acute appendicitis* is inflammation and infection of the appendix. Nonperforated (uncomplicated) appendicitis may be treated with antibiotics and a scheduled appendectomy. A perforated appendix requires emergent surgery to remove the appendix and the surrounding infection.
- Swelling associated with appendicitis causes peritoneal irritation, which progressively worsens as inflammation continues.
- The appendix most likely has ruptured if the patient's pain suddenly stops.

Signs and Symptoms

- Abdominal pain or cramping, usually localized to the right lower quadrant (RLQ)
- Anorexia
- Fever: late sign of ruptured appendix
- Guarding (peritonitis)
- Malaise
- Nausea/vomiting
- Positive Rovsing's sign: pain referred to RLQ when palpating on left lower quadrant (LLQ)
- Signs of hemodynamic instability (tachycardia, hypotension)

Diagnosis

Labs

- Blood cultures before antibiotic administration
- Complete blood count (CBC)
- Comprehensive metabolic panel (CMP)
- Type and screen
- Urinalysis
- Urine pregnancy test

Diagnostic Testing

- Abdominal CT
- Abdominal or pelvic ultrasound

[🧠] **COMPLICATIONS**

Appendicitis can be difficult to diagnose, but an abdominal CT is considered the most reliable test. If treatment is delayed, abscess formation, perforation, and peritonitis can occur. Severe cases can progress to septic shock.

[🤲] **NURSING PEARL**

The PQRST mnemonic is a helpful tool to use to perform a thorough pain assessment:

- **P** (provokes): What provokes the pain? What makes it better or worse?
- **Q** (quality): What does the pain feel like?
- **R** (radiation): Where is the pain located? Does it radiate?
- **S** (severity): How do you rate your pain on a 1–10 scale?
- **T** (time): How long have you had the pain? Does it come and go?

Treatment

- Antibiotic administration
- Intravenous (IV) hydration
- Pain management
- Surgical consultation for subsequent treatment. Nonperforated appendicitis: Start antibiotics, observe, and follow up outpatient for a scheduled appendectomy. Perforated appendicitis: Start IV antibiotics, followed by emergent appendectomy (laparoscopic or open).

Nursing Interventions

- Assess and manage airway, breathing, and circulation.
- Perform a focused abdominal assessment, including signs of peritoneal irritation: verbalizing of pain (e.g., during car ride when going over bumps); pain that starts in abdomen and localizes to RLQ; pain increased in RLQ when palpated on LLQ
- Establish IV access and draw blood for lab tests.
- Position the patient for comfort, usually with hips and knees bent.
- Administer pain medications (see Table A.2).
- Administer antibiotics (see Table A.1).
- Prepare the patient for CT scan.
- Anticipate surgical consultation and prepare the patient for surgery.
- Document patient consent in the chart.
- Keep the patient NPO (nothing by mouth) pending surgery, and record last oral intake.
- Monitor for rapid decline and progression to sepsis.

Patient Education

- Avoid nicotine products.
- Eat a high-fiber diet and limit high-fat, high-sugar foods.
- For possible discharge after nonperforated appendicitis with follow-up consult and a prescription for antibiotics. Continue the whole course of antibiotics even if feeling better. Understand the importance of a follow-up visit and ensure transportation is available. Understand the importance of returning sooner if the pain gets worse, becomes more localized to RLQ, or suddenly stops.

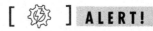 **ALERT!**

A patient who is highly suspicious for a ruptured appendix may go directly to surgery without imaging. This is based on a thorough history and physical exam by the surgeon.

CHOLECYSTITIS

Overview

- *Cholecystitis* is inflammation of the gallbladder; it is usually associated with gallstones blocking the gallbladder duct but can also occur in the absence of stones (acalculous).
- Gallstone obstruction may be intermittent and resolve on its own or may require surgery to prevent gallbladder ischemia and infection.

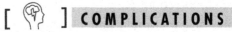 **COMPLICATIONS**

A secondary infection can develop if the cystic duct, the tube that carries bile from the gallbladder, becomes obstructed. *Enterococcus*, *Escherichia coli*, and *Klebsiella* are the most common causative organisms.

Signs and Symptoms

- Pain: sudden onset, usually after eating fried or high-fat foods; located in the epigastrium and/or right upper quadrant (RUQ) and may be referred to the right shoulder or supraclavicular area
- Common bile duct obstruction; bleeding tendencies; clay-colored stools; dark amber urine; pruritus
- Flatulence
- Local and rebound tenderness
- Low-grade fever: 100.4°F (38°C)
- Nausea/vomiting
- Tachycardia

Diagnosis

Labs

- Amylase
- CBC
- CMP
- Lipase
- Urinalysis

Diagnostic Testing

- CT scan
- Gallbladder ultrasound

Treatment

- Control symptoms: pain (see Table A.2); nausea (see Table A.2); fever (see Table A.2).
- Consult with surgery.
- Administer antibiotics (see Table A.1).
- Keep patient NPO.
- Perform fluid resuscitation with crystalloids.

Nursing Interventions

- Administer antibiotics and medications as ordered for pain and nausea.
- Administer IV fluids as ordered.
- Assess and manage airway, breathing, and circulation.
- Establish IV access and draw blood for lab tests.
- Monitor for signs of sepsis.
- Monitor intake/output (I/O), including appearance of stool.
- Perform a focused abdominal assessment.
- Prepare the patient for inpatient admission and/or possible surgical intervention.

Patient Education

- Avoid nicotine products.
- Do not consume alcohol.
- Follow a low-fat, high-fiber diet, and maintain adequate hydration.
- Follow up as suggested by provider, or sooner if the following develops: changed or worsening pain; signs or symptoms of infection.

CIRRHOSIS

Overview

- *Cirrhosis* is cumulative damage to the liver by scarring that may result from autoimmune diseases, chronic alcohol use, hepatitis, medications, or toxins.
- Cirrhosis is not reversible.
- Patients with cirrhosis may experience mild to no symptoms (compensated) to severe symptoms including liver failure (uncompensated).

Signs and Symptoms

- Abdominal pain
- Anorexia
- Ascites
- Bruising
- Edema
- Encephalopathy
- Fatigue
- Itching
- Jaundice
- Nausea
- Varices

Diagnosis

Labs

- Ammonia level
- CBC
- CMP
- Ethyl alcohol (ETOH)
- Hepatitis panel
- Prothrombin time (PT), activated partial thromboplastin time (aPTT)
- Urinalysis

Diagnostic Testing

- Abdominal CT scan
- Hepatic ultrasound

Treatment

- Antibiotics as indicated for secondary infection
- GI consultation for possible inpatient admission and/or surgical procedures, including transjugular intrahepatic portosystemic shunt (TIPS) procedure or endoscopy
- Management of coagulopathies or uncontrolled bleeding
- Removal of excess fluid (diuretics, paracentesis for ascites)
- Treatment/management of hepatic encephalopathy if present (monitor ammonia level and manage with lactulose)
- Treatment/management of hepatorenal syndrome if present (may require dialysis)

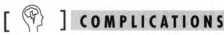 **COMPLICATIONS**

Common complications of cirrhosis include ascites, coagulopathies, encephalopathy, hepatorenal syndrome, peritonitis, portal hypertension, and upper gastrointestinal (GI) bleeding from ruptured esophageal varices.

Nursing Interventions

- Assess and maintain airway, breathing, and circulation, and apply supplemental oxygen as needed to treat ascites-related hypoxia.
- Assess and manage pain as ordered (see Table A.2).
- Establish IV access and draw blood for lab tests.
- Monitor for hemodynamic instability or uncontrolled bleeding.
- Monitor neurologic function to identify signs of encephalopathy.
- Monitor/treat elevated ammonia levels if encephalopathy is present (see Table 5.1 for gastrointestinal medications).
- Monitor urine output if diuretic is given.
- Perform a head-to-toe assessment with focus on the chest and abdomen.
- Prepare for paracentesis if indicated.
- Prepare the patient for possible inpatient admission or surgical intervention.

TABLE 5.1 Gastrointestinal Medications

INDICATIONS	MECHANISM OF ACTION	CONTRAINDICATIONS, PRECAUTIONS, AND ADVERSE EFFECTS
Antacids (aluminum hydroxide)		
• Esophagus • Ulcers	• React with stomach acid to produce aluminum chloride and water • Neutralize stomach acid	• Do not administer at the same time as certain medications. Antacids can affect the absorption of certain medications. • Take with food.
Antibiotics for encephalopathy (rifampin)		
• Encephalopathy	• Believed to reduce ammonia production	• Medication does not treat acute symptoms but is administered to decrease the risk of recurrence of encephalopathic symptoms. • Medication is metabolized by the liver; dose may need to be adjusted based on liver function. • Medication may cause GI upset.
Anticholinergics (dicyclomine hydrochloride)		
• Diverticulitis • IBS	• Antimuscarinic, anticholinergic agents • Relieve GI smooth muscle spasm and decrease contractility	• Medication is contraindicated for severe ulcerative colitis or bowel obstruction. • Consider cumulative effects of all anticholinergic medications a patient may be taking, especially in older adults. • Anticholinergics can cause paralytic ileus. • Medication is indicated for oral or IM use only.
Antidiarrheals (loperamide hydrochloride)		
• Acute diarrhea	• Antipropulsive medication class • Interfere with peristalsis and slow GI motility	• Antidiarrheals can cause serious cardiac arrhythmias. • Do not use for patient with dysentery, infectious gastroenteritis, or pseudomembranous colitis. • Mild side effects include nausea and constipation.
Antivirals (entecavir, ribavirin, peginterferon ALFA-2A)		
• Hepatitis B	• Suppress viral replication	• Monitor liver enzymes. • Use with caution in patients with HIV infection. • Medication may cause peripheral edema, ascites, encephalopathy, or fever (entecavir).

(continued)

TABLE 5.1	Gastrointestinal Medications (continued)	
INDICATIONS	MECHANISM OF ACTION	CONTRAINDICATIONS, PRECAUTIONS, AND ADVERSE EFFECTS
• Hepatitis C	• Ribavirin: antiviral used for multiple viral illnesses; exact mechanism of action unknown • Interferon alfa-2a: binds with leukocytes to stimulate an antiviral and immunomodulatory response	• Antivirals may cause anemia, fever, fatigue, headache, body aches. • Ribavirin is not effective as monotherapy; it is given in conjunction with peginterferon alfa-2a. • Interferon alfa-2a is administered subcutaneously once per week.
H₂ blockers (ranitidine, cimetidine)		
• GERD • Ulcers	• Histamine-type-2 receptor antagonists • Decrease the amount of gastric acid	• Minor side effects include headache and nausea.
Hormones, antidiuretic (vasopressin)		
• GI bleeding	• Parenteral exogenous antidiuretic hormones • Increase blood pressure	• Medication is not approved for intraosseous administration. • Medication requires frequent blood pressure monitoring.
Hormones, glycogenolytic (glucagon)		
• To facilitate examination of upper GI tract • To aid in passage of esophageal foreign body	• Relax muscles of the GI tract	• Medication can cause hyperglycemia. • Minor side effects include headache and nausea. • Do not use in conjunction with anticholinergics.
Laxatives (lactulose)		
• Hepatic encephalopathy	• Promote excretion of ammonia in the stool, reducing blood ammonia levels and improving mental status	• Medication can be mixed with water or juice to improve taste. • Medication can be administered orally or rectally (may be readministered if inadvertently expelled).
Proton pump inhibitors (pantoprazole sodium)		
• GI bleeding • Esophagitis • Ulcers	• Suppress gastric acid secretion by inhibiting the gastric ATPase enzyme pump	• Administer via IV diluted through a dedicated line. • Administer via slow IV push or IV infusion (intermittent or continuous).
Somatostatins (octreotide acetate)		
• Esophageal varices • Nonvariceal upper GI bleeding	• Counteract vasodilation • Decrease blood flow to the liver and GI tract	• Administer via IV (either IV push or intermittent/continuous infusion). • In emergency situations, medication may be administered undiluted (IV push). • Medication can cause bradycardia.

Note: All agents are contraindicated in the presence of hypersensitivity to the medication or one of its components.
ATPase, adenosine triphosphatase; GERD, gastroesophageal reflux disease; GI, gastrointestinal; IBS, irritable bowel syndrome; IM, intramuscular; IV, intravenous.

Patient Education

- Do not drink alcohol.
- Follow a low-sodium diet to minimize fluid retention.
- Follow up with the provider if a fever develops or if increasing abdominal pain, bloating, dark urine, or pale-colored stool occur.
- Seek urgent treatment for increased weakness, dizziness, new signs or symptoms of bleeding, or uncontrolled pain.

DIVERTICULITIS

Overview

- *Diverticulosis* is a condition in which small pouches or sacs form and push outward through weak areas in the wall of the colon.
- *Diverticulitis* occurs when one or a few of the pouches become blocked with stool, allowing bacteria to grow and become inflamed.
- Older age and low-fiber diet have been identified as potential risk factors for developing the condition.

Signs and Symptoms

- Abdominal pain and cramping (typically LLQ pain)
- Anorexia
- Blood in stool
- Changes in bowel habits (usually constipation)
- Fever
- Nausea/vomiting
- Signs of peritonitis (if perforation)

Diagnosis

Labs

- CBC
- CMP
- C-reactive protein (CRP)
- Fecal occult blood (FOB)
- Lactate level
- Stool culture
- Urinalysis

Diagnostic Testing

- Abdominal CT scan
- Abdominal ultrasound
- Barium enema
- Endoscopy

[🌐] **POP QUIZ 5.1**

An older adult patient presents with confusion; pale, jaundiced skin; and distended abdomen. Emergency medical services (EMS) reports a history of cirrhosis. What does the nurse predict is causing the patient's confusion, and what lab test would confirm the cause?

[🧠] **COMPLICATIONS**

Complications of diverticulitis include abscess, bleeding, intestinal obstruction, and perforation. The bleeding can be severe and life threatening if diverticula develop near an artery.

Treatment

- Antibiotic administration (IV progressing to oral)
- Inpatient admission/surgery for severe infection or peritonitis
- NPO status for complete bowel rest or clear liquids for milder cases
- Pain management (anticholinergics to reduce spasms)
- Rehydration with IV fluids

Nursing Interventions

- Administer antibiotics as ordered (see Table A.1).
- Administer crystalloid fluids if ordered (see Table A.3).
- Assess and maintain airway, breathing, and circulation.
- Assess and manage pain as ordered (see Table A.2).
- Establish IV access and draw blood for lab tests.
- Monitor vital signs and assess for fever.
- Perform a focused abdominal assessment.
- Prepare the patient for possible surgical intervention; keep patient NPO.

Patient Education

- Complete full course of antibiotics.
- Do not use nicotine products.
- Once cleared for a full diet, increase/maintain a high fiber intake by consuming fiber-rich foods such as fruits, vegetables, and whole grains.
- Report any signs and symptoms of infection.
- Monitor and seek treatment for blood in stools.
- Seek urgent evaluation of uncontrolled pain.

ESOPHAGITIS

Overview

- *Esophagitis* is inflammation of or damage to the esophagus.
- The causes include gastroesophageal reflux disease (GERD), radiation, and ingestion of a caustic substance.

Signs and Symptoms

- Anorexia/weight loss
- Hoarseness
- Sore throat
- Substernal pain or heartburn
- Upper GI bleeding
- Vomiting

 COMPLICATIONS

If untreated, esophagitis can cause bleeding, difficulty swallowing, scarring, and ulcers. These complications can interfere with oral intake, leading to malnutrition. Barrett's esophagus, another potential complication of long-term esophageal damage, is a risk factor in the development of esophageal cancer.

Diagnosis

Labs

- CBC
- CMP
- FOB
- PT, aPTT
- Type and screen

Diagnostic Testing

- Chest and abdomen CT scan
- EKG
- Endoscopy
- Upper GI series

Treatment

- Symptom management
- Management of pain and inflammation with proton pump inhibitors, histamine blockers, or antacids (see Table 5.1)
- Ruling out of cardiac causes of chest pain
- Treatment of underlying cause
- GI consultation for possible surgical procedures including fundoplication or esophageal dilation

Nursing Interventions

- Administer medications as prescribed (see Table 5.1).
- Assess and manage respiratory signs/symptoms.
- Assess and treat pain (see Table A.2).
- Perform focused GI assessment.

Patient Education

- Avoid foods that exacerbate symptoms (e.g., alcohol, high-fat foods, acidic foods, caffeine-containing foods).
- Consume smaller portions of food throughout the day.
- Do not eat large meals before lying down, and sleep with HOB elevated to 30 degrees.
- Seek urgent evaluation for worsening pain or evidence of GI bleeding.

FOREIGN BODIES

Overview

- *Foreign body obstruction* is the result of a substance or item, such as animal bones, a food bolus, or an inedible item, being lodged in the GI tract.
- Patients with esophageal stricture are at higher risk for obstruction.
- Surgery may be required to retrieve the item.
- Children are at higher risk for foreign body ingestion.

[ ] **COMPLICATIONS**

Ingested foreign bodies may perforate the GI tract, requiring surgery and putting the patient at risk for sepsis.

Signs and Symptoms

- Coughing
- Drooling
- Dysphagia
- Pain related to site of blockage
- Sensation of something stuck in the throat
- Shortness of breath
- Subcutaneous emphysema (if perforation)
- Vomiting

Diagnosis

Labs

- Preoperative labs if needed (basic metabolic panel [BMP], CBC)

Diagnostic Testing

- CT: neck, chest, and/or abdomen
- X-rays: neck, chest, and/or kidneys, ureter, bladder

Treatment

- Admit patient for observation as indicated.
- Endoscopy may be indicated.
- Administer medications such as glucagon to relax smooth muscle in the GI tract (see Table 5.1).
- Perform airway management.
- Refer patient for psychiatric care for intentional ingestion.
- Surgical repair of tissue damage or surgery to retrieve item may be indicated.

Nursing Interventions

- Administer medications as ordered (see Table 5.1).
- Assess/manage airway and respiratory complications.
- Calm pediatric patients, as crying may dislodge foreign body and cause airway obstruction; allow parents to comfort their children.
- Closely monitor psychiatric patients to minimize further self-harm behaviors.
- Position patient in high Fowler's.
- Prepare patient for surgery.

Patient Education

- Childproof the house and keep small items out of reach of children.
- Monitor for any dark, tarry stools or bright red rectal bleeding.
- Monitor stools for the foreign object.
- Seek urgent treatment for respiratory distress or uncontrolled pain.
- When eating, cut food into small, bite-sized portions and chew completely, while being careful to avoid small bones in meat and fish.

[ ]   **ALERT!**

Patients who are unable to swallow secretions due to upper GI blockage are at high risk for aspiration. Airway maintenance, such as intubation and suctioning, may be required.

[ ]   **POP QUIZ 5.2**

A construction worker presents to the ED after accidentally swallowing a screw that they had been holding in their mouth. X-rays reveal that the screw is in the patient's stomach. What should the nurse prepare to do next?

GASTRITIS

Overview

- *Gastritis* is inflammation and irritation of the stomach lining.
- It is usually caused by infectious agents (most commonly *Helicobacter pylori*), excessive alcohol intake, or certain medications, or it is immune mediated; however, the cause is often unknown.

Signs and Symptoms

- Abdominal pain in the middle or upper quadrant
- Anorexia
- Burning sensation in stomach
- GI bleeding (in vomit or stool)
- Nausea/vomiting

Diagnosis

Labs

- CBC
- CMP
- FOB
- Guaiac test of gastric contents
- *H. pylori*
- Immunologic markers

Diagnostic Testing

- Abdominal CT scan
- Chest x-ray (if respiratory distress is present)
- EKG
- Endoscopy
- Gastric biopsy and histology
- Upper GI series

Treatment

- Antibiotics if *H. pylori* infection present (clarithromycin, metronidazole, or amoxicillin commonly prescribed)
- Hydration/nutritional stabilization
- Pain management
- Steps to block/minimize/neutralize effects of stomach acid: antacids, histamine blockers, and proton pump inhibitors

Nursing Interventions

- Administer medications and crystalloid IV fluids as ordered (see Table 5.1 and Table A.3).
- Assess and manage pain (see Table A.2).
- Monitor I/O.
- Perform focused GI assessment.

[🧠] **COMPLICATIONS**

Complications from gastritis include bleeding, dehydration, and poor nutritional intake.

Patient Education

- Avoid the use of alcohol.
- Avoid foods that trigger symptoms.
- Avoid nonsteroidal anti-inflammatory drugs (NSAIDs) if indicated.
- Do not use tobacco products.
- Follow up with GI specialist.
- Monitor and follow up for any signs of GI bleeding, including dark, tarry stools.
- Return for increased pain or decreased ability to eat.

GASTROENTERITIS

Overview

- *Gastroenteritis*, sometimes referred to as "stomach flu," is inflammation and infection of the intestines.
- It is usually viral but can also be caused by bacteria, parasitic agents, or protozoa.

Signs and Symptoms

- Abdominal pain/cramps
- Blood in stool
- Diarrhea
- Fever
- Hyperactive bowel sounds
- Nausea/vomiting

Diagnosis

Labs

- CBC
- CMP
- FOB
- Guaiac test of gastric contents
- Stool culture
- Stool for ova and parasites

Diagnostic Testing

- Likely diagnosed based on physical exam
- Abdominal CT scan or ultrasound helpful in some cases to rule out other conditions

Treatment

- Antibiotic administration, if indicated
- Crystalloid fluid administration to maintain hydration (see Table A.3)
- Symptomatic management

Nursing Interventions

- Administer medications and crystalloid fluids as ordered (see Table A.3 and Table 5.1).
- Assess for signs of dehydration, skin tenting, dry mouth, hypotension, and tachycardia.   ▶

[🧠] **COMPLICATIONS**

Gastroenteritis can cause dehydration and metabolic acidosis due to frequent diarrheal episodes.

Nursing Interventions *(continued)*

- Ensure that the patient is able to tolerate oral fluids before discharge.
- Monitor input/output (I/O).
- Perform focused GI assessment, including oral intake and symptom onset, to determine if contaminated food is the cause.

Patient Education

- Follow up for increased abdominal pain, uncontrolled nausea/vomiting, weakness, or dizziness.
- Keep all kitchen and bathroom surfaces clean.
- Start with a clear liquid diet, advance to the BRAT (bananas, rice, applesauce, toast) diet, and then maintain regular diet as tolerated.
- Stay home until symptoms have resolved for at least 48 hours.
- Wash hands, and clean high-touch surfaces frequently.

[ ] **NURSING PEARL**

Patients prescribed a BRAT diet consume foods that, although they are low in nutrients, are easier for the digestive tract to process. BRAT stands for bananas, rice, applesauce, and toast, which are the primary components of the diet.

GASTROINTESTINAL BLEEDING

Overview

- GI bleeding is categorized by its location, in either the upper or the lower GI tract. The division point is the ligament of Treitz.
- Upper GI bleeding: Risk factors include NSAID or aspirin use, alcohol use, and liver disease. Upper GI bleeding is either variceal or nonvariceal. *Varices* are enlarged venous channels, usually found in the lower part of the esophagus. These veins are dilated secondary to portal hypertension and are usually caused by cirrhosis. The risk of rebleeding is high until the varices are surgically treated. These patients require immediate intervention and close observation. Nonvariceal bleeding occurs when the esophageal or gastroduodenal mucosa erodes into an underlying vein or artery. These erosions are caused by medications, peptic ulcer disease, or prolonged retching and vomiting.
- Lower GI bleeding: Common causes of lower GI bleeding include angiodysplasia, colitis, colon cancer, colonic polyps, diverticulum, or hemorrhoids.

[ ] **COMPLICATIONS**

Patients frequently delay seeking treatment for lower GI bleeding. Prolonged bleeding can result in anemia, hypovolemia, and shock.

Signs and Symptoms

- Abdominal pain
- Anemia
- Ascites
- Dizziness
- Hematemesis (upper GI bleeding)
- Hematochezia (lower GI bleeding)
- Hypovolemia (tachycardia, orthostatic hypotension, and syncope)
- Lethargy/altered mental status
- Melena (lower GI bleeding) ▶

Signs and Symptoms *(continued)*

- Nausea/vomiting
- Pallor or jaundice (esophageal varices)
- Weakness

Diagnosis

Labs

- CBC
- CMP
- FOB
- Guaiac test of gastric contents
- PT, aPTT
- Type and screen

Diagnostic Testing

- Abdominal ultrasound
- Chest, abdomen, and pelvis CT scan
- Chest x-ray
- EKG (to identify cardiac changes or for preoperative clearance)

Treatment

- Airway: Sengstaken–Blakemore, Minnesota, or Linton balloon tube to tamponade variceal bleeding; intubation as indicated by clinical status
- Hemodynamic stability: isotonic fluid resuscitation; serial CBCs to monitor blood counts; blood product transfusions (packed red blood cells (PRBCs), fresh frozen plasma (FFP), and platelets) as indicated; possible massive transfusion protocol depending on patient's condition
- Bleeding: medications to stop or reverse anticoagulation
- Portal hypertension: endoscopy; beta-blockers; urgent GI consultation
- Nonvariceal bleeding: endoscopy; IV proton pump inhibitors
- Lower GI bleeding: colonoscopy; radionuclide imaging
- Observation/monitoring if bleeding is expected after a GI procedure

Nursing Interventions

- Administer crystalloid fluids and blood products as ordered.
- Administer medications as ordered to control bleeding, reverse anticoagulation, and manage portal hypertension as indicated (see Table 5.1).
- Assess/manage airway, breathing, and circulation, and apply supplemental oxygen as indicated.
- Assess and monitor hemodynamic instability and vital signs.
- Establish two large-bore IV lines and draw blood for lab tests.
- Insert/manage nasogastric (NG) tube as indicated.
- Monitor I/O, including characteristics of stool and emesis output.
- Prepare patient for surgical intervention or inpatient admission.

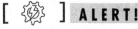 **ALERT!**

Patients with esophageal varices can develop life-threatening complications quickly. They can aspirate blood and develop pneumonia or develop hypovolemic shock from substantial blood loss. Closely monitor these patients and be prepared to maintain their airway and administer blood products emergently.

Patient Education

- Begin smoking cessation program, if needed.
- Seek treatment immediately for any additional bleeding, including black, tarry stools.
- Follow up for increased pallor, weakness, dizziness, or pain.
- If instructed by the provider, stop taking medications that increase risk of bleeding, such as NSAIDs.
- Limit or eliminate alcohol use.

HEPATITIS

Overview

- *Hepatitis* is an acute or chronic liver infection that may lead to cirrhosis or liver failure.
- All hepatitis viruses have an asymptomatic incubation period.
- Hepatitis A is transmitted by the fecal-oral route; it is often associated with contaminated food and water and tends to have mild symptoms that resolve in a couple of weeks.
- Hepatitis B and C are blood-borne viruses with little to no symptoms; they can cause long-term liver damage and are often transmitted sexually, from mother to fetus, or by sharing drug needles.
- Hepatitis C often has no symptoms until the patient enters advanced stages of liver disease. There is no vaccine. More than half of those infected develop chronic conditions such as cirrhosis and cancer.

Signs and Symptoms

- Altered mental status
- Dark-colored urine
- Excessive bleeding
- Fatigue/weakness
- Fever
- Jaundice
- Loss of appetite
- Nausea/vomiting
- Pale-colored stools
- Pain in RUQ

Diagnosis

Labs

- CBC
- CMP
- Coagulation panel
- Drug screen
- Hepatitis panel
- Guaiac test on gastric contents
- FOB
- Urinalysis

[🌐] **POP QUIZ 5.3**

An intoxicated patient presents to the ED complaining of nausea. Soon after arrival, the patient vomits a large amount of frank blood. What is the most appropriate next step?

[🧠] **COMPLICATIONS**

Hepatitis A can cause acute liver failure, also known as fulminant hepatitis. This occurs when the liver does not function quickly enough to repair itself. Patients will show signs of encephalopathy and coagulation problems, which may lead to coma and death if not reversed quickly enough.

Diagnostic Testing
- Abdominal CT scan
- Hepatic ultrasound

Treatment
- Antiviral medications, as indicated, for hepatitis B and C
- Control of symptoms with antiemetics
- IV crystalloid fluids for rehydration
- Management of associated coagulopathies
- Postexposure prophylaxis

Nursing Interventions
- Assess for uncontrolled bleeding or signs of coagulopathies.
- Assess for signs of liver abnormalities, including jaundice and ascites.
- Assess and manage pain (see Table A.2).
- Administer antiviral medications as prescribed (see Table 5.1).
- Encourage rest.
- Establish IV access if indicated, draw blood for lab tests, and administer IV fluids.

Patient Education
- Learn ways to keep the liver healthy, such as by avoiding alcohol, and discuss use of medications with the provider.
- Learn about hepatitis A: Wash hands before eating and after using the bathroom. Keep surfaces clean. Know that traveling to other countries may increase chance of contracting the virus. Use safe food preparation.
- Learn about hepatitis B and hepatitis C: Have all family members get tested for hepatitis B and get vaccinated if they have not been. Know that hepatitis B is not transferred by hugging. Know that pregnant patients should be tested for hepatitis B, as the risk of transmission to the fetus can be reduced by antiviral medications. Know that IV drug users should be tested for hepatitis C, as there is treatment that may be effective if it is detected within the first 2 to 8 weeks. Take antiviral medications as prescribed; to avoid further liver damage, do not stop taking the medication without discussing it with the provider. Use one part bleach to nine parts water for cleaning blood spills.
- Contact the health department to help determine the source of sickness.

HERNIA
Overview
- A *hernia* is a protrusion of the intestine through a weakened area of abdominal wall muscle.
- Common sites for a hernia are umbilical, inguinal, femoral, hiatal, and incisional.
- Contributing factors to developing a hernia are heavy lifting, straining with bowel movement, and congenital defects.

[ ]   COMPLICATIONS

An *incarcerated hernia* occurs when part of the intestine becomes ischemic by strangulation between muscles Manual reduction will be attempted, and if the hernia is not reducible, then surgery will be required.

Signs and Symptoms

- Bloating/belching
- Bulge in the abdomen or groin (becomes more prominent with crying, coughing, or laughing)
- Constipation
- Localized pain (incarcerated hernia)
- Nausea/vomiting

Diagnosis

Labs

- Preoperative labs (CBC, CMP, type, and screen)

Diagnostic Testing

- Abdominal CT scan

Treatment

- Manual reduction for incarcerated hernias
- Surgical repair with postoperative antibiotics if bedside reduction unsuccessful

Nursing Interventions

- Apply a cold pack before attempted reduction, if requested.
- Assess and administer pain/sedation medications and assist with procedure as indicated (see Table A.2).
- Perform a focused abdominal assessment.
- Place an IV if indicated for pain control.
- Position patient supine for bedside reduction (Trendelenburg position for a groin hernia or other positions as requested by provider to facilitate reduction).
- Prepare patient for surgery if indicated.

Patient Education

- Avoid lifting heavy objects or straining to decrease the risk of recurrence.
- Drink adequate fluids.
- Eat a high-fiber diet to avoid constipation.
- Exercise regularly.
- Minimize sneezing and coughing, if possible, to decrease the risk of recurrence.

INFLAMMATORY BOWEL DISEASE

Overview

- *Inflammatory bowel disease* is an umbrella term describing disorders that involve chronic inflammation of the digestive tract: Crohn's disease and ulcerative colitis.
- Crohn's disease usually affects the end of the small intestine and the beginning of the colon but can occur anywhere in the GI tract.
- Ulcerative colitis only affects the colon.

[ ] **COMPLICATIONS**

Patients with Crohn's disease can develop intestinal blockages and fistulas and have an increased risk of colon cancer.

Signs and Symptoms

- Abdominal pain/cramps
- Anorexia ▶

Signs and Symptoms *(continued)*

- Anxiety/stress
- Bloody stools
- Changes in bowel habits: diarrhea, constipation
- Weight loss

Diagnosis

Labs

- CBC
- CMP
- Erythrocyte sedimentation rate
- Stool culture
- Stool for occult blood
- Stool for ova and parasites

Diagnostic Testing

- Abdominal CT scan
- Abdominal x-ray
- Barium enema
- Colonoscopy (part of outpatient diagnostic evaluation)

Treatment

- Antidiarrheal medications
- Anxiety or antidepressant medications, if indicated
- Diet modifications, including bowel rest
- Pain management (see Table A.2)
- Steroids and immunotherapy

Nursing Interventions

- Administer medications as prescribed (see Table 5.1).
- Assess and manage pain (see Table A.2).
- Assess for signs of GI bleeding.
- Monitor I/O, including characteristics of stool.
- Place an IV and administer crystalloid fluids as indicated to maintain hydration status.

Patient Education

- Avoid large quantities of fluids with meals to minimize abdominal distention.
- Avoid nicotine products.
- Exercise regularly.
- Identify and avoid foods and stressful situations that may trigger symptoms.
- Maintain adequate fluid and fiber intake to manage constipation.

INTESTINAL ISCHEMIA

Overview

- Intestinal ischemia develops when blood flow to the intestines is reduced or stopped. ▶

 COMPLICATIONS

If sustained reduced blood flow occurs, or if the blood supply is suddenly and completely disrupted, then necrosis, gangrene will develop.

Overview *(continued)*

- Possible causes include blood clots in the vessels supplying the intestines (mesenteric ischemia), intestinal blockages, hypotension, blood disorders, and medications.
- Previous abdominal surgery is a risk factor for developing this condition.

Signs and Symptoms

- Abdominal pain/cramping (severe pain for mesenteric ischemia)
- Dehydration
- Distention
- Nausea/vomiting
- Stool mixed with blood (late finding)
- Peritonitis (late finding)
- Tachycardia, hypotension (late finding)

Diagnosis

Labs

- Blood cultures before antibiotic administration
- CBC
- CMP
- FOB
- Lactate level
- PT, aPTT
- Type and screen
- Urinalysis

Diagnostic Testing

- Abdominal or pelvic ultrasound
- Angiography
- Chest, abdomen, and pelvis CT scan
- X-rays (acute abdominal series)

Treatment

- Anticoagulation as indicated if underlying cause is related to clotting
- Correction of electrolyte abnormalities
- GI decompression
- Management of hemodynamic instability, including with crystalloid fluid
- Management of sepsis/septic shock
- Ongoing hemodynamic monitoring
- Pain management
- Referral for possible emergent surgical intervention and inpatient treatment

Nursing Interventions

- Administer antibiotics as prescribed (see Table A.1).
- Administer anticoagulation if prescribed.
- Administer crystalloid fluid.
- Apply supplemental oxygen as needed.
- Assess and manage pain (see Table A.2). ▶

Nursing Interventions *(continued)*

- Assess and monitor hemodynamic status and vital signs, as these patients are at high risk for fluid shifts and septic shock.
- Assess and treat for sepsis/septic shock.
- Establish an IV and draw blood for laboratory tests.
- Keep patient NPO.
- Monitor I/O.
- Place and monitor NG tube as indicated.
- Prepare patient for inpatient admission or for transfer to the operating room for surgical intervention.

Patient Education

- Follow prescribed diet to allow intestines time to heal.
- Monitor for a fever or other signs of infection.
- Monitor stool output for adequate quantity and consistency.
- Report increased/uncontrolled pain or uncontrolled vomiting.

OBSTRUCTION

Overview

- Bowel obstructions are classified as mechanical or nonmechanical: A mechanical obstruction results from something found outside or within the intestine that causes a blockage. A nonmechanical obstruction develops when the muscular activity of the intestine decreases (e.g., paralytic ileus).
- Obstructions can cause partial or complete intestinal blockage.
- Signs and symptoms may vary depending upon the location of the obstruction.
- Intussusception is a type of mechanical intestinal obstruction that occurs when the bowel telescopes within itself (Figure 5.1).

Signs and Symptoms

- Abdominal pain: crampy, intermittent, wavelike
- Bowel sounds: Distal: hypoactive or absent; proximal: hyperactive
- Constipation
- Distention
- Flatus
- Hypotension
- Nausea/vomiting
- Stool mixed with fluid/mucus (intussusception)
- Tachycardia

Diagnosis

Labs

- CBC
- CMP ▶

[ ] **COMPLICATIONS**

A complete bowel obstruction can cause ischemia and necrosis. These complications, in turn, can lead to peritonitis and sepsis.

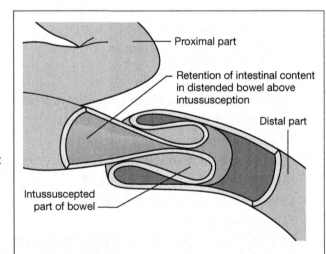

FIGURE 5.1 Intussusception of the bowel occurs when a distal segment of the intestine telescopes over a more proximal segment.

Source: Tkacs, N. C., Herrmann, L. L., & Johnson, R. L. (Eds.). (2021). *Advanced physiology and pathophysiology: Essentials for clinical practice*. Springer Publishing Company.

Labs (continued)
- FOB
- Urinalysis

Diagnostic Testing
- Abdominal CT scan
- Abdominal x-ray

Treatment
- Bowel rest
- Broad-spectrum antibiotic, if indicated
- Conservative management (observation) or surgical intervention
- For symptomatic intussusception: reduction via manual manipulation, enema, or surgical intervention
- IV fluid hydration
- NG tube for stomach decompression
- NPO
- Observation for transient/asymptomatic intussusception, if indicated
- Pain management

Nursing Interventions
- Administer medications as prescribed to manage nausea/vomiting.
- Assess and manage pain (see Table A.2).
- Assess for signs of infection or acute abdomen.
- Establish an IV and draw blood for lab tests.
- Insert and manage NG tube as ordered.
- Perform focused abdominal assessment to monitor for return of bowel sounds and to assess gastric distention.
- Prepare patient for transfer to the operating room or for inpatient admission as indicated.
- Monitor I/O, including characteristics of gastric contents and stool output.
- Monitor vital signs.

Patient Education
- Remain NPO until obstruction is resolved.
- When able to eat, begin with clear liquids and advance diet as tolerated.
- Follow up for any worsening signs/symptoms.
- Monitor/track bowel movements.
- Use stool softeners and other bowel regimens only as prescribed by the provider.

PANCREATITIS

Overview
- *Pancreatitis* is acute inflammation of the pancreas with sudden onset, usually secondary to gallstones blocking the pancreatic duct or to chronic alcohol and/or substance use. ▶

[ ]   COMPLICATIONS

Hemorrhagic pancreatitis may result in a Cullen sign, which is seen by bruising in the periumbilical region. This may be the result of a pseudocyst that ruptures. Pancreatitis can lead to serious, even fatal, complications, including abscess formation, development of pseudocysts, necrosis, and multisystem organ failure. In addition, pulmonary capillary leak syndrome can develop, putting the patient at risk for acute respiratory distress syndrome and multisystem organ failure.

Overview *(continued)*

- It is characterized by the release of activated digestive enzymes into the pancreas and surrounding tissues, causing tissue damage (similar to a chemical burn) and third-space fluid loss.
- Patients can develop multisystem organ failure secondary to inflammatory chemicals secreted throughout the body.

Signs and Symptoms

- Anorexia
- Fever
- Hypoactive or absent bowel sounds
- Hypotension
- Nausea/vomiting
- Pain: sudden onset, dull, in left upper abdomen or epigastrium radiating to back
- Tachycardia
- Tachypnea
- Tenderness: abdominal with guarding

Diagnosis

Labs

- Amylase
- CBC
- CMP
- Lipase
- Lipid panel

Diagnostic Testing

- Abdominal ultrasound
- Chest, abdomen, and pelvis CT scan
- Chest x-ray, if associated with respiratory complications
- Endoscopic retrograde cholangiopancreatography

Treatment

- Crystalloid fluid administration
- IV antibiotics, if indicated
- NG tube (if ileus present)
- NPO or modified diet to manage symptoms
- Pain management
- Steroids if from an autoimmune disease
- Surgery if indicated to relieve pressure/blockage in pancreatic duct

Nursing Interventions

- Administer crystalloid fluids as prescribed.
- Administer medications to decrease nausea/vomiting as ordered (see Table 5.1).
- Apply supplemental oxygen as needed, as these patients are at high risk for respiratory complications.
- Assess and manage pain (see Table A.2).
- Assess for nutritional or electrolyte imbalances.
- Establish a large-bore IV and draw blood for lab tests.
- Follow prescribed diet, keeping patient NPO, if indicated, or on bland or carbohydrate-rich diet.
- Insert/maintain NG tube if prescribed. ▶

Nursing Interventions *(continued)*

- Monitor I/O, including characteristics of gastric/stool content.
- Perform focused abdominal assessment.
- Prepare the patient for surgical intervention or inpatient admission as indicated.

Patient Education

- Begin a smoking cessation program, if needed.
- Follow a low-fat diet to minimize symptoms.
- Limit or stop drinking alcohol.
- Take pancreatic enzymes as prescribed to aid digestion.
- Take vitamin supplement to ameliorate effects of malabsorption.

PERITONITIS

Overview

- *Peritonitis* is an infection of the peritoneum that can be life threatening. Peritonitis as a primary condition (spontaneous bacterial peritonitis) occurs in patients with liver disease or in those undergoing peritoneal dialysis.
- Peritonitis as a secondary condition is related to ruptured or perforated abdominal organs with the release of their contents into the abdominal cavity.

Signs and Symptoms

- Abdominal pain
- Anorexia
- Cloudy dialysis effluent
- Guarding
- Malaise
- Nausea/vomiting
- Signs of hemodynamic instability (tachycardia, hypotension)

Diagnosis

Labs

- Blood cultures before antibiotic administration
- CBC
- CMP
- Dialysis effluent or paracentesis fluid analysis (culture, cell count with differential, Gram stain)
- FOB
- Lactate level
- PT, aPTT
- Type and screen
- Urinalysis

Diagnostic Testing

- Abdominal or pelvic ultrasound
- Chest, abdomen, and pelvis CT scan ▶

[🌐] **POP QUIZ 5.4**

A patient diagnosed with acute pancreatitis is receiving antibiotics, IV fluids, and pain medications. What is a critical complication the nurse should assess for?

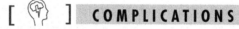 [🧠] **COMPLICATIONS**

Peritonitis is frequently fatal in patients with cirrhosis. These patients should be treated aggressively to prevent septic shock, multisystem organ failure, and death.

Diagnostic Testing (continued)
- EKG
- Paracentesis to determine cause

Treatment
- Assessment/management of sepsis, including broad-spectrum antibiotics
- Management of hemodynamic instability, including crystalloid fluid resuscitation and vasopressors, if indicated
- Therapeutic paracentesis, if indicated, to relieve pressure from ascites
- Surgical intervention, if indicated

Nursing Interventions
- Administer antibiotics as prescribed (see Table A.1).
- Assess and manage pain (see Table A.2).
- Assess for signs of sepsis/septic shock.
- Assess/instruct patient on proper aseptic technique for peritoneal dialysis.
- Assist with culture collection from paracentesis or peritoneal dialysis effluent.
- Initiate at least two large-bore IV lines for crystalloid fluid administration.
- Obtain blood cultures before antibiotic administration.
- Prepare patient and assist with paracentesis if performed.
- Prepare patient for inpatient admission.

Patient Education
- Follow up if pain worsens/returns or if signs and symptoms of infection recur.
- If performing peritoneal dialysis, wash hands thoroughly before and after procedure and maintain strict aseptic technique throughout.
- Take all antibiotics as prescribed.

TRAUMA

Overview
- Abdominal trauma is associated with high morbidity and mortality rates.
- Trauma is either blunt or penetrating and can result in significant blood loss or infection. Blunt trauma: most commonly from a motor vehicle crash; penetrating trauma: from a gunshot or stabbing
- Consider the mechanism of injury and the underlying structures when assessing the patient to help identify potential injuries.
- Abdominal injuries are not limited to the GI tract. Major arteries and veins, as well as genitourinary structures, can also be affected.

[ ] **COMPLICATIONS**

A splenic injury is the most common blunt trauma abdominal injury. Patients with splenic injuries can quickly become hemodynamically unstable as the spleen can store a significant amount of blood. These patients have a significant risk of developing hypovolemic shock.

Signs and Symptoms
- General: bleeding, bruising, hypotension, pain, seat belt sign, tachycardia
- Organ-specific: diaphragm, intestine, liver, pancreas, spleen
- Stomach
- Blood aspiration from NG tube
- Left upper quadrant (LUQ) pain
- Vascular structures   ▶

Signs and Symptoms (continued)

- Hemorrhage
- Shock

Diagnosis

Labs

- CBC
- CMP
- FOB
- Guaiac test of gastric contents
- PT, aPTT
- Type and screen
- Urinalysis

Diagnostic Testing

- Chest, abdomen, and pelvis CT scan
- Diagnostic peritoneal lavage
- Focused assessment with sonography in trauma (FAST) exam
- X-rays (as indicated for associated injuries)

Treatment

- Airway, breathing, and circulation management
- Emergent surgical intervention, if indicated
- Fluid resuscitation followed by blood product administration (PRBCs, FFP, and platelets); massive transfusion protocol may be indicated
- Pain management
- Vasopressors as indicated

Nursing Interventions

- Administer crystalloid fluids and blood products as indicated.
- Assess and manage airway, breathing, and circulation.
- Assess and manage pain (see Table A.2).
- Assist with placement of arterial and central line for hemodynamic monitoring as needed.
- Ensure two large-bore IV lines are placed and draw blood for lab tests.
- Insert indwelling urinary catheter if needed for close monitoring of urine output and if not contraindicated by the presence of genitourinary trauma (urology to place if indicated).
- Insert NG tube as ordered; it is contraindicated in suspected basal skull fracture.
- Maintain airway and apply supplemental oxygen as indicated.
- Monitor vital signs frequently.
- Prepare patient for emergent transfer to the operating room or trauma unit.

Patient Education

- Follow diet and activity guidelines as prescribed.
- Follow up with social worker or other community resources, if needed, to address underlying factors associated with the injuries (e.g., violence or abuse, driving while intoxicated).
- Seek urgent treatment if pain worsens or bleeding occurs (bleeding may be GI or from other wounds).

[ ] **POP QUIZ 5.5**

The nurse is assessing a patient involved in a motor vehicle crash. The patient complains of RUQ pain. The nurse notes RUQ bruising and generalized abdominal rigidity. The patient's pulse is 136 bpm, and blood pressure is 68/30 mmHg. What type of injury should the nurse suspect and treat?

ULCERS

Overview

- *Peptic ulcers* are defects in the gastric or duodenal mucosa that extend through the muscularis mucosae. Ulcers develop and persist due to the acid-peptic activity in gastric juice.
- Peptic ulcer disease is associated with two major factors: *H. pylori* infection and consumption of NSAIDs.
- There are two types of ulcers: duodenal ulcers and gastric ulcers.

Signs and Symptoms

- GI bleeding
- Indigestion
- Feelings of fullness or bloating
- Nausea/vomiting
- Pain: burning, relieved or exacerbated by food

Diagnosis

Labs

- BMP
- CBC
- Noninvasive testing for *H. pylori*

Diagnostic Testing

- Barium swallow
- Chest and abdomen CT scan
- Endoscopy

Treatment

- Pain management
- Medications: proton pump inhibitors, H_2 blockers
- Antibiotics (*H. pylori* infection)

Nursing Interventions

- Administer medications as prescribed (see Table 5.1).
- Assess and treat pain (see Table A.2).
- Monitor for signs of GI bleeding.
- Monitor vital signs.
- Perform focused GI assessment, including nutritional intake.
- Prepare patient for endoscopy if indicated.

Patient Education

- Avoid alcohol and tobacco use.
- Avoid medications that can trigger symptoms, including aspirin, ibuprofen, and naproxen.
- Follow prescribed dietary recommendations, including adequate intake of fruits, vegetables, and fiber.
- Monitor for any signs and symptoms of GI bleeding.
- Take all medications as prescribed.

[🧠] **COMPLICATIONS**

Patients with peptic ulcer disease are at risk for developing GI bleeding. It is estimated that 50% of upper GI bleeding cases are caused by ulcers.

RESOURCES

Almeida, S. (2020). Communicable diseases and organisms in the health care setting. In V. Sweet & A. Foley (Eds.), *Sheehy's emergency nursing: Principles and practice* (7th ed., pp. 181–192). Elsevier.

Andreoni, C. (2013). Pediatric considerations in emergency nursing. In B. Hammond & P. Zimmerman (Eds.), *Sheehy's manual of emergency care* (7th ed., pp. 547–591). Elsevier Mosby.

Bacidore, V. (2020). Abdominal and genitourinary trauma. In V. Sweet & A. Foley (Eds.), *Sheehy's emergency nursing: Principles and practice* (7th ed., pp. 465–476). Elsevier.

Centers for Disease Control and Prevention. (n.d.). *Viral hepatitis*. U.S. Department of Health and Human Services. https://www.cdc.gov/hepatitis/index.htm

Foley, A. (2020). Triage. In V. Sweet & A. Foley (Eds.), *Sheehy's emergency nursing: Principles and practice* (7th ed., pp. 56–67). Elsevier.

Hamm, R. (2020). Pain. In V. Sweet & A. Foley (Eds.), *Sheehy's emergency nursing: Principles and practice* (7th ed., pp. 74–92). Elsevier.

Herrington, A. (2020). Gastrointestinal emergencies. In V. Sweet & A. Foley (Eds.), *Sheehy's emergency nursing: Principles and practice* (7th ed., pp. 260–270). Elsevier.

Prescribers' Digital Reference. (n.d.-a). *Aluminum hydroxide* [Drug information]. https://www.pdr.net/drug-summary/Aluminum-hydroxide-2835.5854

Prescribers' Digital Reference. (n.d.-b). *Dicyclomine-hydrochloride* [Drug information]. https://www.pdr.net/drug-summary/Bentyl-dicyclomine-hydrochloride-1358.24

Prescribers' Digital Reference. (n.d.-c). *Entecavir* [Drug information]. https://www.pdr.net/drug-summary/Baraclude-entecavir-105

Prescribers' Digital Reference. (n.d.-d). *Glucagon* [Drug information]. https://www.pdr.net/drug-summary/Glucagon-glucagon--rDNA-origin--290.2553

Prescribers' Digital Reference. (n.d.-e). *Lactulose* [Drug information]. https://www.pdr.net/drug-summary/Constulose-lactulose-1544.2434

Prescribers' Digital Reference. (n.d.-f). *Loperamide hydrochloride* [Drug information]. https://www.pdr.net/drug-summary/Loperamide-hydrochloride-capsules-loperamide-hydrochloride-2664.2114

Prescribers' Digital Reference. (n.d.-g). *Octreotide acetate* [Drug information]. https://www.pdr.net/drug-summary/Sandostatin-octreotide-acetate-438.1133

Prescribers' Digital Reference. (n.d.-h). *Pantoprazole sodium* [Drug information]. https://www.pdr.net/drug-summary/Protonix-I-V--pantoprazole-sodium-2096.5821

Prescribers' Digital Reference. (n.d.-i). *Peginterferon alfa-2a* [Drug information]. https://www.pdr.net/drug-summary/Pegasys-peginterferon-alfa-2a-2752.3508

Prescribers' Digital Reference. (n.d.-j). *Ranitidine-hydrochloride* [Drug information]. https://www.pdr.net/drug-summary/Zantac-injection-ranitidine-hydrochloride-239.3325

Prescribers' Digital Reference. (n.d.-k). *Ribavirin* [Drug information]. https://www.pdr.net/drug-summary/Copegus-ribavirin-2464.4062

Prescribers' Digital Reference. (n.d.-l). *Rifampin* [Drug information]. https://www.pdr.net/drug-summary/Rifadin-rifampin-1036.2531

Prescribers' Digital Reference. (n.d.-m). *Vasopressin* [Drug information]. https://www.pdr.net/drug-summary/Vasostrict-vasopressin-3644

Wolf, L., & Zimmermann, P. (2013). Abdominal pain and emergencies. In B. Hammond & P. Zimmerman (Eds.), *Sheehy's manual of emergency care* (7th ed., pp. 291–301). Elsevier Mosby.

6 GENITOURINARY EMERGENCIES

FOREIGN BODIES
Overview

- The genitourinary (GU) system is composed of the kidneys, ureters, bladder, urethra, and genital organs. The presence of a foreign body within this system may lead to injury and infection, and surgical removal of the object may be required.
- Foreign bodies in the upper GU tract are often iatrogenic in nature, while foreign bodies in the lower GU tract are often self-inserted for a variety of possible reasons.

[🧠] **COMPLICATIONS**

Foreign bodies in the GU tract frequently require urologic or gynecologic consultations and/or surgical procedures to remove. Additional trauma can occur if the patient attempts to remove the object without seeking medical evaluation. Delays in object retrieval will lead to an increased likelihood of secondary infection.

- Vaginal foreign bodies are commonly encountered in the ED. These items may have been intentionally placed, accidentally dislodged, or placed and then forgotten about. Items may include tampons, dislodged intrauterine devices (IUDs), piercings, or objects used for sexual stimulation.
- Patients may delay seeking treatment due to fear or embarrassment.

Signs and Symptoms

- Abnormal vaginal bleeding
- Abnormal vaginal or penile discharge
- Dysuria
- Hematuria
- Pelvic, genital, abdominal, and/or flank pain
- Urinary retention
- Vaginal discomfort

Diagnosis
Labs

In some cases, objects may be manually removed by the provider and lab tests may not be required; however, the following laboratory tests may be indicated depending on the patient presentation:

- Complete blood count (CBC)
- Renal function tests (blood urea nitrogen [BUN], creatinine, estimated glomerular filtration rate [eGFR])
- Urinalysis
- Urine culture
- Vaginal/cervical cultures

Diagnostic Testing

In some cases, objects may be manually removed by the provider during pelvic or genital examination without the need for radiographic imaging; however, the following diagnostics may be indicated depending on object location and concern for secondary trauma and/or infection: ▶

Diagnostic Testing (continued)

- CT scan (abdomen/pelvis)
- Cystoscopy
- Ultrasound (abdomen/pelvis, vagina)
- X-ray (kidneys, ureters, bladder [KUB])
- Ureteroscopy

Treatment

- Object removal: Often requires surgical intervention, frequently done by ureteroscopic or cystoscopic removal under general anesthesia. Vaginal foreign bodies most often removed by provider during the pelvic examination.
- Antibiotic prophylaxis and/or treatment of secondary infection (see Table A.1)
- Pharmacologic and nonpharmacologic pain management (see Table A.2): warm compresses, soaks, sitz bath, and intermittent ice application to alleviate discomfort associated with genital trauma. Possible oral analgesics and/or topical anesthetics (e.g., topical lidocaine) applied to external genitalia or instilled into the urethra or vagina upon object removal.

Nursing Interventions

- Administer antibiotics as ordered.
- Assess and treat pain as indicated.
- Assess any medical devices within the pelvic or genital area, such as urinary catheters and contraceptive devices such as intrauterine devices (IUDs). Ensure that such devices appear properly placed and inspect upon removal to ensure objects are intact.
- Assess for signs and symptoms of infection including fever, localized pain, and vaginal discharge.
- Assess for urinary retention using bedside bladder scan. Monitor urinary output and assess urine quality, noting any hematuria, cloudiness/sediment, or foul odor.
- Prepare patient for pelvic examination and assist provider with object removal.
- Provide emotional support and referral to sexual assault resources as needed.

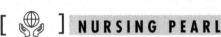

[🌐] **NURSING PEARL**

The nurse should ensure that a private space is available to discuss patient history, acknowledging that fear or embarrassment may prevent the patient from disclosing a history of vaginal or GU foreign body insertion.

Patient Education

- Often, certain foreign bodies within the GYN and GU system are medically necessary. Obtain education regarding the care and maintenance of any medical devices within the GYN system and GU tract, such as urinary catheters, ureteral stents, and IUDs, to prevent infection and secondary trauma.
- Stents may have a string that visibly extends out of the urethra. Do not pull on strings or attempt to dislodge stents.
- IUDs have strings that extend through the cervix into the vaginal canal. Upon insertion, gynecologists typically advise patients to intermittently feel for the presence of strings to ensure that the IUD remains properly placed. Do not attempt to dislodge IUDs.
- Avoid insertion of any object into the urethra. Obtain appropriate resources if self-insertion of objects may be related to a psychiatric condition.
- If using tampons or menstrual cups, keep track of menstrual product usage to ensure that any objects inserted in the vagina are removed. ▶

[📝] **POP QUIZ 6.1**

A young adult patient arrives complaining of pelvic discomfort and abnormal vaginal bleeding. The patient reports having had an IUD placed 6 months ago. The ED provider performs a pelvic examination and is unable to visualize the IUD string extending through the cervix. What further intervention should the nurse anticipate?

Patient Education *(continued)*

- Monitor and report any signs or symptoms of infection, such as dysuria, hematuria, decreased urinary output, fevers, or worsening pain.
- Never manipulate or remove a foreign body without the assistance of a healthcare provider.
- Seek immediate medical care for any object lodged within GU tract.

GENITAL INFECTIONS AND SEXUALLY TRANSMITTED INFECTIONS

Overview

- Infections of genital organs are commonly encountered in the ED and may occur due to a disruption of normal genital flora. Genital infections may also be sexually transmitted.

- Common inflammatory complaints in patients with male genitalia include epididymitis and orchitis. Epididymitis refers to swelling of the epididymis, which may cause testicular pain. Orchitis refers to swelling of the testicles, which may occur with or without concurrent epididymitis (epididymo-orchitis). Potential causes for these conditions include trauma and viral or bacterial infection, including sexually transmitted infections (STIs) such as gonorrhea and chlamydia infection.

- Common inflammatory complaints in patients with female genitalia include vaginitis and candidiasis. Vaginitis may be related to yeast overgrowth, bacterial imbalance, STI such as trichomoniasis, or noninfectious causes such as chemical exposure. Bacterial vaginosis develops from *Gardnerella vaginalis* and *Mycoplasma hominis*. Candidiasis develops secondary to colonization by the *Candida* species of fungi. Trichomoniasis is an STI caused by the protozoan *Trichomonas vaginalis*.

- Some STIs such as syphilis, gonorrhea, and HIV infection can lead to severe complications if left untreated, such as pelvic inflammatory disease, infertility, neurologic manifestations, various types of cancer, and death. STIs may be contracted orally or anally. Many patients with STIs are asymptomatic or have mild symptoms. The expected course of each illness varies depending on the pathogen and exposure. STIs in pregnancy may lead to birth defects and complications such as low birth weight and prematurity, and some infections may pass from the pregnant patient to the fetus. It is important to screen all pregnant patients for STIs.

[🧠] COMPLICATIONS

Untreated STIs cause significant physical and mental complications ranging from localized infections in the GU tract to systemic infection, infertility, and death. Additionally, those with undiagnosed infections may continue to unknowingly spread these conditions.

Signs and Symptoms

- It is likely that there are no symptoms and that the patient is unaware of the STI. Male patients more likely to have asymptomatic presentation of certain STIs. Possible development of long-term sequelae of STIs, such as damage to reproductive system if untreated (even in asymptomatic patients).

- Genital infections include the following: candidiasis; chlamydia infection; gonorrhea; genital herpes (herpes simplex virus [HSV]); human papillomavirus (HPV); HIV infection; hepatitis; syphilis; trichomoniasis.

Diagnosis

Labs

- CBC
- Serum or urine human chorionic gonadotropin (HCG)
- Urinalysis and urine culture (if secondary infection suspected)

[⚙] ALERT!

Although HPV is considered to be the most common STI in the world, there is no HPV screening test available for male patients.

Labs (continued)

- STI screening (may be assessed through serum, urine, or vaginal/cervical, penile, or urethral swab collection, specific to suspected STI)
- Vaginal and/or cervical cultures

Diagnostic Testing

In most cases, imaging is not required for diagnosis of genital infections; however, the following may be indicated depending on patient presentation:

- Abdominal and pelvis CT scan
- Pelvic examination
- Ultrasound: transvaginal or abdominal

Treatment

- Antibiotic, antifungal, and antiviral administration for many infections (see Table A.1): chlamydia—doxycycline; hepatitis C virus (HCV)—direct-acting antiviral therapy; HIV—antiretroviral therapy; gonorrhea—ceftriaxone; syphilis—penicillin G.
- Specific infection prevention or risk/exposure treatment: appropriate vaccinations to lower the risk of certain infections (hepatitis A, hepatitis B, HPV); pre- or postexposure prophylaxis possible for patients before and after HIV exposure (see Table 6.1 for genitourinary medications); proper screening, such as Pap tests to monitor for abnormal cells (cervical cancer/precancerous cells) that may indicate HPV
- Limited treatment options for some STIs, with management focusing on symptom relief: pain management (see Table A.2); no specific treatment available to eradicate HPV; possible medications for treatment of genital warts; no cure for HSV, although certain medications may control lesion outbreaks.
- Counseling/referral to sexual partner(s) to receive treatment

TABLE 6.1 Genitourinary Medications

INDICATIONS	MECHANISM OF ACTION	CONTRAINDICATIONS, PRECAUTIONS, AND ADVERSE EFFECTS
5-Alpha reductase inhibitors (finasteride)		
• Symptomatic treatment of BPH, reducing symptoms, decreasing risk of urinary retention, and decreasing likelihood of requiring surgical interventions such as TURP and prostatectomy	• Act as an analog of testosterone to competitively inhibit type II 5-alpha reductase, thereby inhibiting conversion of testosterone into 5-alpha-dihydrotestosterone, an isoenzyme that stimulates prostate tissue development	• Use with caution in patients with hepatic disease. • Therapy is expected to result in a decreased serum PSA concentration; any increase from baseline PSA in male patients using finasteride should be considered a possible signal of prostate cancer development. • Medication has potential for increased incidence of high-grade prostate cancer.
Alpha-blockers (tamsulosin hydrochloride)		
• Treatment of signs and symptoms of BPH, medical expulsive treatment of renal calculi	• Selective antagonists of alpha-1 receptors, assisting to mediate smooth muscle contraction, causing relaxation of the bladder neck and prostate	• Medication is a sulfa derivative and is contraindicated in patients with sulfa allergy.

(continued)

TABLE 6.1 Genitourinary Medications *(continued)*

INDICATIONS	MECHANISM OF ACTION	CONTRAINDICATIONS, PRECAUTIONS, AND ADVERSE EFFECTS
		• Use with caution in patients with history of hypotension and heart disease, as it may contribute to orthostatic hypotension. • Medication has significant drug-drug interactions; assess interactions with concurrent therapies.
Alpha-1 agonists (phenylephrine)		
• Provide localized vasoconstriction when injected for priapism	• Mediate vasoconstriction through localized stimulation of alpha-adrenergic receptors	• Although localized effect is intended, systemic effects may occur (hypertension, tachycardia, reflex bradycardia, palpitations, and arrhythmias). • Use with caution in patients with cardiac disease. • Medication is contraindicated in patients with poorly controlled hypertension or concurrent use of MAOIs.
Progestins (levonorgestrel)		
• Postcoital emergency contraceptive	• Exact mechanism unclear but appears to either inhibit ovulation or disrupt fertilization and implantation	• Medication must be taken within 72 hours of unprotected intercourse. • Repeat the dose if vomiting occurs within 2 hours of administration. • Medication can cause nausea, abdominal or pelvic pain, and amenorrhea.
Integrase inhibitors (raltegravir)		
• Used in combination with other antiretroviral medications for PEP and treatment of HIV-1 in adult patients	• Inhibit HIV-1 integrase, preventing incorporation of HIV-1 DNA in the host cell genome	• Medication may cause increased serum CK levels, leading to myopathy and rhabdomyolysis; use is contraindicated in patients with a history of elevated CK, rhabdomyolysis, or myopathy. • Medication must be immediately discontinued if rash or hypersensitivity reaction occurs; it may cause Stevens-Johnson syndrome or toxic epidermal necrolysis. • Coadministration with aluminum- or magnesium-containing medications is contraindicated. • Patients should be cautioned that therapy does not prevent all cases of HIV or any other STIs; provide education regarding further measures to reduce STI risk.

(continued)

TABLE 6.1	Genitourinary Medications *(continued)*	
INDICATIONS	**MECHANISM OF ACTION**	**CONTRAINDICATIONS, PRECAUTIONS, AND ADVERSE EFFECTS**
Nucleotide reverse transcriptase inhibitors (emtricitabine/tenofovir)		
• Combination antiretroviral therapy for pre- and postexposure prophylactic treatment to reduce risk of acquiring HIV-1 in at-risk adults	• Emtricitabine: inhibits viral replication by interfering with HIV viral DNA polymerase • Tenofovir: competes with AMP as substrate to inhibit HIV-1 reverse transcriptase	• If used for pre-exposure prophylaxis, patients must be tested for HIV immediately before initiating treatment as well as periodically during ongoing therapy (every 3 months at minimum). • All patients should be tested for hepatitis before initiating therapy; if coinfection is present, severe exacerbation of hepatitis B may occur upon discontinuation. • Patients should be cautioned that therapy does not prevent all cases of HIV or any other STIs; provide education regarding further measures to reduce STI risk. • Lactic acidosis and severe hepatomegaly may occur; if so, treatment should be suspended. • Medication may cause new or worsening renal toxicity and is contraindicated in patients with renal impairment.
Urinary analgesics (phenazopyridine hydrochloride)		
• Symptomatic relief of lower urinary tract discomfort	• Mechanism of action unknown; azo dye provides topical analgesic effect on urinary tract mucosa	• Medication is contraindicated in patients with impaired renal function and in those with G6PD deficiency. • Educate patients that drug causes urine discoloration (red/orange stain). • Use should be limited to 2 days. • Medication may cause GI discomfort; administer with meals

Note: All agents are contraindicated in the presence of hypersensitivity to the medication or one of its components
AMP. adenosine monophosphate; BPH, benign prostatic hyperplasia; CK, creatine kinase; GI, gastrointestinal; G6PD, glucose-6-phosphate dehydrogenase; MAOI, monoamine oxidase inhibitor; PEP, postexposure prophylaxis; PSA, prostate-specific antigen; STI, sexually transmitted infection; TURP, transurethral resection of the prostate.

Nursing Interventions

- Assess gynecologic history, including discussion of plans for STI and pregnancy prevention, if applicable.
- Assess for interpersonal/intimate relationship violence.
- Administer medications, such as antibiotics for bacterial infection, as ordered.
- Assist with pelvic examination and obtaining appropriate cultures. ▶

Nursing Interventions *(continued)*

- Assess/treat pain.
- Provide support and resources to inform sexual partners of STI status and ensure appropriate notification and treatment for possible transmitted infection.
- Instruct on the importance of treatment compliance and follow-up care.

Patient Education

- Disclose STI status to all sexual partners encountered within 60 days of ED visit, and encourage those sexual partners to seek testing as well.
- Follow up with primary care, OB/GYN, and/or infectious disease as appropriate. Receive regular health screenings and appropriate vaccinations (e.g., hepatitis B, HPV). Attend any scheduled outpatient specialist follow-up visits. Patients with chronic disease, such as HIV and hepatitis C, will require further evaluation and more rigorous medication regimens.
- Learn about any prescribed medications and complete the full course of antibiotics if prescribed.
- Avoid sexual activity until treatment has been completed and symptoms have resolved.
- Learn risk factors and STI prophylaxis as applicable. Consider barrier method prophylaxis, limiting number of sexual partners, and inquiring about any potential sexual partner's STI status. Learn about pre- and postexposure prophylaxis for HIV. If at risk, learn about medication and testing as applicable. If at risk, obtain STI screening on a regular basis.
- Seek further evaluation for worsening pain, fever, dysuria, or abnormal bleeding/discharge.

> **[📝] POP QUIZ 6.2**
>
> A patient presents for evaluation of a single, round, painless lesion to the penis approximately 3 weeks after unprotected intercourse with a new partner. What condition would the nurse suspect may be responsible, and what actions would the nurse expect to take to care for this patient?

GENITOURINARY TRAUMA

Overview

- Injury to the GU system frequently occurs in conjunction with abdominal trauma.
- Injuries vary in presentation depending on the structure involved: renal trauma, bladder trauma, female genitalia, male genitalia (Tables 6.2 and 6.3).
- Sexual assault and abuse should be considered as a potential cause in cases of genital trauma. All patients presenting with GU trauma should be screened for possible sexual violence. Refer to the Sexual Assault section for more information.

> **[🧠] COMPLICATIONS**
>
> While most cases of GU trauma are not immediately life threatening, some presentations, such as renal vascular lacerations, can quickly lead to hemodynamic instability and rapid decompensation. It is important to assess for injury to the GU system in all patients presenting with abdominal trauma and/or pelvic fractures.

Signs and Symptoms

- Renal trauma: flank, back, or abdominal pain and/or bruising or discoloration; hematuria, presence of blood at urethral meatus or vaginal introitus; nausea and vomiting
- Bladder trauma: abdominal distention; hematuria, presence of blood at urethral meatus; incontinence; suprapubic/lower abdominal pain and/or bruising or discoloration; painful urination; urinary retention
- Female genital injury: vaginal bleeding/blood at vaginal introitus; vulvar edema/contusions, perineal ecchymosis; painful urination; urinary retention
- Male genital injury: hematuria, presence of blood at urethral meatus; painful urination; scrotal or penile edema and/or contusions, perineal ecchymosis; urinary retention

TABLE 6.2	Renal Injury Scale
Grade I	Nonexpanding subcapsular hematomas without parenchymal laceration and renal contusions
Grade II	Nonexpanding perirenal hematoma extending to retroperitoneum, or laceration of less than 1 cm parenchymal depth of renal cortex without urinary extravasation
Grade III	Laceration greater than 1 cm parenchymal depth of renal cortex without urinary extravasation or collecting system rupture
Grade IV	Laceration involving the renal cortex, medulla, and collecting system, or contained hemorrhage of the main renal artery or vein
Grade V	Complete devascularization or shattering of the kidney

TABLE 6.3	Bladder Injury Scale
Grade I	Intramural hematoma or contusion or partial-thickness laceration
Grade II	Extraperitoneal bladder wall laceration of less than 2 cm
Grade III	Extraperitoneal bladder wall laceration greater than 2 cm or intraperitoneal laceration less than 2 cm
Grade IV	Intraperitoneal bladder wall laceration greater than 2 cm
Grade V	Any bladder wall laceration extending into the bladder neck or ureteral orifice

Diagnosis

Labs

- Basic metabolic panel (BMP)
- CBC
- Coagulation panel
- hCG (serum or urine, for all female patients of childbearing age)
- Type and screen
- Urinalysis

Diagnostic Testing

- Focused assessment with sonography in trauma (FAST) examination prioritized after provider completes primary survey: quickly identifies internal injuries in patients presenting with blunt or penetrating trauma. Assessment includes bedside ultrasound of the heart, right upper quadrant (RUQ), left upper quadrant (LUQ), and pelvis. Further imaging possibly deferred to expedite surgical intervention if severe injury/uncontrolled bleeding identified with initial FAST and patient hemodynamically compromised.
- In hemodynamically stable patients, further imaging possible to investigate GU injury: CT scan (abdomen/pelvis, angiography if indicated); cystography for suspected bladder injury; retrograde urethrography for suspected urethral injury; ultrasound (location dependent on area of suspected injury); x-rays (KUB, hip/pelvis).

[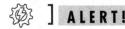] **ALERT!**

If blood is noted at the urinary meatus during the initial trauma evaluation, catheter insertion is often contraindicated because it may worsen injury to the GU system. Consult to urology is indicated.

Treatment

- Management of any uncontrolled bleeding or hemodynamic compromise: Most cases of GU trauma do not cause hemodynamic instability, although stabilizing interventions may be required for some injuries, such as renovascular trauma. In patients with unstable urologic/pelvic trauma, any uncontrolled hemorrhage must be addressed first, and then airway, breathing, and circulatory concerns should be managed. If external hemorrhage is noted or the provider notes concern for hemorrhage upon performing FAST examination, the following may be indicated: pain management; pelvic examination if indicated; sexual assault forensic examination if indicated; stabilization of pelvic fractures with pelvic binder; urgent consultation with urology and gynecology if applicable

Nursing Interventions

- Facilitate or perform sexual assault forensic examination if indicated. (See the Sexual Assault section for further information.) Follow mandatory reporting guidelines for any suspected abuse of children, older adults, or patients with a disability. Conduct psychosocial assessment and provide support and resources as needed.
- Insert urinary catheter if indicated and/or if cleared by urology (contraindicated in certain cases, such as if blood is present at urethral meatus). In some circumstances, urology may place the urinary catheter, depending on injuries sustained.
- Monitor urine output and quality, alerting provider to any hematuria.
- Provide emergent stabilization in accordance with established trauma algorithms (advanced cardiovascular life support [ACLS], trauma nursing core course [TNCC]). Continuously monitor vital signs and hemodynamic status. Prepare patient for transfer to operating room or interventional radiology as indicated for surgical intervention. Assess pain and administer medications, fluids, and blood products as ordered. Apply ice for initial management of testicular or vulvar injuries.

Patient Education

- Avoid sexual stimulation/activity until cleared by urology or gynecology.
- Discuss safe discharge planning and obtain support resources for sexual assault or interpersonal violence survivors.
- Learn about prescribed medications, such as analgesics and antibiotics; nonpharmacologic pain management, such as ice or heat application; and any prescribed activity limitations, such as pelvic rest.
- Learn injury-specific and postsurgical information when indicated, including wound care and necessary follow-up.
- Recognize signs and symptoms of infection and when to return for reevaluation.
- Seek immediate care for any uncontrolled pain, weakness, dizziness, hematuria, decreased urine output, or inability to urinate.

[ ] **NURSING PEARL**

If patient presents with penile amputation, preserve amputated appendage in saline-soaked gauze, placed in a sterile plastic bag and then placed on ice until the patient is received by the surgical team.

[ ] **POP QUIZ 6.3**

The nurse is treating a patient involved in a high-speed motor vehicle crash. When preparing to insert an indwelling urinary catheter to measure the patient's urine output, the nurse notices blood on the urinary meatus. What should the nurse do next?

PRIAPISM

Overview

- *Priapism* is a persistent erection (greater than 4 hours) without sexual stimulation and may be categorized by ischemic and nonischemic causes.
- Ischemic priapism requires prompt treatment to prevent tissue injury and permanent erectile dysfunction. Causes include blood abnormalities such as hypercoagulability and sickle cell disease; certain medications (including antidepressants like trazodone, vasoactive medications, and illicit substances such as cocaine); and some cancers and neurologic disorders.
- Nonischemic priapism is usually related to penile/perineal trauma and often resolves spontaneously.

Signs and Symptoms

- Painful, persistent erection (ischemic)
- Persistent erection with a nontender penis (nonischemic)
- Urinary retention (ischemic and nonischemic)

Diagnosis

Labs

- Nonischemic priapism: often resolves spontaneously; does not require lab testing
- Ischemic priapism: CBC, coagulation panel, hemoglobin S, lactate dehydrogenase, reticulocyte count, urinalysis; urine toxicology

Diagnostic Testing

- Abdominal/pelvic CT scan or MRI to rule out associated conditions (such as malignancy)
- Vascular ultrasound

Treatment

- Nonischemic priapism: Often resolves without intervention. Pain management measures include regional nerve blocks and analgesics.
- Possible relief with conservative management techniques (such as ejaculation, voiding, application of ice to the groin, gentle exercise/ambulation, and application of supplemental oxygen).
- Possible medication administration: pseudoephedrine or terbutaline. Rarely resolves with oral therapy alone.
- Cavernosal blood aspiration: Required in 75% of cases of ischemic priapism. Possible procedural sedation to facilitate aspiration.
- Adrenergic agent injection (such as phenylephrine) may be required if unresolved after aspiration (see Table 6.1).
- Surgical intervention may be required if less invasive methods fail.

Nursing Interventions

- Administer and titrate sedative medications as ordered for procedural sedation.
- Assess and manage pain (pharmacologic and nonpharmacologic therapies). Application of ice for 10 to 20 minutes may assist in managing pain and promote vasoconstriction.
- Assist in facilitating nonpharmacologic methods that promote detumescence. Assist patient to ambulate. Apply supplemental oxygen. Encourage patient to attempt to empty bladder. Provide hydration.   ►

 COMPLICATIONS

Ischemic priapism can lead to necrosis of penile corporal tissue if the condition is not treated emergently. Cellular changes begin to occur within 6 hours of onset, and damage to erectile tissue is considered irreversible within 12 to 36 hours, resulting in permanent sexual dysfunction in 90% of patients.

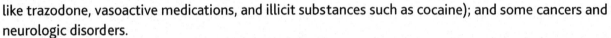 **NURSING PEARL**

Hemoglobin S is an abnormal variant of normal hemoglobin (hemoglobin A) and is found in patients with sickle cell disease. The atypical hemoglobin shape places patients at increased risk for ischemic priapism.

Nursing Interventions *(continued)*

- Assist medical provider as needed to prepare for corporal aspiration.
- Hold certain medications as advised by provider. Some medications (such as phosphodiesterase type 5 inhibitors, alpha-adrenergic receptor antagonists, and certain antipsychotic and antidepressant medications) may lead to a recurrence of symptoms and should be held for a time.

Patient Education

- Avoid sexual stimulation until cleared to resume sexual activity by urology.
- Learn about long-term effects of priapism, including the potential for permanent erectile dysfunction, and discuss treatment options with urology to address these concerns.
- Seek treatment for any recurrence of symptoms, including any sustained erection, painful erection, or erection that occurs without sexual stimulation.
- Seek care for any signs of infection, such as abdominal, pelvic, or genital pain, dysuria, fever, or chills.

RENAL CALCULI

Overview

- Also referred to as "kidney stones," *renal calculi* are mineral deposits that form within the kidney and often cause severe pain and damage to urinary structures as the body attempts to move the stone through the urinary tract.
- Approximately 9% of the population will be diagnosed with a kidney stone in their lifetime, and stones are a leading cause of hematuria. Depending on size and location, most stones can be excreted without intervention.
- Some risk factors include diet, dehydration, urinary stasis or infection, and urine abnormalities such as hypercalciuria and hyperoxaluria.

Signs and Symptoms

- Dysuria
- Fever, chills
- Hematuria
- Nausea, vomiting
- Pain in flank (often unilateral), groin, lower abdomen, or back
- Restlessness and irritability
- Urinary retention, weak or interrupted stream of urine
- Urinary urgency

Diagnosis

Labs

- 24-hour urine collection (urine pH, calcium, citrate, magnesium, oxalate, phosphate, sodium, sulfate, uric acid, and total volume)
- BMP ▶

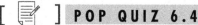
POP QUIZ 6.4

An adult patient with a history of sickle cell trait arrives for evaluation of a persistent erection that began 7 hours ago. What interventions should the nurse anticipate?

COMPLICATIONS

Obstructive calculi can cause altered elimination, infection, or ischemia. While 90% of stones can pass through the urinary tract without invasive measures, surgical intervention may be required to remove or break up large-diameter stones (5 mm or greater).

Labs (continued)

- CBC
- Kidney stone analysis
- Urine culture with sensitivity
- Urinalysis

Diagnostic Testing

Dependent on patient presentation; one or more of the following may be indicated:

- CT scan of the abdomen and pelvis with or without contrast
- KUB x-ray
- Renal ultrasound

Treatment

- Administration of antibiotics and antiemetic medication, if indicated (see Table A.1)
- Facilitation of stone passage with ample hydration using isotonic crystalloid infusion and administration of alpha blocker (tamsulosin) to relax smooth muscle to assist in facilitating stone passage (see Table 6.1)
- Measures to facilitate and monitor stone passage (watchful waiting or surgical intervention if required)
- Pain management, including nonpharmacologic measures, such as repositioning, and pharmacologic measures, such as administration of opioid analgesics and NSAIDs as needed (see Table A.2)
- Preparation for transfer to the operating room if surgical intervention (such as lithotripsy, cystoscopy and ureteroscopy, or percutaneous nephrolithotomy) is necessary

Nursing Interventions

- Assess intake/output (I/O), strain all urine, and evaluate for urinary retention. Observe for hematuria. Alert provider to any increase in bleeding. Report passage of any stones to medical provider.
- Evaluate for signs of infection and monitor hemodynamic status.
- If patient is unable to tolerate oral intake due to nausea/vomiting, administer antiemetic medications as ordered and provide IV fluids to maintain hydration, aiming to achieve urine output of 3,000 to 4,000 mL per 24 hours.
- Monitor pain and administer medications as ordered.
- Promote dietary changes, facilitate ambulation, and encourage oral hydration if applicable.
- Provide patient with a urine strainer and educate patient to strain all urine to collect stones for analysis.

Patient Education

- Learn risk factors for stone recurrence and adhere to appropriate dietary changes as indicated. If stone composition is known, suggested therapies and dietary changes include the following: calcium stones—limited sodium and protein intake, increased fluid intake, prescription of ammonium chloride to acidify urine, thiazide diuretics possibly indicated to treat hypercalciuria; uric acid stones—limited protein intake, low purine diet (limiting or eliminating high-purine foods such as organ meats, red meat, some seafood such as sardines, certain alcohols such as beer and distilled liquors), prescription of xanthine oxidase inhibitor (allopurinol), and addition of vitamin C supplement; cystine stones—limited protein intake, increased fluid intake, increased intake of fruits and vegetables, addition of medication to alkalize urine (potassium citrate); struvite stones—decreased ▶

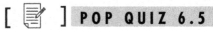

[📝] POP QUIZ 6.5

A patient arrives complaining of severe lower back pai radiating to the groin. The patient's urinalysis is positive fc hematuria. What interventions should the nurse anticipate

Patient Education *(continued)*

sodium intake, increased fluid intake, antibiotic administration and surgical removal often indicated as these stones are most often larger and usually associated with underlying infection.

■ Seek further care for any uncontrolled pain; persistent nausea/vomiting; fever/chills; or urinary changes, such as dysuria, hematuria, or inability to urinate. Some hematuria is to be expected as stones are passed through the urinary tract. Monitor bleeding and return for further care if gross hematuria occurs.

SEXUAL ASSAULT

Overview

■ Patients who have experienced sexual trauma may present to the ED for treatment and forensic examination.

■ The need to provide emergent care of injuries can be complicated by the need to preserve forensic evidence.

■ Some survivors seek care immediately after an assault, while others may disclose sexual trauma to the provider at a later date. Some patients choose not to disclose sexual assault history to their medical provider. Others may be survivors of repeated/chronic sexual abuse and assault.

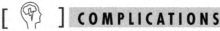

[🧠] COMPLICATIONS

A sexual assault survivor may be exposed to STIs, such as HIV. Patients who have experienced sexual trauma should be tested for infection and provided with postexposure prophylaxis (PEP) medications to reduce the risk of acquiring an STI. Patients should also be offered prophylactic medication to help prevent pregnancy.

The timeline of presentation/disclosure affects likelihood of evidence collection. Under most law enforcement regulations, evidence must be collected within 72 to 96 hours post assault. If the physical examination leads the provider to suspect sexual assault, the patient should be offered appropriate resources and forensic examination if desired.

■ Patients who have experienced sexual assault often suffer physiologic and emotional trauma, as well as secondary trauma in the form of infections, unwanted pregnancy, and chronic psychological effects, such as posttraumatic stress disorder (PTSD).

■ A trained sexual assault nurse examiner, if available, may be called to assess the patient, collect evidence, and provide resources. Patients may choose to undergo sexual assault examination but forgo reporting the encounter to law enforcement. Exceptions exist for populations who fall under mandatory reporting guidelines, such as children and adults with a disability.

[🤲] NURSING PEARL

Patients presenting for evaluation of sexual assault may have knowingly or unknowingly ingested drugs or alcohol. These substances may cause sedation or amnesic effects and limit the patient's ability to recall/report events. Altered mental status may also be caused by head injuries, choking injuries, or psychological responses to trauma, all of which may cause impaired memory and delays in seeking care or reporting events.

Signs and Symptoms

■ Emotional/psychological distress

■ Physical injury, such as lacerations, contusions, genital or rectal injuries, ligature/restraint marks, and signs of choking/strangulation

■ Symptoms associated with STIs, such as vaginal or penile discharge, skin lesions, or dysuria

Diagnosis

Labs

■ Cultures (vaginal, cervical, and/or rectal)

■ Ethyl alcohol level

Labs (continued)

- Pregnancy test (urine or serum)
- STI testing
- Urinalysis
- Urine toxicology

Diagnostic Testing

Depending on patient presentation, any of the following diagnostic tests may be indicated:

- CT scan or x-ray (location dependent on area of suspected injury)
- Forensic examination
- Ultrasound: transvaginal or abdominal, carotid (if choking injury suspected or reported)

Treatment

- Evidence collection/preservation and forensic examination if mandated or desired by patient
- Prophylactic antibiotics, PEP medications for HIV, and emergency contraceptive medications (levonorgestrel) as indicated (see Table 6.1)
- Psychiatry and/or social work consults to provide support and resources
- Reporting to law enforcement in accordance with local reporting mandates
- Stabilizing care of any traumatic injury in accordance with ACLS and TNCC guidelines with consult to OB/GYN, urology, and/or general surgery as necessary for assessment and treatment of severe injuries
- Vaccinations for hepatitis B and HPV per patient request

[⚡] ALERT!

Proper, timely evidence collection is best performed by a trained sexual assault nurse examiner. If a sexual assault nurse examiner is not available, some situations may require the emergency nurse caring for the patient to conduct the examination. The sexual assault examination kit comes with all of the necessary supplies and instructions for evidence collection. Use only the supplies contained in the kit, and document the procedure thoroughly. Maintain possession of the kit until it can be transferred to law enforcement and the chain of custody is documented.

Nursing Interventions

- Administer medications as ordered to treat pain, infection, or other symptoms, such as anxiety and nausea (see Table A.2).
- Assess support and involve family in patient's care if patient desires.
- Ensure that a safe, private space is available to discuss events and conduct examination.
- Facilitate evidence collection. Communicate with patient and sexual assault nurse examiner, if available, to expedite examination. Prior to forensic examination, take steps to preserve evidence while providing care.
- Notify law enforcement per patient request and/or in accordance with local reporting requirements.
- Provide emotional support and resources to maintain safety upon discharge.

Patient Education

- Adhere to postexposure medication regimen, including medication schedule for antibiotic treatment and HIV prophylaxis. Many patients experience nausea while taking PEP. Learn about any PRN antiemetics, if ordered, and seek further care if nausea/vomiting occurs and results in missed doses.
- Use outpatient resources for psychological support. If family will be involved in care, family should seek resources for themselves.
- Communicate with law enforcement regarding investigation of the assault, if applicable.
- Follow up regarding cultures and testing performed. Repeat HIV antibody testing at 4 to 6 weeks and again at 3 months post exposure; repeat HCV antibody testing 4 to 6 months post exposure.
- Seek further care for worsening pain, fever, bleeding/discharge, or dysuria.

TESTICULAR TORSION

Overview

- *Testicular torsion* is a urologic emergency in which the spermatic cord twists, leading to restricted arterial blood flow to the testicle (Figure 6.1).
- Testicular torsion must be identified and corrected emergently as vascular compromise and ischemia can lead to tissue necrosis within 6 to 8 hours.
- Most cases of testicular torsion occur spontaneously, presenting with acute atraumatic unilateral groin pain. In rare cases, torsion may be associated with exertion, trauma, or malignancy.
- Most cases of testicular torsion occur in adolescence, although this condition may present in patients of any age.

Signs and Symptoms

- Abdominal pain
- Nausea and/or vomiting
- Prehn's sign (pain when elevating the scrotum)
- Sudden-onset unilateral groin/testicular pain
- Testicular changes: erythema, edema, hardening, "high-riding" or retracted testicle

Diagnosis

Labs

Emergent intervention may be prioritized over obtaining diagnostic laboratories; however, the following may be indicated:

- Preoperative lab tests; CBC; CMP; coagulation panel; type and screen ▶

[🧠] **COMPLICATIONS**

Prompt identification and treatment of testicular torsion is key in preserving viability of the affected testicle. Compromised testicular circulation can lead to permanent damage within 4 to 6 hours of onset. If untreated, tissue necrosis will necessitate testicular amputation.

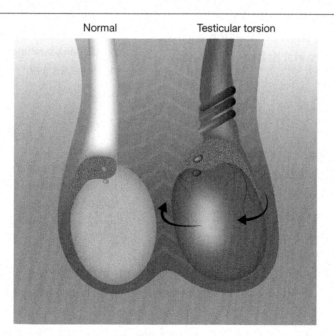

Normal   Testicular torsion

FIGURE 6.1 Testicular torsion.

Source: Gawlik, K. S., Melnyk, B. M., & Teall, A. M. (2020). *Evidence-based physical examination: Best practices for health and well-being assessment.* Springer Publishing Company.

Labs (continued)

- Urinalysis
- Urine culture with sensitivity testing

Diagnostic Testing
Color Doppler ultrasonography

Treatment

- Emergent orchiopexy: must be performed if manual detorsion is unsuccessful
- Orchiectomy if testis is found to be nonviable
- Possible bedside manual detorsion if urologic intervention delayed
- Urgent urologic consultation within 4 to 6 hours of symptom onset to expedite detorsion interventions and prevent complications related to prolonged vascular compromise

Nursing Interventions

- Immediately alert emergency provider of any suspected cases of testicular torsion.
- Assess pain and administer medications as prescribed (see Table A.2).
- Assist medical provider with manual detorsion if attempted.
- Monitor strict urinary output.
- Prepare patient for emergent surgical intervention if indicated.
- Provide emotional support and reassurance while protecting patient's privacy.

Patient Education

- Avoid sexual stimulation until cleared by urology to resume sexual activity.
- Seek emotional support and resources regarding psychosocial impact of physiologic and cosmetic changes and risk for impaired body image.
- Seek immediate care for any recurrence of severe testicular pain, changes such as swelling or hardening of the testis, or signs of infection such as fever/chills, erythema, dysuria, or abdominal pain.

URINARY RETENTION

Overview

- *Urinary retention* is the acute or chronic inability to completely empty the bladder, which may be related to dysfunction of bladder musculature or to obstructive causes, such as prostate enlargement (Figure 6.2) or renal calculi.
- While urinary retention may occur in any patient due to a variety of causes, acute obstructive urinary retention is more likely to occur in male patients between the ages of 60 and 80 years, most often related to an acute exacerbation of prostate enlargement.
- Chronic urinary retention is more likely to be neurologic in nature and is often associated with diabetic neuropathy or spinal injury. However, older patients with benign prostatic hyperplasia (BPH) also commonly experience chronic urinary retention, placing this population at greater risk for the development of urinary infections

[🌐] **NURSING PEARL**

Advanced epididymitis can cause testicular swelling and other changes that resemble testicular torsion. To differentiate between the two conditions, the nurse should consider the onset of the patient's symptoms. *Epididymitis* is an infection that develops gradually, while testicular torsion has a sudden onset.

[📝] **POP QUIZ 6.6**

A teenage patient presents to the ED with a sudden onset of scrotal pain, swelling, and erythema. What condition should the nurse suspect?

[🧠] **COMPLICATIONS**

Urinary retention should be evaluated by assessing post-void residual volumes via bladder ultrasound. A residual volume of 300 mL or greater suggests urinary retention, indicating possible need for catheterization.

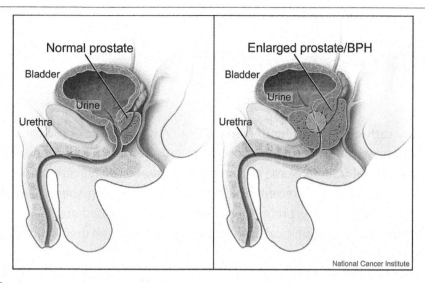

FIGURE 6.2 Normal prostate and benign prostatic hyperplasia.

Source: National Cancer Institute. (n.d.). *Understanding prostate changes: A health guide for men.* https://www.cancer.gov/types/prostate/understanding-prostate-changes

Overview *(continued)*

- Urinary retention increases the likelihood of developing acute renal failure, urinary tract infections (UTIs), and urosepsis.

Signs and Symptoms

- Bladder distention (palpable or detected with ultrasound)
- Dysuria
- Feeling of needing to urinate after completing urination
- Frequent urination in small amounts
- Lower abdominal pain
- Nocturia
- Urgency
- Urinary hesitancy
- Weak or interrupted urinary stream

Diagnosis

Labs

- BMP
- CBC
- Prostate-specific antigen (PSA) (in patients older than 50 years or if enlarged prostate is palpated)
- Urinalysis
- Urine culture with sensitivity testing

Diagnostic Testing

Post-void residual volume obtained by ultrasound alone may be diagnostic; however, the following may be indicated to further investigate retention:

- CT scan (abdomen/pelvis)
- MRI ▶

Diagnostic Testing (continued)

- Voiding cystourethrogram
- Urodynamic testing (cystometry, electromyography)
- Ultrasound

Treatment

- Insertion of a urinary catheter for bladder decompression. Advancement of the catheter may be difficult due to an enlarged prostate or other urologic condition; catheterization may be deferred to urology to minimize urethral/genital trauma. Some circumstances may contraindicate urethral catheterization by the nurse, such as in patients with recent urologic surgery. Ongoing management often involves intermittent catheterization, which is preferred as chronic indwelling catheters increase infection risk. Surgical placement of a suprapubic catheter may be required when urethral catheterization is contraindicated or not possible.
- Treatment of underlying etiology: specialist consultation (e.g., consult to urology for management of obstructive causes, to neurologist for a neurogenic bladder, to oncologist for a malignancy); treatment specific to associated conditions (BPH, UTI, renal failure, malignancy).

[ ] **NURSING PEARL**

Patients with urinary retention related to an enlarged prostate may require placement of a larger coudé catheter with a curved tip to enable the catheter to bypass the prostate and facilitate urinary drainage.

Nursing Interventions

- Administer medications, such as alpha blockers or 5-alpha reductase inhibitors, as prescribed.
- Assess bladder volume using ultrasound and reassess post-void residual volume.
- Assess urine volume and quality, noting any hematuria or foul odor.
- Maintain strict I/O.
- Perform abdominal/GU assessment and discuss voiding pattern with patient.
- Perform urethral catheterization using sterile technique.
- Strain urine if renal calculi suspected.

Patient Education

- If discharged with indwelling catheter: Clean around the insertion site twice daily with soap and water. Ensure catheter is secured to the leg to limit movement and pulling. Keep the drainage bag below waist level and avoid kinking/obstructing tubing. Empty the drainage bag every 3 to 6 hours or when two-thirds full. Use a leg-bag if ambulatory and connect to a standard drainage bag overnight. Seek immediate care for signs of infection, such as fever, pain, or altered mental status. Seek immediate care if catheter dislodges, if urine is leaking around catheter, if urine quality changes (hematuria, gross sediment), or if urine is no longer draining.
- Learn about aseptic intermittent self-catheterization if indicated.
- Seek care if unable to void or if developing signs of infection such as fever, dysuria, altered mental status, increased urinary frequency, flank pain, or suprapubic fullness/discomfort.

URINARY TRACT INFECTIONS

Overview

- UTIs are among the most common infections affecting the GU system, occurring when microorganisms enter the urinary tract. ▶

Overview (continued)

- Infections are classified by location and may be further categorized as complicated versus uncomplicated infections. *Upper UTIs* refer to infection in the kidneys, while *lower UTIs* refer to infection of the bladder and urethra. Uncomplicated UTIs are more likely to occur in female patients and are usually caused by perineal bacteria. Complicated UTIs are more likely to occur in patients with urologic abnormalities and may be related to iatrogenic causes, such as catheterization.
- Urinary infection is responsible for nearly 25% of all cases of sepsis. Nurses must be vigilant for signs of worsening infection, such as the development of systemic symptoms (including altered mental status, fevers, tachycardia, and tachypnea).

[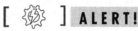] **COMPLICATIONS**

Patients with comorbidities and previous GU conditions, including internal stents or enlarged prostates, are at a higher risk for complicated UTIs. These patients may require multiple antibiotics and hospital admission to treat the infection.

[ ] **ALERT!**

Though it is not considered a classic symptom of UTI, older adult patients with urinary infections often present with altered mental status.

Signs and Symptoms

- Abdominal, suprapubic, and/or flank pain
- Altered mental status
- Cloudy urine
- Dysuria
- Fever, chills
- Foul-smelling urine
- Hematuria
- Nausea, vomiting
- Urinary frequency and urgency
- Urinary retention
- Weakness, lethargy

Diagnosis

Labs

Dependent on presentation; minor symptoms may require little to no laboratory testing, while severe or broad symptoms may require a more thorough workup.

- Blood cultures (if urosepsis is suspected)
- BMP
- CBC
- hCG (urine or serum, if applicable)
- PSA (if applicable)
- Screening for STI (genital cultures, HIV antibody testing, rapid plasma reagin (RPR), hepatitis panel)
- Urinalysis
- Urine culture with sensitivity testing

Diagnostic Testing

Radiographic imaging is often not required for diagnosis of urinary or genital complaints; however, more severe symptoms may require the following:

- CT scan of the abdomen and pelvis
- X-ray: KUB
- Ultrasound: abdominal, transvaginal, or scrotal

Treatment

- Antibiotic therapy indicated (see Table A.1): Most uncomplicated UTIs can be managed in the outpatient setting, treated with a brief course of oral antibiotics. Complicated UTIs are more likely to recur, and treatment becomes more challenging if drug-resistant pathogens have invaded the urinary tract.
- Antipyretics (such as acetaminophen; see Table A.2)
- Fluid resuscitation with isotonic crystalloid, if indicated
- Pain management, such as a limited course of phenazopyridine hydrochloride for topical analgesia of the urinary tract mucosa (see Table 6.1)

Nursing Interventions

- Administer antibiotics as ordered.
- Assess voiding pattern and evaluate for urinary retention.
- Continually reassess readiness for Foley catheter removal and discontinue catheter as soon as appropriate.
- Institute fall precautions for all patients, especially older adults.
- Monitor for signs of worsening infection.
- Monitor I/O.
- Monitor vital signs, especially noting for fever, hypotension, or tachycardia.
- Perform catheterization as indicated for specimen collection using aseptic technique. Depending on institutional guidelines, this may involve replacing a long-term indwelling catheter before specimen collection.
- Provide perineal care and proper catheter care if indicated.

[⚡] **ALERT!**

Catheter-associated UTIs (CAUTIs) are the most common hospital-acquired infections. Reducing unnecessary catheterizations, using proper sterile technique, and removing indwelling catheters as soon as possible all assist in reducing rates of CAUTI.

Patient Education

- Follow proper perineal hygiene practices and infection prevention. Void after intercourse. Female patients should always wipe skin from front to back after voiding. Use only gentle soaps when cleansing; female patients should avoid douching.
- Follow up regarding urine culture results.
- If long-term indwelling catheter is used, follow proper cleansing and catheter care. Wash hands before touching the catheter. Use mild soap and water to cleanse the genital area. Continue cleaning the catheter itself from where it enters the body down to where it connects to the drainage bag. Dry the skin and the catheter itself. Ensure that the catheter is reattached to a securing device to limit catheter movement and prevent shearing.
- Maintain adequate hydration and nutrition.
- Learn about any prescribed medications and complete the full course of antibiotics.
- Learn reasons to return for further evaluation, such as increasing pain, fever, dysuria, hematuria, or difficulty voiding.

[📝] **POP QUIZ 6.7**

An older adult patient with a chronic indwelling urinary catheter presents to the ED with flank pain, fever, and altered mental status. What should the nurse suspect as the most likely cause of the patient's symptoms? What diagnostic tests should the nurse anticipate?

RESOURCES

Alawamlh, O., Goueli, R., & Lee, R. K. (2018). Lower urinary tract symptoms, benign prostatic hyperplasia, and urinary retention. *Medical Clinics of North America*, *102*(2), 301–311. https://doi.org/10.1016/j.mcna.2017.10.005

Aune, D., Mahamat-Saleh, Y., Norat, T., & Riboli, E. (2018). Body fatness, diabetes, physical activity and risk of kidney stones: A systematic review and meta-analysis of cohort studies. *European Journal of Epidemiology*, *33*(11), 1033–1047. https://doi.org/10.1007/s10654-018-0426-4

Bacidore, V. (2020). Abdominal and genitourinary trauma. In V. Sweet & A. Foley (Eds.), *Sheehy's emergency nursing: Principles and practice* (7th ed., pp. 465–476). Elsevier.

Bansal, A., Yadav, P., Kumar, M., Sankhwar, S., Purkait, S., Jhanwar, A., & Singh, S. (2016). Foreign bodies in the urinary bladder and their management: A single-centre experience from North India. *International Neurourology Journal*, *20*(3), 260–269. https://doi.org/10.5213/inj.1632524.262

Baxter, C. (2020). Renal and genitourinary emergencies. In V. Sweet & A. Foley (Eds.), *Sheehy's emergency nursing: Principles and practice* (7th ed., pp. 271–279). Elsevier.

D'Alessandro, C., Ferraro, P. M., Cianchi, C., Barsotti, M., Gambaro, G., & Cupisti, A. (2019). Which diet for calcium stone patients: A real-world approach to preventive care. *Nutrients*, *11*(5), 1182. https://doi.org/10.3390/nu11051182

Erlich, T., & Kitrey, N. D. (2018). Renal trauma: The current best practice. *Therapeutic Advances in Urology*, *10*(10), 295–303. https://doi.org/10.1177/1756287218785828

Fedrigon, D. C., Jain, R., & Sivalingam, S. (2018). Current use of medical expulsive therapy among endourologists. *Canadian Urological Association Journal*, *12*(9), E384–E390. https://doi.org/10.5489/cuaj.4978

Han, H., Segal, A. M., Seifter, J. L., & Dwyer, J. T. (2015). Nutritional management of kidney stones (nephrolithiasis). *Clinical Nutrition Research*, *4*(3), 137–152. https://doi.org/10.7762/cnr.2015.4.3.137

Howe, A. S., Vasudevan, V., Kongnyuy, M., Rychik, K., Thomas, L. A., Matuskova, M., Friedman, S. C., Gitlin, J. S., Reda, E. F., & Palmer, L. S. (2017). Degree of twisting and duration of symptoms are prognostic factors of testis salvage during episodes of testicular torsion. *Translational Andrology and Urology*, *6*(6), 1159–1166. https://doi.org/10.21037/tau.2017.09.10

Hudnall, M., Reed-Maldonado, A. B., & Lue, T. F. (2017). Advances in the understanding of priapism. *Translational Andrology and Urology*, *6*(2), 199–206. https://doi.org/10.21037/tau.2017.01.18

Lachance, C. C., & Grobelna, A. (2019). *Management of patients with long-term indwelling urinary catheters: A review of guidelines*. Canadian Agency for Drugs and Technologies in Health.

Levey, H. R., Segal, R. L., & Bivalacqua, T. J. (2014). Management of priapism: An update for clinicians. *Therapeutic Advances in Urology*, *6*(6), 230–244. https://doi.org/10.1177/1756287214542096

Lin, B. B., Lin, M. E., Huang, R. H., Hong, Y. K., Lin, B. L., & He, X. J. (2020). Dietary and lifestyle factors for primary prevention of nephrolithiasis: A systematic review and meta-analysis. *BMC Nephrology*, *21*(1), Article 267. https://doi.org/10.1186/s12882-020-01925-3

Mellick, L. B., Sinex, J. E., Gibson, R. W., & Mears, K. (2019). A systematic review of testicle survival time after a torsion event. *Pediatric Emergency Care*, *35*(12), 821–825. https://doi.org/10.1097/PEC.0000000000001287

Muneer, A., Alnajjar, H. M., & Ralph, D. (2018). Recent advances in the management of priapism. *F1000Research*, *7* (F1000 Faculty Rev), Article 37. https://doi.org/10.12688/f1000research.12828.1

Pal, D. K., Biswal, D. K., & Ghosh, B. (2016). Outcome and erectile function following treatment of priapism: An institutional experience. *Urology Annals*, *8*(1), 46–50. https://doi.org/10.4103/0974-7796.165717

Podolej, G. S., Babcock, C., & Kim, J. (2017). Emergency department management of priapism [digest]. *Emergency Medicine Practice*, *19*(1 Suppl Points and Pearls), S1–S2. https://www.ebmedicine.net/topics/hepatic-renal-genitourinary/priapism-emergency/pearls

Prescribers' Digital Reference. (n.d.-a). *Emtricitabine/tenofovir disoproxil fumarate* [Drug information]. https://www.pdr.net/drug-summary/Truvada-emtricitabine-tenofovir-disoproxil-fumarate-164.5884

Prescribers' Digital Reference. (n.d.-b). *Phenazopyridine hydrochloride* [Drug information]. https://www.pdr.net/drug-summary/Pyridium-phenazopyridine-hydrochloride-3457

Prescribers' Digital Reference. (n.d.-c). *Phenylephrine hydrochloride* [Drug information]. https://www.pdr.net/drug-summary/Vazculep-pheylephrine-hydrochloride-3539.412

Prescribers' Digital Reference. (n.d.-d). *Raltegravir* [Drug information]. https://www.pdr.net/drug-summary/Isentress-raltegravir-360.3365

Prescribers' Digital Reference. (n.d.-e). *Sofosbuvir/velpatasvir* [Drug information]. https://www.pdr.net/drug-summary/Epclusa-sofosbuvir-velpatasvir-3922

Prescribers' Digital Reference. (n.d.-f). *Tamsulosin hydrochloride* [Drug information]. https://www.pdr.net/drug-summary/Flomax-tamsulosin-hydrochloride-2893.5649

Prieto, J. A., Murphy, C. L., Stewart, F. &, Fader, M. (2021). Intermittent catheter techniques, strategies and designs for managing long-term bladder conditions. Cochrane Database of Systematic Reviews, (10). Article CD006008. https://doi.org/10.1002/14651858.CD006008.pub5

Quallich, S. (2013). Genitourinary emergencies. In B. Hammond & P. Zimmerman (Eds.), *Sheehy's manual of emergency care* (7th ed., pp. 353–360). Elsevier Mosby.

Richards, J. R., & McGahan, J. P. (2017, April). *Focused assessment with sonography in trauma (FAST) in 2017: What radiologists can learn. Radiology, 283*(1), 30–48. https://doi.org/10.1148/radiol.2017160107

Rodríguez, D., Thirumavalavan, N., Pan, S., Apoj, M., Butaney, M., Gross, M. S., & Munarriz, R. (2020). Epidemiology of genitourinary foreign bodies in the United States emergency room setting and its association with mental health disorders. *International Journal of Impotence Research, 32*(4), 426–433. https://doi.org/10.1038/s41443-019-0194-z

Runyon, M. S. (2021, April 5). Blunt genitourinary trauma: Initial evaluation and management. *UpToDate.* https://www.uptodate.com/contents/blunt-genitourinary-trauma-initial-evaluation-and-management

Sandhu, M. S., Gulati, A., Saritha, J., & Nayak, B. (2018). Urolithiasis: Comparison of diagnostic performance of digital tomosynthesis and ultrasound. Which one to choose and when? *European Journal of Radiology, 105*, 25–31. https://doi.org/10.1016/j.ejrad.2018.05.017

Serlin, D. C., Heidelbaugh, J. J., & Stoffel, J. T. (2018). Urinary retention in adults: Evaluation and initial management. *American Family Physician, 98*(8), 496–503. https://www.aafp.org/pubs/afp/issues/2018/1015/p496.html

Song, P. H., & Moon, K. H. (2013). Priapism: current updates in clinical management. *Korean Journal of Urology, 54*(12), 816–823. https://doi.org/10.4111/kju.2013.54.12.816

Tan, E., Ahluwalia, A., Kankam, H., & Menezes, P. (2019). Urinary catheterization 1: indications. *British Journal of Hospital Medicine, 80*(9), C133–C135. https://doi.org/10.12968/hmed.2019.80.9.C133

7 GYNECOLOGIC AND OBSTETRIC EMERGENCIES

ABNORMAL VAGINAL BLEEDING

Overview

- Vaginal bleeding is considered abnormal if bleeding is too frequent, infrequent, excessively heavy (menorrhagia), or light.
- Abnormal vaginal bleeding also includes bleeding occurring at unusual times (between periods, after sex, during menopause) and inconsistent or irregular menstrual cycles (cycle length varying by more than 7–9 days).
- Vaginal hemorrhage is characterized by sustained periods of excessive vaginal bleeding, which may occur secondary to a variety of causes, including gynecologic disorders, trauma, malignancies, and blood disorders. Saturation of more than 8 pads or 12 tampons per day is usually considered excessive bleeding.
- Absence of vaginal bleeding (amenorrhea) may be related to malnutrition, disordered eating, increased physiologic or psychological stress, or excessive weight loss or exercise.
- If an underlying cause cannot be identified, the patient may be diagnosed with dysfunctional uterine bleeding.

Signs and Symptoms

- Abdominal pain
- Abdominal/pelvic cramping
- Change in pattern of vaginal bleeding
- Excessive bleeding/hemorrhage showing signs related to acute blood loss, possibly including the following: dizziness; hypovolemia; pallor; shortness of breath; tachycardia; weakness

Diagnosis

Labs

- Complete blood count (CBC)
- Comprehensive metabolic panel (CMP)
- Coagulation panel
- Pregnancy test (serum or urine)
- Sexually transmitted infection (STI) testing, if indicated
- Thyroid panel
- Type and screen
- Urinalysis

[ ] **COMPLICATIONS**

Excessive vaginal bleeding can lead to hemodynamic instability. Volume resuscitation with fluids and blood products is often indicated. If hemodynamic stability is not achieved, administration of intravenous (IV) or intramuscular (IM) conjugated estrogen may be indicated to help decrease vaginal bleeding. In these situations, urgent gynecologic consultation is advised.

[ ] **NURSING PEARL**

It can be difficult to determine how much blood loss has occurred through vaginal bleeding. When assessing the patient, ask how many sanitary pads/tampons have been used in a specific time frame to indicate rate and amount of bleeding.

[🌀] **ALERT!**

Always obtain a pregnancy test for patients of childbearing age. Dysfunctional bleeding can make it difficult to track menstrual cycles and may confound signs of pregnancy, early miscarriage, or pregnancy complications.

Diagnostic Testing

- Abdominal CT scan
- Endometrial biopsy
- Hysteroscopy
- Pelvic examination, including cervical examination and Pap test
- Ultrasound: transvaginal, abdominal, and/or pelvic

Treatment

- Estrogen administration to regulate bleeding (see Table 7.1)
- Infusion of isotonic crystalloid solution or blood products to achieve hemodynamic stabilization. Depending on the patient's clinical status, initiate massive transfusion protocol per institutional guidelines. ▶

TABLE 7.1 Obstetric Medications

INDICATIONS	MECHANISM OF ACTION	CONTRAINDICATIONS, PRECAUTIONS, AND ADVERSE EFFECTS
Antifibrinolytics (tranexamic acid)		
• Reduce bleeding in patients experiencing vaginal/postpartum hemorrhage	• Act as a hemostatic agent, binding to plasminogen, thereby inhibiting the breakdown of fibrin clots	• Medication carries an increased risk for thrombotic events. • Nausea/vomiting and diarrhea may occur, as well as visual changes such as blurriness. • Vital signs and blood loss must be continually monitored; hypotension may occur with rapid infusion.
Antimetabolites (methotrexate)		
• Halt development of ectopic trophoblast in unruptured ectopic pregnancy	• Antagonize folate to prevent nucleic acid synthesis, thereby preventing cellular division	• Medication is contraindicated in patients who are breastfeeding. • Medication requires follow-up for repeat serum hCG levels and reevaluation to ensure ectopic pregnancy does not rupture; repeat dose may be required. • Patients must be advised to discontinue all folic acid supplements and avoid NSAIDs and alcohol. • Medication can cause GI upset, including nausea, vomiting, and diarrhea.
Corticosteroids (betamethasone)		
• Prophylaxis against neonatal respiratory distress	• Stimulate production and release of surfactant to accelerate fetal lung development	• Medication is most often administered as two IM injections 12–24 hours apart while interventions are under way to slow or halt preterm labor. • Some evidence suggests a higher incidence of fetal cleft lip if used in first trimester of pregnancy.
Electrolytes (calcium gluconate)		
• Hypermagnesemia	• Act as antidote for magnesium sulphate toxicity • Direct antagonist of magnesium at neuromuscular junction	• There is a risk for severe tissue necrosis with extravasation; observe closely for IV patency/signs of extravasation during infusion. • There is a risk for cardiac arrhythmia; maintain cardiac monitoring throughout infusion.

(continued)

TABLE 7.1 Obstetric Medications *(continued)*

INDICATIONS	MECHANISM OF ACTION	CONTRAINDICATIONS, PRECAUTIONS, AND ADVERSE EFFECTS
Electrolytes (magnesium sulfate)		
• Prevention and control of seizures in preeclampsia, tocolytic when used in preterm labor	• CNS depressants that act as anticonvulsants • Lower blood pressure and reduce cerebral vasospasm through vasodilation • Act as smooth muscle relaxant to decrease uterine contractility in preterm labor	• Prior to administration, the nurse must assess baseline maternal vital signs, fetal heart rate, deep tendon reflexes, clonus, bilateral breath sounds, and urinary output. • Patients must be assessed for signs of magnesium toxicity. • Infusion must be discontinued if signs of toxicity occur (visual changes, decreased level of consciousness, paralysis, loss of DTRs, respiratory depression). • Calcium gluconate is indicated for reversal of magnesium toxicity.
Estrogens (conjugated estrogens)		
• Control of prolonged dysfunctional uterine bleeding	• Reduce elevated gonadotropin levels and cause proliferation of the endometrium and increased uterine tone	• Medication increases risk for thrombotic events such as stroke and DVT. • Long-term use increases risk of breast cancer and dementia. • Medication may cause elevated triglycerides and hypertension.
Immune globulins (RhoGAM)		
• Rh isoimmunization prophylaxis in Rh-negative patients	• Appears to prevent interaction between the antigens and the patient's immune system	• Medication is contraindicated in Rh-positive patients and in patients with high risk for hemolysis. • Medication can cause chills or fever. • Medication should be administered in emergency situations when there is not enough time to determine the patient's Rh status.
Oxytocic hormones (oxytocin)		
• Labor augmentation (inevitable or incomplete abortion) • Postpartum bleeding	• Stimulate uterine smooth muscle contraction	• Medication causes more frequent, intense contractions; may cause uterine hypertonicity • Adverse effects include maternal nausea and vomiting, maternal bradycardia and hypotension, and fetal bradycardia (often as a result of hypertonicity). • Medication is contraindicated for eclampsia. • Medication is not indicated for prolonged uterine atony.
Prostaglandins (misoprostol)		
• Uterotonic agent used in termination of pregnancy	• Bind to smooth muscle to promote uterine contractility and cervical ripening to facilitate expulsion of products of conception	• Abortifacient medication; should not be used in patients with desired, viable intrauterine pregnancy • Medication has a risk for uterine rupture if used in third trimester. • Medication may cause fever/chills, abdominal pain, and diarrhea. • Medication may be administered orally or vaginally.

(continued)

		CONTRAINDICATIONS, PRECAUTIONS,
INDICATIONS	MECHANISM OF ACTION	AND ADVERSE EFFECTS

TABLE 7.1 Obstetric Medications *(continued)*

Vitamins (folic acid)

• Dietary supplement recommended during pregnancy • Hyperemesis gravidarum • Neural tube defect prophylaxis	• Essential vitamin required for nucleic acid synthesis to enable DNA replication in the developing fetus	• Daily oral dosage is recommended for those of childbearing age before, during, and after pregnancy. • Deficiency of folic acid may lead to neural tube defects. • It is especially important to supplement in patients with hyperemesis gravidarum as they are likely taking in little to no folic acid nutritionally.

Note: All agents are contraindicated in the presence of hypersensitivity to the medication or one of its components.
CNS, central nervous system; DTRs, deep tendon reflexes; DVT, deep vein thrombosis; GI, gastrointestinal; hCG, human chorionic gonadotropin; IM, intramuscular; IV, intravenous; NSAIDs, nonsteroidal anti-inflammatory drugs.

Treatment *(continued)*

- Identification and treatment of any secondary infections
- Management with birth control/hormone therapy
- Referral to appropriate specialist to treat underlying cause (OB/GYN, oncology, hematology)
- Treatment with surgical procedures including uterine artery embolization, endometrial/uterine ablation, or hysterectomy

Nursing Interventions

- Administer crystalloid IV infusion or blood products as ordered.
- Administer medications as ordered, such as analgesics and oral or IV estrogen.
- Assess and manage pain (see Table A.2).
- Assist provider and patient to prepare for pelvic exam. Encourage patient to void before exam, if possible, and promote comfort during evaluation.
- Ensure patient adheres to fall precautions if weakness, dizziness, or signs of hemodynamic instability are present.
- Monitor hemodynamic status, frequently reassess vital signs, and estimate blood loss. Alert provider to any increased bleeding or change in vital signs. Draw serial CBCs per provider orders to monitor blood counts. Monitor quantity of vaginal bleeding by tracking pad usage and saturation.
- Perform focused abdominal assessment, including gynecologic history.

Patient Education

- Discuss any activity limitation, such as pelvic rest if prescribed.
- Follow up with OB/GYN and report changes in bleeding amount or frequency.
- Seek emergent evaluation if severe bleeding, dizziness/lightheadedness, weakness, shortness of breath, or worsening pain is experienced. ▶

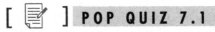 **POP QUIZ 7.1**

A young adult patient reports an abnormal pattern vaginal bleeding, stating that their cycles have been varyir in duration from 20 to 40 days. What are some factors th may be related to irregular vaginal bleeding?

Patient Education *(continued)*

- Track menstrual cycles and monitor patterns and quantity of bleeding, reporting any abnormality to OB/GYN upon follow-up.

ABRUPTIO PLACENTAE

Overview

- Abruptio placentae occurs when the placenta prematurely separates from the uterine wall.
- This is a common cause of painful bleeding in late pregnancy.
- The degree of abruption and presenting symptoms can range from mild to severe.
- There is a significant association with maternal and fetal morbidity and mortality
- Risk factors include abdominal trauma, advanced maternal age, multiparity, preeclampsia, and hypertension.

[🧠] **COMPLICATIONS**

Complications of abruptio placentae for the pregnant patient include coagulopathy, hemorrhagic shock, uterine rupture, or organ failure. Fetal distress and/or demise can also occur.

Signs and Symptoms

- Abdominal and/or back pain
- Fetal distress
- Uterine contractions
- Uterine pain and rigidity (hypertonic uterus)
- Vaginal bleeding: may be absent to severe

Diagnosis

Labs

- CBC
- CMP
- Coagulation panel
- Type and screen

Diagnostic Testing

- Pelvic examination
- Ultrasound

Treatment

- Administration of blood products, as needed
- Administration of RhoGAM (if patient is Rh negative; see Table 7.1)
- Consult with OB emergently
- Continuous fetal heart rate monitoring
- Maternal hemodynamic instability management
- Preparation for immediate Cesarean section, if indicated

Nursing Interventions

- Assess hemodynamic status (e.g., heart rate, blood pressure, urine output, blood loss).
- Assess vital signs frequently.
- Insert two large-bore IV lines and administer crystalloid fluids, preferably lactated Ringer's solution, to maintain urine output above 30 mL/hr (see Table A.3). ▶

Nursing Interventions *(continued)*

- Keep the patient warm and provide supplemental oxygen, as needed.
- Obtain serial CBCs to monitor blood counts.
- Perform fetal monitoring.
- Perform focused maternal assessment.
- Prepare for emergent transfer to labor and delivery.
- Quantify blood loss by counting pad usage. Notify the blood bank so blood products are prepared if needed.

Patient Education

- Discuss activity restrictions as prescribed, such as pelvic rest and bed rest.
- Discuss lifestyle modification to promote healthy gestation. Seek support and resources regarding smoking cessation and substance use counseling, if needed; Recognize the importance of adequate nutrition and hydration.
- Monitor for signs and symptoms of infection, such as fever and chills. Seek urgent evaluation if symptoms of infection occur.
- Notify provider and seek emergent evaluation if worsening pain or bleeding occur.
- Patients with abruption are at a higher risk for abruption in a subsequent pregnancy. Follow up with the OB/GYN provider to discuss modifiable risk factors to decrease the risk of abruption with future pregnancies.

ECTOPIC PREGNANCY

Overview

- An ectopic pregnancy occurs when the fertilized ovum implants anywhere other than the uterus, such as the fallopian tube, ovary, or abdominal cavity.
- Risk factors include a history of salpingitis or pelvic inflammatory disease (PID), a history of surgery in the fallopian tubes, or previous ectopic pregnancy.

Signs and Symptoms

- Abdominal/pelvic pain
- Hypovolemia (if ruptured), which may present with the following: tachycardia, hypotension, compromised perfusion, loss of consciousness
- Kehr's sign (if ruptured)
- Vaginal bleeding

Diagnosis

Labs

- CBC
- CMP
- Coagulation panel
- Human chorionic gonadotropin (hCG; quantitative)
- Type and screen
- Urinalysis

 POP QUIZ 7.2

A patient who is 37 weeks' pregnant presents with a sudden onset of severe abdominal pain and vaginal bleeding. What is the priority intervention for the nurse?

 COMPLICATIONS

Ectopic pregnancies are one of the leading causes of maternal death. If ectopic pregnancy is not diagnosed promptly, the developing sac can rupture and cause substantial hemorrhaging, which may be life-threatening.

 NURSING PEARL

In a typical intrauterine pregnancy, beta-hCG is expected to double every 48 to 72 hours until serum levels reach 10,000 to 20,000 mIU/mL. In an ectopic pregnancy, beta-hCG levels rise at a slower rate, so serum quantitative hCG is lower than expected per estimated gestation.

Diagnostic Testing
- Pelvic examination
- Ultrasound (transabdominal and/or transvaginal)

Treatment
- Limited population of patients with ectopic pregnancy: may be managed expectantly if risk for rupture appears unlikely and hCG levels are closely monitored. Development of the gestational sac expected to cease without intervention. Pregnancy potentially reabsorbed by body.
- hCG levels: lower levels may require a single dose of IM methotrexate; higher levels may indicate need for two doses (see Table 7.1). Patients receiving methotrexate must be willing to comply with post-treatment follow-up and have access to emergency medical services (EMS) within a reasonable time frame in case of a ruptured fallopian tube. Surgery (salpingostomy or salpingectomy) indicated if there is hemodynamic instability or signs of rupture.

Nursing Interventions
- Administer medications, such as methotrexate, as ordered (see Table 7.1).
- Assess and manage pain as indicated; monitor for sudden changes in pain that can indicate rupture (see Table A.2).
- Assess and monitor for signs of hemodynamic stability.
- Consider the initiation of fetal heart rate monitoring, if indicated with patient clinical status.
- Monitor vital signs frequently.
- Perform OB/GYN assessment and patient history, including pregnancy history and last missed period.
- Provide emotional support to the patient and family.

Patient Education
- Ensure appropriate follow-up for any necessary repeat hCG testing or additional doses of methotrexate. It is important to be willing and able to comply with post-treatment follow-up and have access to EMS within a reasonable time frame if taking methotrexate.
- Follow activity restrictions as prescribed, such as pelvic rest and lifting restrictions.
- If receiving methotrexate, learn immunosuppressive effects and relevant contraindications and lifestyle changes. Discontinue any folic acid–containing supplements, such as prenatal vitamins, and limit folic acid–rich foods (such as certain legumes, fruits, and vegetables) as folic acid limits the effectiveness of methotrexate therapy. Avoid intercourse, excessive sun exposure, nonsteroidal anti-inflammatory drugs (NSAIDs), and alcohol while receiving medication and during postmedication monitoring period for methotrexate.
- Monitor for reasons to return for emergent evaluation, such as increased bleeding or abdominal/pelvic pain, or if any signs of infection develop, such as fever and chills.

EMERGENT DELIVERY
Overview
- There are three stages of labor: stage 1—onset of contractions to complete cervical dilation; stage 2—complete dilation to delivery; stage 3—delivery of fetus to delivery of placenta. ▶

 COMPLICATIONS

Umbilical cord prolapse occurs when the umbilical cord exits the cervical os before the fetus. The cord can become compressed, which obstructs fetal circulation. If this occurs, the goal is to restore circulation by relieving pressure on the cord by either repositioning the patient or manipulating the fetus. An emergent Cesarean section may be necessary.

Overview (continued)

- A patient who presents to the ED in labor must be quickly assessed to determine if delivery will occur in the ED or if the patient can be safely transferred to the obstetric unit.

Signs and Symptoms

- Uterine contractions
- Vaginal discharge/bleeding
- Infant crowning (second stage)
- Urge to push (second stage)

Diagnosis

Labs

- CBC
- Coagulation panel
- hCG
- Infection testing, such as group B streptococcus, syphilis, HIV, and hepatitis (if screening was not obtained during prenatal care or if patient is determined to be high risk)
- Type and screen
- Urinalysis

Diagnostic Testing

- Pelvic examination and assessment to confirm delivery is imminent
- Fetal monitoring
- Ultrasound

Treatment

- Physical examination to determine that the patient is not in false labor and that delivery is imminent
- Pharmacologic and nonpharmacologic pain management, as indicated (see Table A.2)
- High-flow supplemental oxygen as needed for fetal or maternal distress
- Emergent delivery in the ED if unable to transfer to an obstetric unit

Nursing Interventions

- Perform rapid obstetric assessment: quickly assess the patient's delivery history, medical history, and gestational age.
- Prepare the patient and the immediate area for emergent delivery (if unable to transfer patient to obstetric unit, notify OB services and pediatric services to respond to the ED).
- Assist with patient positioning.
- Perform frequent maternal-fetal assessment.
- Monitor patient's vital signs.
- Monitor fetal heart rate.
- Assess and monitor duration, frequency, and quality of contractions. ▶

[ ] **ALERT!**

Fetal heart tones that remain outside normal limits (120–160 bpm) for any prolonged period of time indicate fetal distress. Place the patient on the left side, administer oxygen, and prepare the patient for delivery.

[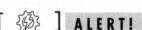] **ALERT!**

In the event the nurse must deliver the fetus without provider present, the nurse must support and monitor both the patient and the fetus. The nurse provides support for the fetus's head while the shoulders are delivered. Once the shoulders have passed, the body will be expelled quickly. Using a bulb syringe, the nurse must first suction the newborn's mouth and then the nose to clear the airway and stimulate breathing. Additional stimulation will be provided by drying the newborn with a towel, helping to promote spontaneous breathing. Finally, the nurse will clamp the umbilical cord in two places at least 6 inches from the umbilicus and cut when it has stopped pulsating. If sterile equipment is not available to cut the cord, this should be delayed.

Nursing Interventions *(continued)*

- Assess and manage pain control and comfort measures.
- Administer infection prophylaxis if indicated.
- Provide support.
- If time allows, provide perineal care, such as a warm compress and perineal massage with a lubricant to soften and stretch the perineum to reduce perineal trauma during birth.
- Include the support of family presence.

Patient Education

- Arrange appropriate follow-up with OB/GYN for routine obstetric care post discharge.
- Follow orders for pelvic rest, often prescribed for 4 to 6 weeks to allow for healing and limit risk for postpartum infection.
- Learn about expected bleeding versus signs of postpartum hemorrhage and return for evaluation of increased vaginal bleeding or worsening abdominal/pelvic pain.
- Recognize signs of postpartum infection, such as fever, chills, and foul-smelling vaginal discharge, and return for evaluation of any suspected infection.
- Recognize any symptoms of postpartum depression and anxiety. Learn about mental health resources to use upon discharge if such symptoms occur, consulting case management or social work if needed. Call 911 or seek emergent evaluation if significant mood disturbances or thoughts of harm to self or newborn occur.
- Discuss plans for infant feeding, providing support and education regarding lactation, and/or provide guidance and resources regarding formula feeding. Discuss infant nutritional needs (hunger cues, expected intake, expected output) and ensure follow-up with pediatrician has been arranged to continue to monitor infant growth and development. Discuss potential contraindications for breastfeeding such as certain medications. Ensure that any prescribed or over-the-counter medications are safe for breastfeeding. Learn about potential breastfeeding complications such as latching issues, issues with milk supply, engorgement, or clogged ducts, and return for evaluation if signs and symptoms of mastitis occur. Recognize expected breast changes and follow up with lactation consultant if needed.
- Learn about infant care and be prepared to meet all infant needs such as feeding, warmth, rest, and comfort. Consider family/social support system to assist in caring for infant, as well as any available resources for childcare. Request consultation to case management or social work where appropriate. Discuss home environment and infant safety, including education regarding safe sleep practices. Monitor for signs of infant distress. Bring infant to ED for emergent evaluation of any signs of distress, such as increased work of breathing, poor urine output, abnormal skin color, fevers, lethargy, or inconsolability.

HYPEREMESIS GRAVIDARUM

Overview

- *Hyperemesis gravidarum* is the most severe form of pregnancy-related nausea and vomiting, characterized by severe, intractable vomiting, which often necessitates hospitalization due to electrolyte disturbance. ▶

[ ] **COMPLICATIONS**

Hyperemesis gravidarum can cause electrolyte imbalances and weight loss, both of which can hinder fetal growth and development. Additionally, patients with this condition are at greater risk for preterm labor.

Overview *(continued)*

■ Hyperemesis gravidarum can cause severe adverse physical and psychological effects.

Signs and Symptoms

■ Anorexia
■ Hypovolemia, which may present as decreased urine output; dehydration, which may involve dry mucous membranes, extreme thirst, fatigue, confusion; dizziness; generalized weakness; increased urine concentration
■ Nausea
■ Orthostatic hypotension
■ Severe, persistent vomiting
■ Weight loss exceeding 5% of prepregnancy body weight

Diagnosis

Labs

■ CBC
■ CMP
■ Urinalysis

Diagnostic Testing

■ EKG
■ Ultrasound to assess fetal status

Treatment

■ Antiemetic administration, using caution to minimize side effects in respect to fetal development
■ Crystalloid fluid administration
■ Diet: slowly advanced to minimize risk for fluid and electrolyte shifts related to refeeding syndrome
■ Electrolyte replacement as indicated based on laboratory values
■ Laboratory tests to assess for hypophosphatemia, hypokalemia, and other electrolyte abnormalities
■ May require admission to antepartum unit for fetal monitoring, depending on available resources and severity of maternal condition
■ Vitamin and mineral (such as folic acid) replacement (see Table 7.1)

Nursing Interventions

■ Administer IV fluids for hydration.
■ Administer medications to manage nausea/vomiting.
■ Initiate continuous fetal monitoring, if available.
■ Perform frequent maternal assessment.
■ Monitor laboratory work and vital signs for complications related to fluid and electrolyte shifts.
■ Monitor intake/output (I/O) and notify provider if patient is not maintaining a minimum urine output greater than 30 mL/hr.
■ Provide emotional support and reassurance.
■ Reintroduce diet as tolerated.

Patient Education

- Discuss strategies for increasing oral intake and minimizing vomiting. Discuss symptom history to identify foods, smells, and activities that may trigger symptoms. Drink small amounts of fluids frequently throughout the day. Eat as soon as feeling hungry, or even before. Eat foods high in protein and carbohydrates and avoid spicy, greasy, or acidic foods. Eat frequent small meals, and snack often. Remain upright for 1 hour after eating. Use alternatives for drinking liquids, such as popsicles and gelatin dessert.
- Learn about any prescribed antiemetic medications.
- Return for evaluation if unable to tolerate any oral intake despite taking as-needed medications as prescribed, or if worsening symptoms develop, such as weakness and dizziness or abdominal pain.
- Take prenatal vitamins and folic acid as prescribed to maintain adequate nutrition and reduce symptoms.

NEONATAL RESUSCITATION

Overview

- Resuscitation is required when the usual means of stimulating the neonate post delivery fails. Drying the infant generally provides adequate stimulation to encourage spontaneous respiration in the neonate.
- It is indicated for neonates who are bradycardic, apneic, or hypoxic, and/or unresponsive or minimally responsive.
- Assess neonates at delivery and 5 minutes post delivery using the Apgar scale (Table 7.2).
- An Apgar score of 4 to 6 indicates a moderately depressed neonate, and a score of 3 or less indicates a severely depressed neonate.

Signs and Symptoms

- Bradycardia (less than 100 bpm)
- Cyanosis
- Depressed or absent ventilatory rate
- Flaccid
- No spontaneous movement

[ ]   **COMPLICATIONS**

It is not unusual for infants to need some suctioning and stimulation after delivery, but the need for prolonged resuscitation efforts can indicate congenital or delivery-related complications.

[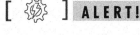]   **ALERT!**

Point-of-care blood glucose testing may be used to obtain rapid blood glucose values before CMP results are available.

[⊕]   **NURSING PEARL**

Additional laboratory testing is often performed 24 hours post delivery to screen the newborn for a variety of rare, potentially deadly congenital conditions. This may include testing for phenylketonuria, homocystinuria, maple syrup urine disease, galactosemia, congenital adrenal hyperplasia, sickle cell disease, and medium chain acyl-CoA dehydrogenase deficiency.

TABLE 7.2 Apgar Score

	0	1	2
Appearance (color)	Blue, pale	Pink body, blue extremities	Pink
Pulse (heart rate)	Absent	Less than 100 bpm	Greater than 100 bpm
Grimace (muscle tone)	Limp	Some flexion	Good flexion
Activity (reflex irritability)	Absent	Some motion	Good motion
Respiratory effort	Absent	Weak cry	Strong cry

Diagnosis

Labs

- CBC
- CMP

Diagnostic Testing

- Chest x-ray

Treatment

- Initial stabilization by clearing airway if necessary
- Neonate warming, drying, and stimulating (drying the infant, suctioning secretions, and using warming lights during resuscitation efforts)
- Ventilation assistance and oxygen if apneic, gasping, or bradycardic
- Continuous positive airway pressure (CPAP) or intubation (if indicated)
- Chest compressions (if heart rate falls below 60 bpm)
- Administration of IV epinephrine if the heart rate remains below 60 bpm despite adequate ventilation and chest compressions (see Table 2.1)

Nursing Interventions

- Administer medications as ordered or per neonatal resuscitation algorithm.
- Assess cardiac and respiratory status.
- Closely monitor the newborn's temperature to prevent hypothermia.
- Perform continuous pulse oximetry and EKG monitoring.
- Perform resuscitation interventions as indicated.
- Provide support to the patient.

Patient Education

- Identify signs of infant distress such as increased work of breathing, abnormal skin color, abnormal temperature (fever or hypothermia), lethargy, or inconsolability, and seek emergent evaluation if signs of distress are noted.
- Remember that the infant cannot maintain their body temperature independently and should always be kept warm.
- Use safe sleep practices. Nothing should be kept in the crib with a sleeping infant. Infant should be dressed and kept in a warm environment rather than under coverings like blankets.
- Learn how to use bulb syringe to clear secretions from the infant's mouth and nose as needed to keep airways patent.

 NURSING PEARL

It is vital that each step of neonatal resuscitation be performed sequentially, as subsequent resuscitative efforts are dependent on the success of previous steps. For example, the mouth must be suctioned before the nose because infants are obligate nose-breathers; if the nares are suctioned first, this may trigger a gasp that may cause the infant to aspirate secretions that have yet to be cleared.

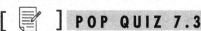 **POP QUIZ 7.3**

After delivery, a newborn is warmed and stimulated to cry. The nurse assesses the newborn's heart rate and finds it is 90 bpm. What should the nurse do next?

 COMPLICATIONS

A ruptured corpus luteal cyst causes bleeding that is usually self-limiting but can at times progress to hemorrhaging and hypovolemic shock. Intraperitoneal irritation can also occur in these patients.

OVARIAN CYST

Overview

- *Ovarian cysts*, fluid-filled sacs originating in an ovary, occur in approximately 20% of patients and may or may not cause related symptoms; they often resolve without intervention. ▶

Overview *(continued)*

- Cysts can be differentiated based on what point during the menstrual cycle they develop and/or the composition of the cyst. Follicular cysts (most common) develop during the first 2 weeks of the menstrual cycle. Blood-filled corpus luteal cysts develop during the luteal phase of the menstrual cycle. Hemorrhagic cysts occur when a blood vessel in the cyst wall ruptures. A dermoid cyst is a germ cell neoplasm containing tissue including fat, skin, hair, and teeth.
- As cysts grow, the likelihood of developing severe complications, such as ovarian torsion, increases. Torsion occurs when the supporting ligaments of the ovary become twisted, impairing blood flow, and leading to necrosis. Patients often experience unilateral lower abdominal or pelvic pain, which may be constant or intermittent. Patients are likely to experience more severe pain, fevers, and nausea/vomiting as the organ becomes necrotic. Emergent detorsion is required, often performed via laparoscopic surgery. If blood flow can be successfully restored, the ovary can be salvaged; however, the ovary may need to be surgically removed if the organ has become necrotic.

Signs and Symptoms

- Abdominal/pelvic pain
- Hemodynamic instability (if ruptured)
- Peritoneal irritation (if ruptured)
- Vaginal bleeding

Diagnosis

Labs

- CBC
- Pregnancy test (serum or urine)
- Type and screen (if bleeding suspected)
- Urinalysis (if dysuria present)

Diagnostic Testing

- CT scan: abdomen and pelvis
- Pelvic examination, if indicated
- Ultrasound: transvaginal or abdominal

Treatment

- Many uncomplicated ovarian cysts resolve without intervention, although patients may seek treatment for pelvic pain. Patients may require pain management via pharmacologic (NSAIDs) and nonpharmacologic (heat application) means (see Table A.2). Patients with recurrent cysts should be advised to follow up with OB/GYN for further testing and treatment. Patients may benefit from outpatient follow-up for ongoing therapy with oral contraceptives to help prevent cyst recurrence.
- Cyst rupture is considered complicated if blood loss is significant enough to cause hemodynamic instability, or if fever and leukocytosis occur, and when malignancy is suspected. Complicated cases often require inpatient admission for management and control of ongoing hemorrhage, treatment of secondary infection, and/or surgical consultation to remove a cyst or a whole ovary.

Nursing Interventions

- Administer IV fluids as ordered; blood product administration may be indicated for heavy blood loss.
- Administer antibiotics if infection suspected. ▶

Nursing Interventions *(continued)*

- Alert provider to any increase in blood loss or signs of hemodynamic instability, such as tachycardia and/or hypotension.
- Assess and manage pain.
- Communicate with provider about any suspected presentation of ovarian torsion as evidenced by unilateral lower abdominal or pelvic pain (increased risk if patient has known adnexal mass).
- Perform focused abdominal assessment with gynecologic history.

Patient Education

- Establish regular care with OB/GYN.
- Learn about any pain medications, such as narcotic and non-narcotic analgesics. Discuss nonpharmacologic pain control methods, such as heat application.
- Learn about symptoms of cyst rupture, which is often described as sudden-onset sharp pain potentially followed by vaginal bleeding. Seek urgent evaluation if pain or bleeding continues to worsen.
- Monitor symptoms and seek treatment for any signs of infection, such as fever or chills.

 POP QUIZ 7.4

The nurse triages a young adult patient with a known histo of ovarian cysts presenting with right-sided abdomir pain and heavy vaginal bleeding. The patient's vitals a temperature 98.4°F (36.9°C), pulse 130 bpm, respirations breaths/min, and blood pressure 90/60 mmHg. The seru pregnancy test is negative. What is the priority interventi for this patient?

PELVIC INFLAMMATORY DISEASE

Overview

- *PID* is an inflammatory disorder of the female upper reproductive organs.
- PID most commonly develops from the spread of STIs (*Neisseria gonorrhoeae* and *Chlamydia trachomatis*) from the lower genital tract. It can also develop from microorganisms introduced to the upper reproductive tract via uterine procedures.
- Risk factors for PID include STIs, high-risk sexual behavior or unsafe sexual practices, intrauterine device (IUD) use, and poor genital hygiene practices, such as frequent vaginal douching.

COMPLICATIONS

Patients with PID are at increased risk for infertility a are more likely to develop complications such as ectop pregnancy due to chronic inflammation and scarring of t fallopian tubes. If PID goes untreated, there is a high risk permanent damage to the reproductive structures.

Signs and Symptoms

- Many cases of PID are not diagnosed in the acute phase of infection because symptoms can be mild or vague.
- Patient presentation may include the following: abdominal/pelvic pain; abnormal vaginal bleeding or discharge; dyspareunia; dysuria.

Diagnosis
Labs

There are no lab tests specific to diagnosing PID. The determination is based on the assessment of symptoms, physical exam, and review of the patient's history. However, the following tests may be helpful in assessing for associated causes or conditions:

- CBC
- hCG (urine or serum)

Labs (continued)

▪ STI screening: Note that cervical swabs for *Neisseria gonorrhoeae* and *Chlamydia trachomatis* may not be reliable in detecting infection of the upper reproductive tract.

▪ Urinalysis

Diagnostic Testing

There are no diagnostic tests specific to PID. However, the following imaging studies may be used to assist in determination of a PID diagnosis:

▪ Abdominal CT scan

▪ Abdominal MRI

▪ Laparoscopy

▪ Pelvic examination

▪ Ultrasound: transvaginal or abdominal

Treatment

▪ Patients with chronic pelvic pain and dyspareunia: possible consult to pelvic physical therapy.

▪ Possible combination of pharmacologic (narcotic or non-narcotic medications such as NSAIDs) and nonpharmacologic therapies (such as heat application).

▪ Recommended combination of antibiotic therapies, beginning with IM or IV antibiotic treatment before transitioning to oral therapy (see Table A.2). Mild to moderate PID may trial a single dose of IM ceftriaxone or cefoxitin with a course of oral doxycycline and metronidazole for 14 days; if no clinical improvement is demonstrated within 72 hours, IV treatment may be considered. Moderate to severe infection should be treated with IV therapy for 24 to 48 hours while assessing for clinical improvement that demonstrates readiness to transition to oral antibiotics for 14 days; protocol includes administration of ceftriaxone, cefotetan, or cefoxitin in combination with doxycycline or metronidazole. Patients with moderate to severe infection and abscess formation will require hospital admission to administer repeat antibiotic doses and monitor for improvement.

▪ Recommended pelvic rest until antibiotic treatment complete.

[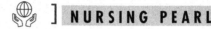] **NURSING PEARL**

While procedures like transvaginal ultrasound and pelvic CT are easily accessed in the emergency setting and can be helpful in identifying signs of PID, such as fluid-filled fallopian tubes or tubo-ovarian abscess, laparoscopy is the standard of care for diagnosis of PID. Although this is an invasive procedure requiring general anesthesia, it is considered the best way to identify structural changes associated with PID, such as fallopian tube adhesions. MRI is the next preferred diagnostic tool for PID, lthough there may also be limitations in accessing MRI on an emergent basis.

Nursing Interventions

▪ Administer medications as ordered, such as antibiotics and analgesics.

▪ Assist provider in performing pelvic examination and providing emotional support to patient during procedure.

▪ Monitor for signs of worsening infection, such as fever, chills, and increased abdominal/pelvic pain, and report any change in condition to provider.

▪ Perform focused abdominal assessment and obtain gynecologic history, including history of any gynecologic medical procedures, sexual health practices, and any previous screening for STIs, if applicable.

[ ] **ALERT!**

Patients with PID are likely to experience more severe pain or discomfort during pelvic examination.

Patient Education

▪ Complete the full course of antibiotics as prescribed.

▪ Follow provider recommendation for pelvic rest until antibiotic therapy is complete. ▶

[ ] **POP QUIZ 7.5**

What information should a nurse reinforce when giving discharge instructions to a patient diagnosed with PID?

Patient Education *(continued)*

- Follow up with OB/GYN for routine gynecologic exams and ongoing treatment of any chronic complaints, including chronic pelvic pain and fertility concerns.
- Inform all recent sexual partners of any STI diagnosis and advise them to avoid any further sexual encounters until STI screening is completed. Practice STI prevention and safe sexual practices to decrease risk of contracting STIs.
- Learn about any pain medications, such as narcotic and non-narcotic analgesics. Discuss nonpharmacologic pain control methods, such as heat application.

PLACENTA PREVIA

Overview

- Placenta previa describes the placenta's proximity to the cervical os: close to (marginal previa); partially (partial previa); completely (complete previa).

Signs and Symptoms

- Vaginal bleeding (usually bright red and painless)
- Uterine contractions

Diagnosis

Labs

- CBC
- CMP
- Coagulation panel
- Type and screen

Diagnostic Testing

- Ultrasound

[ ] **COMPLICATIONS**

Patients with placenta previa are at high risk for hemorrhage, although bleeding is not always present. The bleeding may be obvious or completely internal. Pelvic exams are contraindicated because manipulation of the area could cause uncontrolled bleeding. Risk factors include previous uterine surgeries, advanced maternal age, and cigarette smoking or cocaine use.

Treatment

- Fetal heart rate monitoring
- Immediate Cesarean delivery, if indicated for active labor, sustained fetal heart decelerations unresponsive to resuscitative measures, or severe and persistent vaginal bleeding
- IV fluids to maintain hemodynamic stability and adequate urine output
- Management dependent on clinical status; may be asymptomatic or have active hemorrhage
- Transfusion of blood products in patients with active bleeding

Nursing Interventions

- Administer IV fluids and/or blood products as indicated based on patient's clinical status.
- Assess and monitor bleeding.
- Assess and monitor maternal vital signs and hemodynamic status.
- Monitor input and output.
- Prepare for delivery, if necessary.

Patient Education

- Follow physician recommendation for pelvic rest, recognizing that any sexual activity may cause bleeding. ▶

Patient Education *(continued)*

- Learn risk factors for developing placenta previa, including repeat Cesarean sections, previous history of the condition, smoking tobacco, and history of multiple pregnancies or being pregnant with more than one fetus at a time.
- Monitor abdominal pain/cramping and seek emergent evaluation for any sustained contractions, worsening pain, or bleeding.

POSTPARTUM HEMORRHAGE

Overview

- *Postpartum hemorrhage* is defined as bleeding of more than 500 mL immediately after delivery or up to 6 weeks postpartum.
- This is a common complication caused by uterine atony, retained products of conception, or vaginal/cervical tears.

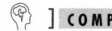 **COMPLICATIONS**

Uterine atony can interfere with *involution*, the process during which the uterus returns to its prepregnant state. Continued atony can cause a life-threatening hemorrhage.

Signs and Symptoms

- Abdominal pain and cramping
- Boggy or relaxed uterus
- Heavy vaginal bleeding (clots may be present)
- Signs of hemodynamic instability

Diagnosis

Labs

- CBC
- Coagulation panel
- Type and screen

Diagnostic Testing

- Focused abdominal/pelvic examination
- Ultrasound

Treatment

- Administration of blood products if indicated for anemia and uncontrolled bleeding
- Dilation and curettage and/or laceration repair, if indicated
- Estrogen or tranexamic acid administration, as indicated (see Table 7.1)
- Fundal massage to improve uterine tone
- Management of hemodynamic instability, including crystalloid fluid resuscitation and administration of vasopressors
- Oxytocin administration to promote hemostasis (see Table 7.1)
- Pain management

Nursing Interventions

- Administer medications as ordered.
- Assess hemodynamic status and monitor for symptoms of shock.   ▶

Nursing Interventions *(continued)*

- Assist the provider during the placement of an arterial or central line if indicated for hemodynamic monitoring and administration of vasopressors.
- Draw serial CBCs to monitor blood counts.
- Initiate two large-bore IV lines for crystalloid fluid or blood product administration.
- Monitor I/O.
- Monitor uncontrolled hemorrhage with continued reassessment of bleeding amount and quality (track pad usage).
- Monitor vital signs frequently.
- Perform fundal massage to encourage the uterus to contract and to prevent further hemorrhage; this can be performed more frequently depending on the rate of bleeding.
- Reassess vital signs frequently.

Patient Education

- Adhere to any activity limitations, such as pelvic rest and lifting restrictions.
- Monitor for any signs of infection, such as fever, malodorous bleeding or discharge, or worsening pain, and to return for evaluation if these symptoms occur.
- Recognize that although bleeding may continue, blood loss should decrease over time.
- Track bleeding through monitoring the number of saturated pads per day and seek care urgently for any sustained increased bleeding or passage of large clots, or any symptoms of worsening blood loss, such as dizziness, weakness, or shortness of breath.

POSTPARTUM INFECTION

Overview

- Infection in the postpartum period is responsible for a significant portion of maternal mortality worldwide, including infections associated with vaginal or Cesarean delivery and infections related to breastfeeding.
- Risk for infection in the postpartum period can be associated with a variety of factors: Trauma to the abdominal wall, reproductive organs, and genitourinary structures during the birthing process places the patient at increased risk for infection. Infection is more common in patients who have undergone Cesarean delivery, as well as in patients with certain conditions such as premature rupture of membranes, chorioamnionitis, or maternal colonization with group A or B streptococcus. Retained products of conception, such as placental tissue, can become necrotic, causing an infection that may progress to sepsis if retained products are not removed.
- While there are many postpartum infections, common infections that may be encountered in the ED are as follows: endometritis, mastitis, perineal infection, septic pelvic thrombophlebitis, surgical site infection, urinary tract infection.

[🧠] **COMPLICATIONS**

Necrotizing fasciitis is a very rare but extremely serious potential complication that may occur in the postpartum period. This infection can commonly develop within the abdomen, pelvis, or perineum, causing rapid subcutaneous necrosis, which is often fatal. Necrotizing fasciitis may have a similar appearance to cellulitis or wound infection upon initial presentation; however, it should be suspected if the patient is experiencing severe pain disproportionate to localized inflammation with any signs of systemic illness.

Signs and Symptoms

- Potential for any untreated infection to progress to systemic illness, which is more likely to occur during postpartum period; signs of systemic illness accompanying any condition may include the following: diarrhea, dizziness, fatigue, fever, hypotension, nausea and/or vomiting, tachycardia
- Endometritis: fever, foul-smelling lochia, uterine tenderness, vaginal bleeding
- Mastitis: fever; purulent discharge (may or may not be present); unilateral breast edema, erythema, and tenderness
- Perineal infection: fever; perineal edema, erythema, and pain; wound drainage
- Septic pelvic thrombophlebitis: fever unresolved after 3 to 5 days of broad-spectrum antibiotic treatment of endometritis; leukocytosis; persistent pelvic pain
- Surgical site infection: fever, peri-incisional erythema, incisional pain, wound drainage
- Urinary tract infection (UTI): dysuria, hematuria, increased frequency/urgency to void and/or foul-smelling urine; pelvic/suprapubic or low back pain

Diagnosis

Labs

While each of these conditions is distinct, laboratory evaluation for a suspected postpartum infection is likely to include the following:

- Blood cultures
- CBC
- CMP
- Coagulation panel
- Lactic acid
- Urinalysis and urine culture
- Vaginal and/or wound cultures

Diagnostic Testing

Depending on the suspected source of infection, the following diagnostics may be indicated:

- CT scan: chest, abdomen, and pelvis
- Pelvic examination
- Ultrasound: abdominal, renal, pelvic, and breast

[ ]   **NURSING PEARL**

Leukocytosis may be an unreliable indicator of potential infection in the immediate postpartum period as patients are expected to experience marked leukocytosis (20,000–30,000/µL) for the first 24 hours after delivery, and white blood cell counts remain elevated for up to 1 week.

Treatment

- Treatment specific to infection source; antibiotic used dependent on organism(s) most likely causing infection (see Table A.1)
- Endometritis: A combination of clindamycin and gentamicin is indicated with addition of ampicillin or vancomycin if indicated per results of endometrial culture; IV antibiotics will continue until fever is reduced and leukocytosis resolves before transitioning to oral antibiotics. If evidence of retained products of conception is found, dilation and curettage is needed to remove retained tissue. If no improvement is evident within 3 to 5 days of treatment, diagnosis of septic pelvic thrombophlebitis should be considered.
- Mastitis: Antibiotic therapy with a penicillin or cephalosporin is indicated. Continued feeding with unaffected breast, and pumping then discarding milk from affected breast, is recommended to prevent milk stasis/engorgement. Self-massage of inflamed areas may improve milk flow and prevent stasis. ▶

Treatment *(continued)*

Warm compresses improve circulation to the area and may assist in relieving discomfort. If an abscess develops, incision and drainage is required.

- Perineal infection: Most often, this can be treated with oral antibiotics and proper wound care/cleansing. Wound irrigation may be needed, particularly after toileting. If abscess formation occurs, incision and drainage may be required to promote healing.

- Septic pelvic thrombophlebitis: Triple antibiotic treatment is recommended with ampicillin, gentamicin, and clindamycin. Continue IV treatment until improvement is evidenced by decreased fever and improved leukocyte count. The decision may then be made to transition to oral antibiotics. Anticoagulation is also recommended in most cases, often using enoxaparin subcutaneous injection for 2 weeks.

- Surgical site infection: Dependent on severity of infection, a single antibiotic therapy may be indicated, such as vancomycin, or triple antibiotic coverage may be required (often a combination of clindamycin, gentamicin, and ampicillin). Specific care may be required depending on surgical wound complications; the site may need to be irrigated, drained, or debrided, and interventions such as a wound vacuum may be required.

- UTI: Dependent on severity of infection and location (upper vs. lower urinary tract), oral or IV antibiotic therapy may be indicated. IV fluids may be required to maintain adequate hydration. Refer to the UTI section in Chapter 6 for additional information.

Nursing Interventions

- Administer antibiotics and pain medications as ordered.
- Assess the breasts and note any inflammation, swelling, warmth, and redness.
- Conduct psychosocial assessment and provide emotional support.
- Monitor I/O.
- Monitor vital signs frequently. Alert provider to any signs or symptoms of sepsis, noting changes in vital sign trends such as increasing temperature and heart rate or decreasing blood pressure. Continuous cardiac monitoring and pulse oximetry should be conducted for all patients with severe infection, significant bleeding, or hemodynamic instability, and for patients at risk for thrombosis.
- Perform focused OB assessment, monitoring quantity and quality of bleeding, noting uterine tone and providing fundal massage to promote uterine contractility and expulsion of any retained products.
- Perform perineal care and assess the skin for any erythema, open wounds, or foul-smelling drainage.
- Promote activity/ambulation as tolerated. Maintain bedrest if indicated (as in cases of hemodynamic instability).

Patient Education

- Complete the entire course of any prescribed antibiotics.
- Follow recommendations for pelvic rest to prevent infection.
- Follow wound care instructions for perineal trauma or episiotomy repair.
- If using sitz baths, thoroughly clean equipment between each use to prevent infection.
- Maintain adequate hydration and nutrition to optimize healing.
- Patients with surgical wounds should understand wound care and follow up to ensure incisional healing. Seek immediate evaluation of wound redness, drainage, dehiscence, or severe pain. ▶

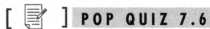 **POP QUIZ 7.6**

What education should the nurse provide to a patient diagnosed with mastitis?

Patient Education *(continued)*

- Patients with mastitis should continue feeding with unaffected breast. Pump and discard milk from affected breast. Use self-massage techniques and warm compresses.
- Recognize signs of infection, such as worsening pain, fever, inflammation or erythema, foul-smelling urine, or lochia, and return for evaluation of any worsening condition.
- Understand anticoagulation administration and associated bleeding precautions if prescribed anticoagulant therapy.

PREECLAMPSIA, ECLAMPSIA, HELLP SYNDROME

Overview

- *Preeclampsia* is a hypertensive disorder of pregnancy that can occur from 20 weeks' gestation up to 6 weeks postpartum. This condition is diagnosed when a patient with gestational hypertension develops signs of organ injury, such as damage to the liver or kidneys as evidenced by proteinuria or elevated liver enzymes. New-onset gestational hypertension is diagnosed when systolic pressure remains over 140 mmHg and diastolic pressure remains over 90 mmHg with two blood pressure readings 4 to 6 hours apart. *Preeclampsia* is a serious condition that can result in poor maternal outcomes, such as the progression to eclampsia (development of seizures), stroke, renal injury, hepatic injury, and heart failure, as well as severe fetal complications, such as intrauterine growth restriction, placental abruption, and fetal demise.

 COMPLICATIONS

Treatment for hypertensive disorders of pregnancy is essential. Eclampsia is an immediate, life-threatening condition for the pregnant patient and fetus. HELLP syndrome also causes life-threatening complications such as coagulopathies, hepatic and splenic hemorrhage, intracranial bleeding, and organ failure. Delivery is often the definitive treatment for these conditions if the patient is over 34 weeks' gestation or if the patient's condition continues to deteriorate The patient must be stabilized (airway management; fluid resuscitation likely including blood products) and prepared for an emergent Cesarean section. On rare occasions, these complications can develop or continue post delivery.

- HELLP syndrome, considered to be a possible variant of preeclampsia, is characterized by organ damage and is associated with significant mortality. HELLP is an acronym for the diagnostic criteria of the syndrome: **H**emolysis, **E**levated **L**iver enzymes, and **L**ow **P**latelets. HELLP may quickly progress to cause irreversible organ damage and maternal and/or fetal death, with potential complications including disseminated intravascular coagulation, cerebral hemorrhage, and hepatic or splenic rupture. HELLP can mimic other serious conditions, including hemolytic-uremic syndrome, thrombotic thrombocytopenia purpura, and chronic renal failure. HELLP syndrome usually affects multiparous patients in the third trimester of pregnancy.

Signs and Symptoms

- Hypertension
- HELLP and preeclampsia/eclampsia: distinct conditions; symptoms secondary to organ damage are shared consequence of both diagnoses. Characteristic symptoms of hepatic, renal, and neurologic damage: decreased urine output, edema, epigastric pain, headache, proteinuria, visual disturbance, uncontrolled bleeding, seizures.

Diagnosis

Labs

While laboratory abnormalities are used to diagnose preeclampsia and HELLP syndrome, eclampsia is based on clinical diagnosis. The following may be indicated during the initial workup:

- CBC
- CMP
- Magnesium level
- Type and screen
- Urinalysis
- 24-hour urine collection (to check for proteinuria)

Diagnostic Testing

Diagnostic imaging may be used to investigate organ damage with the following:

- EEG
- Ultrasound
- X-ray or CT scan (more likely to be used if condition occurs in postpartum period)

Treatment

- Definitive treatment: may include induced delivery or emergent Cesarean section
- Administration of blood products if patient has low platelets and/or active bleeding
- Antihypertensive medications such as IV labetalol to assist in controlling hypertension and minimizing organ damage
- Anticonvulsant medication of choice in preeclampsia and HELLP syndrome: magnesium sulfate infusion to relax smooth muscle and prevent seizures (see Table 7.1). Close monitoring required to ensure therapy adequate to prevent seizures but avoid magnesium toxicity. Possible discontinuation of magnesium and calcium gluconate administration to reverse effects of magnesium (see Table 7.1).
- Continuous fetal heart monitoring, if possible, with transfer to labor and delivery/antenatal unit expedited if fetal monitoring not available in emergency setting
- Possible required fluid restriction or limited use of IV fluids to maintain hydration to prevent further complications, such as pulmonary edema

Nursing Interventions

- Adhere to seizure precautions by decreasing environmental stimuli, having suction available, and proactively padding bed rails.
- Conduct continuous monitoring specific to administration of magnesium sulfate, including assessment of deep tendon reflexes, level of consciousness, maternal and fetal heart rate, and observation and auscultation of respirations.
- Continually monitor maternal and fetal status; if unable to provide continuous fetal monitoring in ED, assist to expedite transfer to antenatal unit. Administer supplemental oxygen to minimize risk for fetal distress. Assist provider in placement and monitoring of arterial line for continuous blood pressure monitoring. Patient may require admission to ▶

 ALERT!

The following criteria are used to diagnose HELLP syndrome: lactic dehydrogenase ≥600 IU/L, aspartate aminotransferase >70 IU/L, and platelet count <100,000 cells/μL.

 ALERT!

If the patient shows signs and symptoms of magnesium toxicity, including absent deep tendon reflexes, respiratory rate less than 12 breaths/min, urine output less than 30 mL/hr, or signs of fetal distress, discontinue magnesium infusion and administer calcium gluconate IV as ordered or per protocol.

Nursing Interventions *(continued)*

critical care unit or antenatal unit for intensive monitoring and treatment. Perform continuous maternal cardiac monitoring and pulse oximetry.

- During postictal period, place patient in left lateral recumbent position, continue to provide supplemental oxygen/ventilatory support if needed, and continue suctioning secretions as needed.
- If a seizure occurs, alert emergency provider and ensure patient safety by preventing injury. If possible, monitor airway and prepare for interventions to ventilate if needed (bag-valve-mask, preparation for intubation), and prevent aspiration by suctioning secretions/emesis as needed.
- Monitor I/O. Place indwelling catheter, if indicated, for strict output monitoring.
- Perform head-to-toe assessment with focused OB evaluation, noting and alerting provider to any bleeding, abdominal pain, headache, visual changes, contractions, or other complications, such as absence of fetal movement.
- Prepare for emergent delivery if indicated.

Patient Education

- Discuss signs of fluid retention and report any increase in swelling to face or limbs (especially hands) or weight gain greater than 3 to 5 lb in less than 1 week.
- For patients with mild preeclampsia who are cleared to resume limited activity, take seizure precautions such as driving and swimming/bathing limitations to reduce the risk of seizure-related injury until cleared by provider.
- If ordered, check blood pressure daily and report any elevated blood pressure readings. Ensure familiarity with blood pressure readings and competence using automated cuff at home.
- Recognize signs and symptoms of hypertensive disorders of pregnancy.
- Seek emergent treatment for severe headache, visual disturbances, epigastric or right upper quadrant pain, and any other concerning symptoms, such as weakness or bleeding.

PRETERM LABOR

Overview

- Preterm labor occurs when contractions cause cervical dilation after 20 weeks and before 37 weeks of gestation. Experiencing more than 6 to 8 contractions per hour before 37 weeks' gestation is indicative of preterm labor. Preterm labor may occur spontaneously or be medically induced due to maternal or fetal health concerns, such as hypertensive emergencies of pregnancy or fetal distress. It may be triggered by trauma, placental abruption, hypoxia, or hypovolemia.
- If the underlying cause cannot be treated, medication to prevent or halt labor may be necessary.

Signs and Symptoms

- Abdominal or pelvic pressure
- Abdominal pain/cramping
- Back pain
- Cervical change (dilation and/or effacement) ▶

 COMPLICATIONS

Preterm labor may result in fetal demise. Infants born before 24 weeks' gestation are not considered viable. Preterm infants who have not achieved enough organ development to thrive outside the womb will require specialized care in a neonatal intensive care unit to survive.

 ALERT!

Preterm labor may be missed in an unconscious trauma patient. Always assess for contractions and ruptured membranes in these patients.

Signs and Symptoms *(continued)*

- Uterine contractions
- Vaginal bleeding and/or ruptured membranes

Diagnosis

Labs

- CBC
- CMP
- Fetal fibronectin, if positive, indicates increased risk of premature birth
- Type and screen
- Urinalysis

Diagnostic Testing

- Fetal monitoring
- Pelvic examination
- Ultrasound

Treatment

Treatment is generally guided by gestation and progression of labor.

- Patients who have reached 34 weeks' gestation: admittance to labor and delivery unit; fetal monitoring for a period of 4 to 6 hours with intermittent cervical checks to assess dilation and effacement. Patients not experiencing progression of labor with reassuring fetal nonstress test with ruled-out complications such as premature rupture of membranes and abruptio placentae.
- Patients who have yet to reach 34 weeks' gestation are at increased risk for fetal complications. Require tocolytic medications to allow time for interventions to promote fetal lung development and protect the fetus from contracting any potential maternal infection during labor.
- Patients experiencing preterm labor with cervical dilation greater than 3 cm: tocolytic medication, usually magnesium sulfate (see Table 7.1) for 48 hours; antibiotics for prophylaxis against group B streptococcus; betamethasone to promote release of surfactant to accelerate fetal lung development (see Table 7.1) and protect against fetal intracranial hemorrhage; magnesium sulfate for neuroprotection

Nursing Interventions

- Perform focused OB assessment, noting any signs/symptoms of preterm labor, such as contractions/ pelvic cramping, low back pain, or rupture of membranes. Collect OB history, including gestational age. Assess contraction frequency, duration, and intensity. Palpate uterus for firmness and approximate fetal size and position. Assess for uterine tenderness upon palpation. Assist provider with pelvic exam to assess cervical dilation and effacement. Conduct continuous fetal monitoring; if unable to place monitoring in ED, facilitate expedited transfer to labor and delivery unit. If delivery is imminent, assist provider and prepare for emergent delivery.
- Assess maternal vital signs and administer supplemental oxygen as needed.
- Initiate IV access for administration of medications and crystalloid fluids if indicated.
- Administer medications, such as tocolytics, steroids, and antibiotics, as ordered.

Patient Education

- Follow activity limitations as prescribed, including specific instruction regarding pelvic rest or bed rest as ordered.
- If contractions occur, record onset and duration of any contractions.

[📝] **POP QUIZ 7.7**

A young adult patient at 36 weeks' gestation is light exercising at home and begins to experience contractior What steps should the patient take upon experienci contractions?

Patient Education *(continued)*

- Drink fluids, attempt to empty bladder, and lie on left side while continuing to monitor any ongoing contractions.
- Return for evaluation if more than five contractions occur at regular intervals within an hour, or if bleeding or rupture of membranes occurs.
- Learn risk factors for preterm labor, such as previous history of early labor, history of certain uterine conditions such as oligohydramnios, placenta previa, abnormal uterine shape, or other factors such as nicotine use.

SPONTANEOUS/THREATENED ABORTION

Overview

- *Spontaneous abortion*, also known as a miscarriage, is fetal demise that occurs naturally and is the leading cause of nonmenstrual vaginal bleeding among those of childbearing age.
- Up to 20% of all known pregnancies are spontaneously aborted, most often related to chromosomal abnormalities.
- A threatened abortion is characterized by symptoms of possible impending miscarriage, which has not yet occurred—the cervical os either is slightly open or remains closed.
- Products of conception that are not fully expelled by the uterus after a fetal demise (incomplete abortion) can cause significant bleeding and become necrotic, leading to infection (septic abortion). Interventions may be required to remove retained tissue.

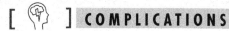 **COMPLICATIONS**

Fetomaternal hemorrhage that occurs during spontaneous abortion has the potential to cause Rh sensitization in an Rh-negative patient. RhoGAM administration can help to prevent fetal demise in subsequent pregnancies.

Signs and Symptoms

- Abdominal or pelvic pain
- Vaginal bleeding, passage of clots and tissue

Diagnosis

Labs

- CBC
- hCG: urine, serum quantitative, or qualitative (if pregnancy is known, a serum quantitative test is indicated)
- Type and screen

Diagnostic Testing

- Doppler assessment of fetal heart tones
- Pelvic examination
- Transvaginal ultrasound

Treatment

- Urgent evaluation/treatment for pregnant patients of less than 20 weeks' gestation with emergent findings, including hemorrhage with hemodynamic instability and/or infection with evidence of sepsis. Possible required emergent surgical intervention to remove products of conception, which contribute to uncontrolled bleeding and/or sepsis.
- Rapid treatment with broad-spectrum antibiotics if concern for sepsis (see Table A.1). ▶

Treatment *(continued)*

- Options of expectant, medication, and surgical management for clinically stable patients with pregnancy loss. Consideration of maternal preferences and values in medical decision-making. Expectant management of spontaneous abortion. Medication management: often misoprostol (see Table 7.1). to promote expulsion of retained products of conception. Surgical management: may be required for cases of retained products of conception, including dilation and curettage and uterine aspiration.

Nursing Interventions

- Administer blood products as ordered. Notify blood bank if emergent blood release is required.
- Administer crystalloid fluid and antibiotics as ordered.
- Administer RhoGAM within 72 hours if the patient is Rh negative.
- Assist provider with pelvic examination.
- Initiate peripheral venous access and draw blood for lab tests, prioritizing CBC and type and screen for any patients with uncontrolled bleeding.
- Monitor amount and quality of bleeding, frequently reassessing vital signs and placing patient on continuous monitoring, if indicated, for signs of hypovolemia that may progress to hemodynamic instability.
- Perform focused OB/GYN assessment, to include pregnancy history, last menstual period, and onset/duration of bleeding. Patient values and preferences regarding pregnancy should also be discussed.
- Provide counseling and emotional support.

Patient Education

- Adhere to physician recommendation for pelvic rest, often prescribed for a period of greater than 2 weeks after miscarriage, for prevention of bleeding and infection.
- Review information regarding miscarriage, understanding that some miscarriages occur without explanation. Understand factors that increase occurrence of miscarriage, such as use of substances like nicotine, cocaine, and alcohol, as well as falls and abdominal injury.
- Patients with expectant or medical management of spontaneous abortion should understand expected passage of blood and tissue. Return for evaluation of severe bleeding, pain, or signs of infection such as fever and foul-smelling discharge.
- Seek out psychosocial support and realize that feelings of grief after pregnancy loss are normal. Obtain resources for pregnancy loss support and seek immediate care for any severe mood disturbance or thoughts of harm to self or others.

TRAUMA DURING PREGNANCY

Overview

- In cases of traumatic injury during pregnancy, the best treatment for the fetus is often focused on optimal resuscitation of the pregnant patient.
- Leading causes of traumatic injury in pregnancy include motor vehicle crashes, falls, and interpersonal violence.
- Physiologic changes of pregnancy should be considered when performing the trauma assessment.

 COMPLICATIONS

If the maternal resuscitation efforts fail, an emerge postmortem Cesarean section may be considered. Becau the fetus has already experienced prolonged hypoxia an circulatory compromise, these are usually unsuccessful an must be performed immediately after the patient's death.

Overview *(continued)*

The gravid uterus displaces abdominal organs as the pregnancy progresses, elevating the diaphragm, increasing maternal respiratory rate, and placing the uterus at risk for blunt and penetrating abdominal trauma. Patient blood volume increases by up to 50%, causing hemodynamic changes and skewing normal values expected upon laboratory analysis. Pregnant patients can lose over a liter of blood before showing symptoms of hypovolemia; in these situations, fetal distress may be the first indicator of maternal hypovolemia.

Signs and Symptoms

- Abdominal pain/contractions
- Fetal heart tones less than 120 bpm and greater than 160 bpm
- Injury-specific signs and symptoms
- Vaginal bleeding/discharge

Diagnosis

Labs

- CBC
- CMP
- Coagulation panel
- Type and screen
- Kleihauer-Betke urinalysis

Diagnostic Testing

- Fetal monitoring
- Pelvic examination to assess for ruptured membranes, if indicated
- Ultrasound
- X-rays depending on injuries (shield abdomen)

[ ] **NURSING PEARL**

The Kleihauer-Betke test is used to quantify fetal blood in maternal circulation, helping detect transplacental hemorrhage and uterine injury. A positive Kleihauer-Betke test is indicative of an increased risk for preterm labor.

Treatment

- Hemodynamically unstable patients: stabilizing treatment of the pregnant patient prioritized before interventions to monitor and treat fetus. Assess and treat hemodynamic instability with crystalloid fluids, vasopressors, and blood products. Additional vascular access, such as placement of a central line or arterial line for invasive hemodynamic monitoring, may be required. FAST ultrasound, conducted by the emergency provider, may need to be altered depending on gestation due to physiologic changes of pregnancy, and may not be reliable in detecting issues such as placental abruption. Signs of preterm/term labor may be missed in the unconscious trauma patient; uterine assessment/palpation, cervical assessment to observe for dilation and effacement, and fetal monitoring should all be used to assess for signs of labor and the need to prepare interventions to deliver the fetus while prioritizing patient stabilization.

[ ] **ALERT!**

When treating a patient who is greater than 20 weeks' gestation, position body slightly toward the left to keep the uterus from compressing the vena cava and restricting blood flow. If the patient is on a backboard, simply place towels underneath to prevent compromised perfusion.

- If concern for neck/spinal injury: cervical collar and backboard to maintain immobilization. Gravid uterus may compress the inferior vena cava when the patient is fully supine. Backboard should be supported to tilt the patient to the left, displacing pressure from the uterus.
- Injury-specific treatment, such as appropriate imaging, splinting, and wound care: may require consults to orthopedics, obstetrics, and other specialties as indicated based on injuries. For most cases (even ▶

Treatment *(continued)*

minor trauma): admission to antenatal unit for fetal monitoring/nonstress test to investigate for signs of fetal distress after maternal injury.

■ Preterm labor: may occur secondary to trauma; emergent Cesarean section possible depending on patient/fetal condition.

Nursing Interventions

■ Change dressings when soiled and provide wound care as needed.

■ Insert at least two large-bore IV lines, drawing labs for priority CBC and type and screen, and initiating fluid resuscitation as ordered.

■ Maintain cervical spine precautions until spinal injury is cleared. Assist to position patient with backboard tilted to prevent circulatory complications related to the gravid uterus.

■ Monitor I/O. Place a urinary catheter using sterile technique, if indicated.

■ Monitor vital signs frequently, placing patient on continuous pulse oximetry and cardiac monitoring as indicated. Apply supplemental oxygen to maintain SpO_2 greater than 95%.

■ Perform continuous fetal monitoring. If unable to conduct fetal monitoring in the ED, assist to expedite transfer to antenatal/labor and delivery unit.

■ Perform obstetric assessment, including estimation of gestational age and assessment for bleeding, cramping, uterine firmness or tenderness, and abdominal or back pain.

■ Perform trauma assessment, including assessment/stabilization of airway, breathing, and circulation.

■ Prepare patient for surgery or immediate delivery if indicated.

Patient Education

■ Adhere to any activity restrictions, including pelvic rest or bed rest as prescribed.

■ Discuss signs and symptoms of infection, such as fever and wound discharge, and recognize reasons to return for further evaluation, such as bleeding or worsening pain.

■ Follow wound care instructions, as needed. Follow up as ordered.

■ Understand that trauma may prompt the onset of labor. Rest, limit strenuous activity and lifting, and maintain adequate hydration; monitor for any contractions. If contractions occur, note onset and duration and seek care if experiencing greater than five contractions at regular intervals over the course of an hour, or if any bleeding, rupture of membranes, or severe pain occurs.

RESOURCES

Aloizos, S., Seretis, C., Liakos, N., Aravosita, P., Mystakelli, C., Kanna, E., & Gourgiotis, S. (2013). HELLP syndrome: Understanding and management of a pregnancy-specific disease. *Journal of Obstetrics and Gynaecology, 33*(4), 331–337. https://doi.org/10.3109/01443615.2013.775231

American College of Surgeons. (2018). *ATLS advanced trauma life support.* Author.

American Heart Association. (2016). *Textbook of neonatal resuscitation* (7th ed.). American Academy of Pediatrics.

Belfort, M. A., Clark, S. L., Saade, G. R., Kleja, K., Dildy, G. A. 3rd, Van Veen, T. R., Akhigbe, E., Frye, D. R., Meyers, J. A., & Kofford, S. (2010). Hospital readmission after delivery: evidence for an increased incidence of nonurogenital infection in the immediate postpartum period. *American Journal of Obstetrics and Gynecology, 202*(1), 35.e1–35. e357. https://doi.org/10.1016/j.ajog.2009.08.029

Bianco, A., Roccia, S., Nobile, C. G., Pileggi, C., & Pavia, M. (2013). Post-discharge surveillance following delivery: The incidence of infections and associated factors. *American Journal of Infection Control, 41*(6), 549–553. https://doi.org/10.1016/j.ajic.2012.06.011

Dalton, E., & Castillo, E. (2014). Postpartum infections: A review for the non-OBGYN. *Obstetric Medicine, 7*(3), 98–102. https://doi.org/10.1177/1753495X14522784

De Wals, P., Tairou, F., Van Allen, M. I., Uh, S. H., Lowry, R. B., Sibbald, B., Evans, J. A., Van den Hof, M. C., Zimmer, P., Crowley, M., Fernandez, B., Lee, N. S., & Niyonsenga, T. (2007). Reduction in neural-tube defects after folic acid fortification in Canada. *New England Journal of Medicine, 357*(2), 135–142. https://doi.org/10.1056/NEJMoa067103

Jordan, K. (2020). Obstetric and gynecologic emergencies. In V. Sweet & A. Foley (Eds.), *Sheehy's emergency nursing: Principles and practice* (7th ed., pp. 279–296). Elsevier.

Kim, C., Barnard, S., Neilson, J. P., Hickey, M., Vazquez, J. C., & Dou, L. (2017). Medical treatments for incomplete miscarriage. *Cochrane Database of Systematic Reviews, (1), Article* CD007223. https://doi.org/10.1002/14651858.CD0
07223.pub4

McParlin, C., O'Donnell, A., Robson, S. C., Beyer, F., Moloney, E., Bryant, A., Bradley, J., Muirhead, C. R., Nelson-Piercy, C., Newbury-Birch, D., Norman, J., Shaw, C., Simpson, E., Swallow, B., Yates, L., & Vale, L. (2016). Treatments for hyperemesis gravidarum and nausea and vomiting in pregnancy: A systematic review. *Journal of the American Medical Association,. 316*(13), 1392–1401. https://doi:10.1001/jama.2016.14337

Poole, J., & Thompson, J. (2013). Obstetric emergencies. In B. Hammond & P. Zimmerman (Eds.), *Sheehy's manual of emergency care* (7th ed., pp. 483–495). Elsevier Mosby.

Prescribers' Digital Reference. (n.d.-a). *Calcium chloride* [Drug information]. https://www.pdr.net/10--Calcium-Chloride-calcium-chloride-3148.2572

Prescribers' Digital Reference. (n.d.-b). *Folic acid* [Drug information]. https://pdr.net/drug-summary/Folic-Acid-Injection-folic-acid-24035

Prescribers' Digital Reference. (n.d.-c). *Methotrexate* [Drug information]. https://www.pdr.net/drug-summary/Methotrexate-Tablets-methotrexate-1797.8191

Prescribers' Digital Reference. (n.d.-d). *Oxytocin* [Drug information]. https://www.pdr.net/drug-summary/Pitocin-oxytocin-1966

Prescribers' Digital Reference. (n.d.-e). *Rhogam* [Drug information]. https://www.pdr.net/drug-summary/MICRhoGAM-RhoGAM-rho-D--immune-globulin--human--1617 ets-terbutaline-sulfate-1659.2088

Roberts, D., & Dalziel, S. (2006). Antenatal corticosteroids for accelerating fetal lung maturation for women at risk of preterm birth. *Cochrane Database of Systematic Reviews*, (3), CD004454. https://doi.org/10.1002/14651858.CD004454.pub2

Turner, J. V., Agatonovic-Kustrn, S., & Ward, H. (2015). Off-label use of misoprostol in gynaecology. *Facts, Views and Vision in ObGyn, 7*(4), 261–264. https://www.ncbi.nlm.nih.gov/pmc/articles/PMC5058416

Uzan, J., Carbonnel, M., Piconne, O., Asmar, R., & Ayoubi, J. M. (2011). Pre-eclampsia: Pathophysiology, diagnosis, and management. *Vascular Health and Risk Management, 7*, 467–474. https://doi.org/10.2147/VHRM.S20181

Yokoe, D. S., Christiansen, C. L., Johnson, R., Sands, K. E., Livingston, J., Shtatland, E. S., & Platt, R. (2001). Epidemiology of and surveillance for postpartum infections. *Emerging Infectious Diseases, 7*(5), 837–841. https://doi.org/10.3201/eid0705.010511

8 MENTAL HEALTH EMERGENCIES

ABUSE/NEGLECT

Overview

- Abuse and neglect may refer to emotional, physical, or spiritual harm; financial exploitation; or failure to provide for a vulnerable party's physiologic and/or psychological needs. Examples include child or elder abuse, intimate partner violence, and human trafficking. It may be difficult to detect these situations in the ED.
- Providing patients with a safe, private environment is key when obtaining an accurate history. Patients may present a fabricated history of events due to fear of their abuser, mistrust of the caregiver, or failure to identify their situation as an incident of abuse or neglect.
- Neglect includes abandonment, inadequate supervision, and the caregiver not meeting physical and emotional needs.
- *Medical neglect* refers to the failure to provide appropriate healthcare for a dependent.
- Sustained neglect can result in injury, malnutrition, and failure to thrive.
- *Elder abuse* occurs when a person in a position of trust either intentionally acts to induce harm or fails to act, thereby causing harm to an adult older than 60 years.
- *Intimate partner violence* includes physical, emotional, financial, or sexual violence enacted by a current or former intimate partner.
- *Human trafficking* is the trade of persons for sexual purposes (forced prostitution, marriage, or pornography) or labor purposes (forced work at low wages in agriculture, food services, and other industries).

[🧠] **COMPLICATIONS**

Children who are abused or neglected are more likely to later misuse alcohol, smoke tobacco, use illicit drugs, experience depression and other psychological conditions, or commit suicide. They are also at increased risk for many adverse health events, including development of heart disease, asthma, stroke, and diabetes.

Signs and Symptoms

- Inconsistent history of illness/injury, discrepancies in provided history from patient and caregiver or intimate partner, inability to provide explanation of injury, and/or unreasonable delay in seeking healthcare
- Wounds, such as lacerations, abrasions, bite marks, or burns
- Contusions, particularly those in various stages of healing and/or isolated to one part of the body, such as bilateral arms/wrists, or patterned injury/marks shaped like fingers/hands, belts/sticks, or other objects
- Swelling or bruising pattern that may indicate use of restraints or ligature injury (wrists, ankles, or neck)
- Fractures (may be new, old, or a combination, and in various stages of healing; particularly suspicious if evidence of multiple older untreated fractures is discovered)
- Poor hygiene, poor dentition, attire inappropriate for weather

Signs and Symptoms *(continued)*

- Psychological complaints, such as depression and anxiety
- Vaginal or rectal pain, infections, or injury
- Failure to maintain or gain weight per expectations, chronic dehydration, and failure to thrive

Diagnosis

Labs

There are no lab tests specific to diagnosing abuse and neglect. However, the following tests may be indicated to diagnose underlying/related illnesses:

- Complete blood count (CBC)
- Comprehensive metabolic panel (CMP)
- Coagulation panel
- Urinalysis
- Sexually transmitted infection (STI) testing

Diagnostic Testing

- Radiographic imaging (CT, x-ray, and ultrasound) as needed for underlying or related illnesses or injuries
- Pelvic examination and/or forensic examination if indicated or needed for legal purposes/law enforcement or if desired by patient

Treatment

- Careful history (obtained in private, with patient separated from caregiver or intimate partner if possible)
- Thorough physical examination unless a forensic examination will be completed during same visit
- Ruling out organic causes for signs and symptoms
- Injury-specific treatment, which may include consultations to specialty services, medication management, procedures, or surgical intervention
- Documentation of all injuries and findings
- Referrals for resources and interventions as indicated
- Mandatory reporting guidelines for all suspected abuse and neglect cases

 NURSING PEARL

Abuse and neglect cannot be identified through lab tests and imaging alone, as there may be no abnormal findings. A thorough history and physical examination may provide sufficient findings for the diagnosis.

Nursing Interventions

- Provide opportunity for privacy in assisting to separate patient from potential abuser during examination.
- Obtain a thorough history and perform a complete head-to-toe assessment.
- Screen all patients for potential abuse.
- Maintain a respectful and nonjudgmental tone with patients.
- Assess pediatric growth and development.
- Report all suspected child abuse and neglect cases to local authorities; follow state guidelines for cases involving adults.
- Arrange referrals for follow-up and additional resources as indicated.
- Be aware of local law regarding mandatory reporting. Some states have laws that may allow the victim to ask law enforcement not to be notified.

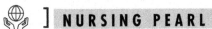 **NURSING PEARL**

Separating the patient from the potential abuser is an essential first step when obtaining an accurate history and thorough examination. Patients may be reluctant to answer questions honestly in the presence of the potential abuser.

Patient Education

- Call 911 or a local hotline for emergency situations.
- Contact organization to obtain resources and connect with others for support and assistance in recovery.
- Identify friends, family members, or community resources that can provide support and resources as needed.
- Families should monitor and report any concerning changes in a child's behavior or health to the patient's provider.

AGGRESSIVE/VIOLENT BEHAVIOR

Overview

- Agitation caused by a variety of medical or psychiatric conditions can escalate into aggressive/violent behavior.
- Acute agitation may be a symptom of many emergent health conditions; the emergency care team is obligated to provide thorough assessment for medical clearance before diagnosing a psychologic cause of aggression.
- The emergency care team should assess all patients for risk of violence and attempt to facilitate therapeutic communication, provide diversionary activities, provide appropriate medication, and enact de-escalation techniques before a situation results in violence.
- The use of physical or chemical restraints should be a last resort.

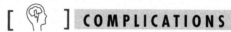

[🧠] **COMPLICATIONS**

Violent behavior places patients and caregivers at risk for injury. Agitation and threats of violence should be addressed proactively, and de-escalation of the agitated patient should be prioritized to reduce incidences of violence in the ED.

Signs and Symptoms

- Violent or threatening statements or actions toward self or others
- Restlessness, pacing, increased vocalization/volume and use of profanity or threatening language, aggressive gestures, and impulsive behavior
- Compromised reality checking (such as with patients experiencing dementia and delirium, hallucinations and/or delusions, de-realization, and/or de-personalization)
- Signs of intoxication or substance use

Diagnosis

Labs

There are no lab tests specific to diagnosing aggressive and violent behavior. However, the following tests may be indicated to diagnose underlying/related illnesses:

- CBC
- CMP
- Thyroid-stimulating hormone (TSH)
- Ethyl alcohol (ETOH) level
- Urine drug screen
- Urinalysis

Diagnostic Testing

- Head CT scan to rule out underlying emergent medical condition
- X-rays as indicated for related injuries

Treatment

- Thorough evaluation to rule out possible emergent medical causes of behaviors
- De-escalation through diversionary techniques, by limiting external stimuli, and by facilitating therapeutic communication
- All threats to be taken seriously
- Ensuring safety of patients and staff by isolating violent patients in an area where potential hazards can be removed
- Visualization of the patient using 1:1 observation, if indicated
- Medical or physical restraints if the patient does not respond to prior interventions and patient or staff harm is imminent (see Table 8.1)
- Inpatient psychiatric admission if indicated

TABLE 8.1 Psychosocial Medications		
INDICATIONS	MECHANISM OF ACTION	CONTRAINDICATIONS, PRECAUTIONS, AND ADVERSE EFFECTS
Antidepressants, MAOIs (phenelzine sulfate)		
• Nonselective monoamine oxidase A and B inhibitor used for treatment-resistant depression; may be used off-label for anxiety disorders	• Irreversibly bind to and inhibit monoamine oxidase, which in turn increases concentration of selected neurotransmitters, including epinephrine, norepinephrine, and dopamine	• Medication is contraindicated in patients with liver disease. • Patients must avoid food containing large amounts of tyramine, tryptophan, and/or caffeine. • Medication can cause orthostatic hypotension, syncope, and blurred vision. • Medication can cause tremors, myoclonia, hyperreflexia, and paresthesia.
Antidepressants, miscellaneous (bupropion hydrochloride)		
• Used for the treatment of depression; also used for management of ADHD and smoking cessation	• Mechanism of action not fully understood but appear to selectively inhibit dopamine reuptake • Produce moderate anticholinergic effects	• Medication can cause insomnia, headache, and GI upset. • Medication is contraindicated in patients with seizure history or those taking MAOIs. • Antidepressant activity can occur within 1 week of initiation of therapy, but full effects may not be seen until 4 weeks of therapy.
Antidepressants, SNRIs (duloxetine)		
• Used to treat depression and generalized anxiety disorder; also indicated for diabetic peripheral neuropathy, fibromyalgia, and chronic pain	• Inhibit reuptake of serotonin and norepinephrine; exact mechanism unknown	• Avoid abrupt discontinuation if possible; taper gradually to discontinue. • Do not administer with MAOIs. • Use with caution in the presence of liver disease or alcohol use • Medication can cause nausea, constipation, weight loss, and headaches. • Use with caution in older adults, who can be more susceptible to falling from orthostatic hypotension and syncope associated with the medication.

(continued)

TABLE 8.1 Psychosocial Medications *(continued)*

INDICATIONS	MECHANISM OF ACTION	CONTRAINDICATIONS, PRECAUTIONS, AND ADVERSE EFFECTS
Antidepressants, SSRIs (fluoxetine)		
• Used for the treatment of depression, panic disorder, PTSD, and anxiety disorder	• Enhance actions of serotonin with decreased binding to histaminergic, muscarinic, and alpha-adrenergic effects	• Medication has fewer sedative, anticholinergic, and cardiovascular effects than other antidepressants. • Medication can cause insomnia, headaches, and GI symptoms. • Avoid abrupt discontinuation of the drug to prevent withdrawal symptoms.
Antidepressants, tricyclic (amitriptyline hydrochloride)		
• For the treatment of depression, social phobia, or panic disorder; additional uses for neuropathy, migraine prophylaxis, insomnia	• Exact mechanism unknown but decrease reuptake of norepinephrine and serotonin; also produce strong anticholinergic activity	• Do not use with MAOI inhibitors. • Medication can cause orthostatic hypotension and dry mouth. • Medication can cause drowsiness, lethargy, and memory impairment. • Toxicity (acute or chronic) causes CNS depression and cardiac arrhythmias and can be life-threatening.
Antipsychotic, atypical (risperidone)		
• For the treatment of schizophrenia and bipolar disorder; also used to manage severe behavioral issues and aggression in certain conditions, including dementia	• Exact mechanism unknown but believed to block dopamine to manage symptoms; also strong alpha antagonist activity	• Injection: IM or subcutaneous administration only • Medication can cause CNS depression and tardive dyskinesia. • Medication can cause hypotension, dizziness, and reflex tachycardia.
Antipsychotic, typical (haloperidol)		
• Injection used for immediate management of acute agitation/psychosis in hospital settings; oral or injection forms used for schizophrenia and Tourette's disorder	• Exact mechanism of action unknown but believed to block dopamine receptors in the mesolimbic pathway • Weak anticholinergic effects and weak affinity for alpha-1 and histamine-1 receptors	• Medication can cause extrapyramidal symptoms including dystonic reactions such as torticollis, akathisia, and blepharospasm (blinking or other eye movements). • Medication can cause dry mouth and drowsiness. • IM form is used for acute situations or long-term medication administration.
Benzodiazepines (lorazepam)		
• Used for the short-term management of anxiety and agitation, the treatment of status epilepticus, and procedural sedation	• Acts on the limbic, thalamic, and hypothalamic regions of the CNS to produce CNS depression ranging from sedation, hypnosis, and skeletal muscle relaxation to anticonvulsant activity and coma	• Medication is a Schedule IV controlled substance. • To administer IV push, dose must be diluted with an equal volume of diluent and be administered slowly at a rate not to exceed 2 mg/min. • Medication is not recommended for CNS-depressed patients because it causes additional CNS depression. • Avoid coadministration with opioids if possible to decrease the risk of respiratory depression. • Monitor patient for drowsiness and more severe signs of CNS depression.

(continued)

TABLE 8.1 Psychosocial Medications *(continued)*

INDICATIONS	MECHANISM OF ACTION	CONTRAINDICATIONS, PRECAUTIONS, AND ADVERSE EFFECTS
Mood stabilizers (lithium carbonate, valproic acid)		
• Lithium: treatment of bipolar disorder • Valproic acid: used for seizures but also used for severe behavioral disturbances	• Lithium: exact mechanism of action related to antimanic and antidepressant actions is unknown but believed to interfere with the synthesis, storage, release, and reuptake of monoamine neurotransmitters; also enhances the uptake of tryptophan and increases the synthesis/release of serotonin • Valproic acid: believed to increase brain concentrations of gamma-aminobutyric acid, which is an inhibitory neurotransmitter	• The acute antimanic effect of lithium occurs in 5–10 days, and the full therapeutic effect is seen within 21 days. • Lithium requires close monitoring to maintain therapeutic levels and avoid nephrotoxicity. • Side effects of lithium include nausea, vomiting, fatigue, and dizziness. • Side effects of valproic acid include GI symptoms, drowsiness, and thrombocytopenia.

Note: All agents are contraindicated in the presence of hypersensitivity to the medication or one of its components.
ADHD, attention deficit hyperactivity disorder; CNS, central nervous system; GI, gastrointestinal; IM, intramuscular; IV, intravenous; MAOIs, monoamine oxidase inhibitors; PTSD, posttraumatic stress disorder; SNRIs, serotonin-norepinephrine reuptake inhibitors; SSRIs, selective serotonin reuptake inhibitors.

Nursing Interventions

- Remove the patient to an appropriate location to maintain patient and staff safety.
- Remain calm and speak to the patient using simple language.
- Attempt to establish a therapeutic relationship.
- Maintain visual and situational awareness of the patient at all times.
- Facilitate de-escalation of the patient's behavior.
- Apply and monitor use of physical restraints as indicated and follow institutional protocols. Perform regular circulatory and neurovascular checks to restrained extremities. Provide assistance with oral intake and toileting as needed. Assess skin integrity per facility protocol to decrease the risk of complications related to restraint use or immobility. The patient may require a 1:1 sitter depending on facility protocol for the type of restraints required to maintain patient safety. Patients in restraints are at increased risk for injury and death. Careful observation and frequent reassessment are necessary.

[ ] **ALERT!**

De-escalating a potentially violent patient can take time but is frequently successful if approached in the correct manner.

- Ensure the environment is safe for the patient and staff involved.
- Speak calmly and objectively to the patient in a normal tone of voice.
- Encourage conversation and attempt to form an alliance.
- Listen to what the patient has to say and respond in a respectful manner.
- Incorporate active listening into the conversation; use reflection to help the patient identify underlying feelings. Nonverbal communication can help the nurse establish a therapeutic relationship.
- If possible, stand next to or offset to the patient to appear less threatening.
- Safety comes first. Do not attempt de-escalation alone and always stand between the patient and the door.

Patient Education

- Use behavioral strategies to manage anger and stress, which may include physical exercise and relaxation techniques (deep breathing, meditation, yoga), journaling, or art.
- Limit alcohol and other substance use.
- Take regular medications as prescribed.

ANXIETY/PANIC DISORDER

Overview

- *Anxiety* is a normal response to many situations. Anxiety can result from a variety of conditions including mental disorders, medications, and substance use. Anxiety involves fear and worry accompanied by a heightened physiologic response, with symptoms ranging from mild to severe.
- An anxiety disorder is diagnosed when anxiety occurs outside a situational context; is pervasive, causing the patient to alter their normal activities; or involves disproportional or continuous signs and symptoms.
- *Posttraumatic stress disorder (PTSD)* is an anxiety disorder that can develop in response to a traumatic event.
- *Panic disorders* involve at least three panic attacks that occur within 3 weeks.
- A *panic attack* occurs when a patient experiences a sudden onset of fear or impending doom accompanied by at least four of the physical symptoms listed in the following Signs and Symptoms section.

Signs and Symptoms

- Excessive worry
- Fear
- Intrusive thoughts
- Shortness of breath
- Chest pain/palpitations
- Abdominal discomfort
- Avoidant behaviors
- Chills or heat sensations
- Depersonalization (the belief that one's body is surreal)
- Diaphoresis
- Dizziness
- Nausea
- Paresthesia
- Perception of altered reality
- Sleep disturbances
- Tremulousness
- Flashbacks/hallucinations (PTSD)

[📝] **POP QUIZ 8.1**

What is the first step the nurse should take to respond to an agitated patient who is shouting and hitting the side of the stretcher?

[ ] **COMPLICATIONS**

Some medical conditions may mimic or involve symptoms of anxiety or panic attacks, making it difficult to determine if the symptoms are related to medical or a psychological condition. To reduce the risk of life-threatening medical complications, emergent medical causes of symptoms of anxiety should always be ruled out.

[⚡] **ALERT!**

Many patients in respiratory distress may have anxiety due to the sensation of air hunger. Those experiencing a myocardial infarction or anaphylaxis may also have considerable anxiety, which should be considered a symptom. These conditions should be considered in the diagnostic workup.

Diagnosis

Labs

There are no lab tests specific to diagnosing anxiety and panic disorder. However, the following may be helpful to rule out underlying medical etiology:

- CBC
- CMP
- ETOH level
- TSH
- Urine drug screen

Diagnostic Testing

There are no diagnostic tests specific to anxiety and panic disorder. However, the following may be indicated to rule out underlying medical etiology:

- EKG
- CT scan
- Chest x-ray

Treatment

- Assess for suicidal or homicidal ideation.
- Rule out an underlying medical cause for the anxiety symptoms.
- Administer supplemental oxygen as needed for tachypnea or tachycardia.
- Provide therapeutic communication.
- Administer antianxiety medications.

Nursing Interventions

- Assess patient for potential for violence.
- Establish rapport with the patient.
- Use therapeutic communication techniques.
- Perform a focused psychosocial assessment.
- Perform a respiratory assessment and administer supplemental oxygen as needed to maintain oxygen saturation greater than 95%.
- Assess and monitor vital signs.
- Instruct on measures to decrease and manage anxiety regardless of cause.
- Refer to online or in-person counseling or treatment options, if indicated.

Patient Education

- Practice good health habits: get adequate sleep, eat a variety of foods, and exercise.
- Follow up with a counselor, social worker, or other community resource to talk about anxiety and how to manage it.
- Identify ways to relax and relieve stress. These may include meditation, deep breathing, yoga, journaling, or art.

 NURSING PEARL

Part of a psychosocial assessment involves evaluating a patient's mental status to determine how well their brain receives and processes information. Assess the patient's level of consciousness and their ability to maintain attention. Assess the patient's affect. Observe the patient's behavior to determine if they are appropriate for the situation. Ask open-ended questions to evaluate the patient's judgment and language comprehension and to observe their speech pattern.

 POP QUIZ 8.2

What priority interventions should the nurse perform for the patient who is having signs and symptoms of acute anxiety?

BIPOLAR DISORDER

Overview

- *Bipolar disorder* is a mood disorder characterized by periods of depression and mania or hypomania.
- The timing and severity of the patient's mood swings distinguish bipolar disorder from other mood disorders.
- Bipolar disorder is differentiated into types based on presenting symptoms: *Bipolar I disorder* involves at least one manic and one depressive episode. *Bipolar II disorder* involves at least one depressive episode and one hypomanic episode. *Cyclothymic disorder* involves milder cyclical mood swings. *Bipolar disorder, unspecified* involves some signs and symptoms, but diagnostic criteria may not be present or may be caused by other conditions.
- Patients are more likely to seek treatment when they are depressed compared with when they are experiencing mania.
- Patients with bipolar disorder are at high risk for suicide; approximately 50% of these patients have attempted suicide at least once.

[🧠] **COMPLICATIONS**

During manic periods, patients may demonstrate extreme impulsivity. This increases the risk for self-harm or violence toward others.

Signs and Symptoms

- Mania: excitement; impulsivity; pressured speech; racing thoughts; agitation; changes in libido; delusional thinking; disinhibition; impaired judgment; irritability; sleep pattern disturbances
- Depression: feelings of sadness, worthlessness, and hopelessness; suicidal ideations; sleep pattern disturbances; fatigue; agitation; changes in libido; impaired judgment; irritability; weight change

Diagnosis

Labs

- Laboratory tests as indicated to rule out underlying medical conditions: CBC; CMP; TSH; ETOH level
- Lithium level, if applicable (normal range 0.6–1.0 mmol/L; increased symptoms can occur if levels are subtherapeutic)
- Urinalysis
- Urine drug screen

Diagnostic Testing

As indicated to rule out underlying medical conditions (e.g., head CT scan)

Treatment

- Assess for suicidal or homicidal ideations.
- Maintain a safe environment for both manic and depressive states.
- Rule out an underlying medical condition.
- Administer medications as needed to control symptoms (see Table 8.1).
- Assess/manage lithium levels.
- Use physical restraints if all other interventions to maintain safety are unsuccessful.
- Admit to a psychiatric unit as indicated.

Nursing Interventions

- Assess for suicidal or homicidal ideations.
- Provide a safe environment for the patient by removing any potentially harmful objects from the room.
- Decrease environmental stimuli.
- Establish a therapeutic relationship. ▶

Nursing Interventions *(continued)*

- Ask focused questions to elicit information but minimize a manic patient's verbal discourse.
- Perform a focused psychosocial assessment.
- Medicate as needed to manage symptoms.
- Assess laboratory values, specifically monitoring lithium levels, if indicated.
- Offer nourishment as indicated for patient's condition. Manic symptoms: Offer high-calorie finger foods to meet the body's elevated caloric requirements. Depressive symptoms: Encourage oral intake if patient's appetite is decreased.
- Apply physical restraints if all other attempts to maintain patient safety have been unsuccessful.

Patient Education

- Call 911 or return to the ED if experiencing suicidal thoughts.
- Take all medications as prescribed even if symptoms improve.
- Report medication side effects so the medications can be adjusted, but do not stop taking the medications.
- Exercise regularly to help manage symptoms of depression.
- Learn the importance of maintaining good sleep hygiene practices.
- Avoid alcohol and drug use, which can disguise symptoms and interfere with prescribed medications.

DEPRESSION

Overview

- *Depression* is characterized by prolonged periods of depressed mood, most often related to a chemical imbalance.
- It can be difficult to diagnose, as a patient can have mild symptoms resulting from a specific situation or trigger, or severe symptoms consistent with a mood disorder.
- A depressive mood disorder is diagnosed when the patient experiences at least five symptoms over a 2-week period.

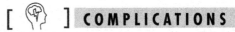 **COMPLICATIONS**

Depressed patients are at risk for abusing drugs or alcohol in an attempt to alleviate their symptoms. Additionally, patients with depression tend to have thoughts of self-harm including self-mutilation and suicide.

Signs and Symptoms

- Depressed mood
- Difficulty thinking
- Fatigue
- Feelings of worthlessness
- Loss of interest in usual activities
- Recurrent thoughts of death
- Change in appetite and weight (markedly increased or decreased)
- Change in sleep patterns (too much or too little)
- Psychomotor agitation or retardation

Diagnosis

Labs

There are no lab tests specific to diagnosing depression. However, the following may be indicated to rule out underlying medical conditions:

- CBC
- CMP ▶

Labs (continued)

- ETOH level
- TSH/thyroid panel
- Urinalysis
- Urine drug screen

Diagnostic Testing

- EKG
- Head CT scan to rule out an underlying medical condition

Treatment

- Assessment/treatment of suicidal ideations or attempts
- Ruling out of underlying medical condition
- Assessment/treatment of any electrolyte abnormalities and nutritional deficits
- Medications to manage symptoms (e.g., anxiety, depression, and insomnia; see Table 8.1)
- Referrals for continued outpatient treatment
- Admittance to a psychiatric unit, as indicated

Nursing Interventions

- Perform a focused psychological assessment.
- Assess for alcohol or drug use.
- Maintain a safe environment for the patient.
- Establish a therapeutic relationship.
- Administer crystalloid fluids or nutritional supplements as indicated.

Patient Education

- Call 911, return to the ED, or contact a support group (virtual, phone, or in person) for any suicidal thoughts.
- Learn the importance of taking medications as prescribed, even if feeling better.
- Perform regular exercise and maintain good sleep and hygiene practices to help manage symptoms of depression.
- Maintain a nutritious diet and follow any special diet instructions from a dietitian.

[ ] **POP QUIZ 8.3**

A nurse triages a patient who reports poor appetite and difficulty sleeping. Additional questioning reveals that the patient feels hopeless and overwhelmed with the situation. What is the priority for this patient?

HOMICIDAL IDEATION

Overview

- *Homicidal ideation* is thought of harming or killing another person or group of people.
- Risk factors for acting on homicidal ideations include anxiety, fear, cognitive impairment, impulsive behavior, fixed beliefs, and delusional thoughts.
- As with suicidal ideations, a specific and well-thought-out plan increases the risk that the patient will act on homicidal thoughts.
- Follow state requirements for mandatory reporting of these situations.

[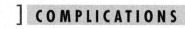] **COMPLICATIONS**

A patient who expresses homicidal thoughts with a detailed plan to act on them is at higher risk for following through on their threats.

Signs and Symptoms

- Expression of a desire to harm or kill another person or group
- Agitation/anger
- Violent behavior
- Impulsive behavior
- Intoxication/substance use

Diagnosis

Labs

There are no lab tests specific to diagnosing homicidal ideation. However, the following may be indicated to rule out underlying medical conditions:

- CBC
- CMP
- ETOH level
- Urinalysis
- Urine drug screen

Diagnostic Testing

- Radiographic imaging as indicated to rule out an underlying medical cause

Treatment

- Ruling out of underlying medical conditions
- Strategies to de-escalate violent/aggressive patients, including diversionary techniques, minimizing external stimuli, and establishing a therapeutic relationship
- Maintenance of patient and staff safety
- Anxiolytics or antipsychotics, as indicated
- Admission for psychiatric treatment, as indicated
- Mandatory reporting per state guidelines

Nursing Interventions

- Assess for the presence of a plan and the patient's intent to implement the plan.
- Assess for accompanying suicidal ideations.
- Observe and maintain situational awareness of the patient at all times.
- Implement elopement precautions per facility protocol.
- Implement appropriate strategies to maintain safety of the patient and staff.
- Establish a therapeutic relationship with the patient.
- Remove all potentially dangerous objects from the patient's room.
- Use communication techniques to de-escalate the situation.
- Conduct a focused psychosocial assessment.
- Administer medications as ordered.

Patient Education

- Follow up with mental health resources as arranged.
- Identify a person or persons to talk to and share feelings with on an ongoing basis.
- Call 911, community resources, or a friend or family member if feelings recur.
- Take all medications as prescribed even if symptoms improve.
- Identify ways to reduce and manage stress.

[ ]   COMPLICATIONS

Acute psychosis requires immediate treatment based on th_ underlying cause to prevent complications. These patient_ are at risk for self-harm or violent behavior. Psychosi_ can affect all areas of a patient's life, causing a significar_ impact at work, at school, and in relationships. If untreate_ psychosis can lead to a point at which the patient can r_ longer take care of themselves properly or communicat_ effectively with others; it can progress to permaner_ neurologic damage.

PSYCHOSIS
Overview
- *Psychosis* is a condition characterized by disordered thoughts and altered perceptions of reality.
- It can be caused by mental or physical disorders (dementia, intracranial tumor, medication, or substance use).
- Maintaining patient safety is essential until symptoms are managed.

Signs and Symptoms
- Delusions
- Disordered thinking
- Disorganized speech
- Hallucinations

Diagnosis
Labs
There are no lab tests specific to diagnosing psychosis. However, the following may be indicated to rule out an underlying medical cause:
- CBC
- CMP
- ETOH level
- TSH/thyroid panel
- Urinalysis
- Urine drug screen

Diagnostic Testing
- Head CT scan
- Other diagnostic testing as indicated to rule out underlying medical conditions

Treatment
- Antipsychotic medications, if indicated (see Table 8.1)
- Maintaining a safe environment
- Restraints as a last resort
- Ruling out any organic cause
- Treatment of underlying cause if identified
- Continued psychiatric treatment

Nursing Interventions
- Maintain patient safety by removing potentially dangerous objects from the room.
- Implement 1:1 monitoring with a sitter as indicated.
- Decrease external stimuli.
- Form a therapeutic relationship.
- Perform a focused psychosocial assessment.
- Reorient patient to reality (as patient's condition allows).
- Acknowledge that hallucinations are real to the patient but not actually occurring.
- Help identify triggers for the hallucinations.
- Help identify ways to de-escalate the patient when hallucinations occur, such as music therapy or deep breathing.

Patient Education

- Call 911 or return to the ED if suicidal or homicidal thoughts or other unsafe situations occur.
- Follow up with community providers and resources for continued treatment.
- Identify a person or group for ongoing support if not returning to a psychiatric facility.
- Allow caregivers to administer and monitor medication regimens as applicable.
- Follow up as instructed to monitor medication effectiveness and the presence of side effects.

SITUATIONAL CRISIS

Overview

- A *situational crisis* is an ineffective coping response to an event, usually an event outside the patient's control.
- It develops from personal situations, such as death of a loved one or job loss, as well as from larger situations, such as a pandemic or a natural disaster.

Signs and Symptoms

- Report of stressful feelings
- Anxiety
- Anger
- Despair
- Hopelessness
- Sleep pattern disturbances
- Suicidal or homicidal ideations
- Violent thoughts or behaviors
- Substance use
- Changes in diet and nutrition
- Changes in weight

Diagnosis

Labs

There are no lab tests specific to diagnosing situational crisis. However, the following may be indicated to rule out an underlying medical etiology:

- CBC
- CMP
- Urinalysis
- Urine drug screen

Diagnostic Testing

- As indicated to rule out underlying medical conditions

Treatment

- Risk assessment for self-harm or suicidal ideation
- Safe environment
- Ruling out of underlying medical conditions
- Anxiolytic medication as indicated (see Table 8.1) ▶

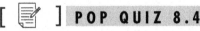 **POP QUIZ 8.4**

What is the nurse's priority when assessing a patient who is aimlessly wandering around the room and talking incoherently?

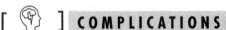 **COMPLICATIONS**

Feelings of anxiety, fear, and apprehension are all part of the normal response to an adverse situation. However, if unrecognized or not addressed, these feelings can escalate and limit the patient's ability to think clearly with sound judgment. If not treated, the patient can become overwhelmed and detached from others. This can lead to self-harm or violent behavior toward others.

Treatment *(continued)*

- Additional mental health treatment, as indicated
- Social work, case management, or community support groups to assist with modifiable risk factors for situational crises

Nursing Interventions

- Assess for suicidal or homicidal ideations.
- Perform a focused psychosocial assessment.
- Remove potentially hazardous objects.
- Establish a relationship with the patient and use therapeutic communication to listen and provide support.

Patient Education

- Follow up for further treatment and community assistance as arranged.
- Identify friends and family members to talk to and obtain support from throughout the situation.
- Seek emergent care for any thoughts of suicide.

SUICIDAL IDEATION

Overview

- Assess all patients for suicidal ideations, as they can be present in patients with various complaints, including mental disorders, substance use, physical abuse, chronic illness, or recent loss.
- Risk factors can be categorized as biologic (family history, disordered neurotransmitter exchange); psychological (feelings of guilt, revenge, or hopelessness); environmental (external influence that combines with internal feelings); cultural (religious beliefs, family values).
- The seriousness of a patient's suicidal ideations is reflected in the specificity of their thoughts as well as the feasibility of their plan. Certain factors, including history of previous suicide attempts, presence of impulsive behaviors, and feelings of hopelessness/helplessness, also increase the risk that the patient will act on their thoughts.

 COMPLICATIONS

Suicide is a leading cause of death in the United States and a leading cause of patient safety events in healthcare facilities. All patients should be screened for suicidal thoughts regardless of chief complaint or diagnosis. Suicidal ideations can occur at any time with any patient.

Signs and Symptoms

- Thoughts of suicide
- Plan for carrying out suicide
- Giving away possessions
- Wishing they could go to sleep and not wake up
- Stating they feel suicidal
- Feelings of depression
- Aggressive behavior
- Anger
- Substance use
- Violent behavior

Diagnosis

Labs

There are no lab tests specific to diagnosing suicidal ideation. However, the following may be indicated to rule out an underlying medical cause:

- CBC
- CMP
- ETOH level
- TSH
- Urinalysis
- Urine drug screen

Diagnostic Testing

- As indicated to rule out an underlying medical cause

Treatment

- Suicide risk assessment using a standardized suicide risk scale per facility guidelines (such as the Columbia-Suicide Severity Rating Scale)
- Safe environment with 1:1 sitter per institutional protocol
- Frequent or continuous direct observation based on suicide risk and facility protocol
- Treatment for any underlying medical conditions
- Medications to manage associated symptoms (see Table 8.1)
- Inpatient psychiatric admission or involuntary hold (per state guidelines) as indicated

Nursing Interventions

- Assess the patient's risk of suicide and implement any facility-specific precautions based on assigned risk (including but not limited to placing the patient in a certain treatment area and placing the patient in certain, easily identifiable clothing such as a special gown).
- Clear the patient's room of potentially harmful objects.
- Notify the dietary department to provide finger foods and disposable trays only.
- Maintain frequent or continuous direct observation based on the patient's suicide risk and institutional protocol.
- Establish a therapeutic relationship with the patient.
- Assess and facilitate family presence and support if helpful to the patient.

Patient Education

- Call 911, a community hotline, or a designated support person, or return to the ED if thoughts recur.
- Contact a suicide prevention organization for additional resources and ongoing support.

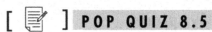 **POP QUIZ 8.5**

A patient with depression expresses a wish to "end the struggle." How should the nurse respond?

RESOURCES

Dillahunty, A. (2020). Abuse and neglect. In V. Sweet & A. Foley (Eds.), *Sheehy's emergency nursing: Principles and practice* (7th ed., pp. 607–630). Elsevier.

Manton, A. (2013). Mental health emergencies. In B. Hammond & P. Zimmerman (Eds.), *Sheehy's manual of emergency care* (7th ed., pp. 505–519). Elsevier.

Pritts, W. (2020). Behavioral health emergencies. In V. Sweet & A. Foley (Eds.), *Sheehy's emergency nursing: Principles and practice* (7th ed., pp. 582–593). Elsevier.

Prescribers' Digital Reference. (n.d.-a). *Amitriptyline hydrochloride* [Drug information]. https://www.pdr.net/drug-summary/Amitriptyline-Hydrochloride-amitriptyline-hydrochloride-1001.5733

Prescribers' Digital Reference. (n.d.-b). *Bupropion hydrochloride* [Drug information]. https://www.pdr.net/drug-summary/Wellbutrin-bupropion-hydrochloride-237

Prescribers' Digital Reference. (n.d.-c). *Duloxetine* [Drug information]. https://www.pdr.net/drug-summary/Cymbalta-duloxetine-288

Prescribers' Digital Reference. (n.d.-d). *Fluoxetine hydrochloride* [Drug information]. https://www.pdr.net/drug-summary/Fluoxetine-Hydrochloride-fluoxetine-hydrochloride-24302

Prescribers' Digital Reference. (n.d.-e). *Haloperidol* [Drug information]. https://www.pdr.net/drug-summary/Haldol-haloperidol-942.4581

Prescribers' Digital Reference. (n.d.-f). *Lithium carbonate* [Drug information]. https://www.pdr.net/drug-summary/Lithobid-lithium-carbonate-757.1126

Prescribers' Digital Reference. (n.d.-g). *Lorazepam* [Drug information]. https://www.pdr.net/drug-summary/Ativan-Injection-lorazepam-996.5972

Prescribers' Digital Reference. (n.d.-h). *Phenelzine sulfate* [Drug information]. https://www.pdr.net/drug-summary/Nardil-phenelzine-sulfate-462

Prescribers' Digital Reference. (n.d.-i). *Risperidone* [Drug information]. https://www.pdr.net/drug-summary/Risperidone-risperidone-3120.8240

Prescribers' Digital Reference. (n.d.-j). *Valproic acid.* [Drug information]. https://www.pdr.net/drug-summary/Depakene-valproic-acid-979.5705

ENDOCRINE EMERGENCIES

ADRENAL EMERGENCIES

Overview

- *Addison's disease*, or primary adrenal insufficiency, is the result of the adrenal glands not producing enough cortisol and aldosterone.
- A failing adrenal system usually results from an autoimmune process that causes cortisol and aldosterone levels to decrease. This creates a chain reaction that may cause hypovolemia, hypotension, hypoglycemia, and hyperkalemia. Patients are at risk of adrenal crisis if steroid medication is abruptly discontinued. Acute addisonian crisis, or adrenal crisis, is a result of physical stress, such as injury, infection, or illness. It is an endocrinologic emergency that is due to an acute deficiency of the adrenal hormone cortisol, requiring immediate recognition and treatment.
- *Cushing syndrome* usually results from prolonged exposure to glucocorticoids, either endogenous or exogenous (e.g., prednisone). Patients often develop a characteristic appearance due to increased adipose tissue in certain locations, such as the face, neck, and above the clavicles. In contrast to Addison's disease, patients with Cushing syndrome often develop hyperglycemia, hypernatremia, hypokalemia, and hypertension. Cushing disease is a subset of Cushing syndrome and specifically refers to an excess of cortisol caused by a pituitary tumor.
- *Pheochromocytoma* is a rare catecholamine-secreting adrenal tumor and is associated with significant complications, such as new-onset type 2 diabetes, cardiomyopathy, myocardial infarction, and stroke. Patients may present with a sudden-onset hypertensive emergency, often with palpitations, diaphoresis, anxiety, and headache. Symptoms may be triggered by physiologic stressors such as illness, use of certain medications or substances such as stimulants, or dietary tyramine intake, with episodes typically occurring suddenly and resolving quickly, usually within 15 minutes.
- Risk factors for adrenal emergencies can include abrupt cessation of long-term steroid therapy, damage to or surgical removal of the adrenal glands, damage to the pituitary glands, physiologic stress, infection, and blunt abdominal trauma.

Signs and Symptoms

- Primary adrenal insufficiency (Addison's disease): abdominal pain; dehydration; diarrhea; fatigue; hyperpigmentation (often to skinfolds and mucous membranes); hypoglycemia; hypotension; nausea and vomiting; unintended weight loss; weakness ▶

[🧠] **COMPLICATIONS**

Complications of adrenal emergencies include arrhythmias, altered mental status and decreased level of consciousness, hypotension, myocardial infarction, cardiomyopathy, glucose intolerance, osteoporosis, fractures, impaired immune response, prolonged wound healing, and death.

Signs and Symptoms *(continued)*

- Cushing syndrome: ecchymosis; glucose intolerance; hirsutism; hypertension; immunosuppression; lethargy; menstrual changes (irregularity, amenorrhea); sexual dysfunction (decreased libido, erectile dysfunction); striae; weight gain (truncal weight gain with abnormal fat distribution)
- Pheochromocytoma: anxiety; diaphoresis; headache; hypertension; pallor; palpitations; tachycardia

Diagnosis

Labs

- Complete blood count (CBC)
- Comprehensive metabolic panel (CMP): hypoglycemia, hyponatremia, and hyperkalemia may be found in patients with Addison's disease. Hyperglycemia, hypernatremia, and hypokalemia may be found in patients with Cushing syndrome.
- Serum cortisol level
- Urinalysis (UA)
- 24-hour urine collection: Elevated urine cortisol (50–100 µg/24 hr) is diagnostic for Cushing syndrome. Significantly elevated urine metanephrines may be indicative of pheochromocytoma.

Diagnostic Testing

- CT scan of adrenals to confirm and localize the tumor for pheochromocytoma
- Abdominal MRI
- EKG

 NURSING PEARL

Additional testing, which is valuable in the diagnosis of adrenal dysfunction (although it is more likely to be pursued by endocrinology upon admission or outpatient referral), includes adrenal antibody screening, serum adrenocorticotropic hormone (ACTH), aldosterone, and cortisol (serum or saliva) testing. An elevated ACTH and serum cortisol level may indicate Cushing syndrome. Low aldosterone with an elevated ACTH and detected adrenal antibodies may suggest Addison's disease.

Treatment

- Manage adrenal crisis with the following therapies: steroids, such as dexamethasone (see Table A.4); fluid resuscitation; vasopressors, if needed for refractory hypotension
- Search for and treat underlying cause and rule out sepsis.
- Admit patient to the hospital (often critical care) for continued monitoring and treatment.
- Treat Cushing syndrome: Lower serum cortisol with medications such as oral metyrapone (Table 9.1). Taper discontinuation of glucocorticoids secondary to long-term corticosteroid treatment. Treat electrolyte imbalances. Perform surgical intervention as required to excise pituitary tumor.
- Monitor patients with pheochromocytoma and administer medications to control blood pressure and heart rate. Surgical removal of tumor is definitive treatment. Alpha-adrenergic medications, such as phentolamine, may be used to manage symptoms before surgery (see Table 9.1).

Nursing Interventions

- Immediately assess blood glucose for any patient presenting with adrenal disease or altered mental status/decreased level of consciousness (LOC). Alert the emergency provider and follow treatment protocols for hypoglycemia, if present.
- Perform head-to-toe assessment and discuss past medical history, including any prescribed medications or recently discontinued medications.
- Assess vital signs and place patient on continuous cardiac monitoring, noting any abnormal cardiac rhythm or blood pressure. Immediately alert provider if there are signs of emergent conditions, such as adrenal crisis or hypertensive emergency.
- Apply supplemental oxygen to maintain SpO_2 greater than 94%. ▶

TABLE 9.1 Medications for Various Medical Emergencies

INDICATIONS	MECHANISM OF ACTION	CONTRAINDICATIONS, PRECAUTIONS, AND ADVERSE EFFECTS
Antihistamines (e.g., diphenhydramine)		
• Treatment of allergic reaction • Anaphylaxis	• Competitively inhibit the effect of histamine on H1 receptor sites in the GI tract, large blood vessels, and bronchial muscle, reducing symptoms of hypersensitivity such as itching and edema.	• Caution in patients regarding sedating effects; sedative properties may be amplified when taken in conjunction with other CNS depressants • Contraindicated in asthma and COPD • Certain conditions exacerbated by anticholinergic effects; use with caution in patients with conditions such as close-angle glaucoma, bladder obstruction/urinary retention. • Other adverse effects: seizures, confusion, hemolytic anemia, agranulocytosis, dermatitis, constipation, and blurred vision
Antimetabolites (e.g., hydroxyurea)		
• Treatment of abnormally shaped hemoglobin in patients with sickle cell disease	• Promote the production of hemoglobin F in sickle cell disease, decreasing the propensity of sickled cells to form clots.	• Wear gloves and use caution when handling medication; those who are pregnant or may become pregnant should not handle this medication. • Female patients must use effective contraception while taking this medication; discontinue if patient plans to become pregnant within 3 months. • May use bone marrow suppression and myelosuppression. • Live vaccines are contraindicated while taking hydroxyurea due to risk for infection.
Antithyroid agents (e.g., propylthiouracil)		
• Hyperthyroidism	• Interfere with endogenous synthesis of thyroid hormone by inhibiting incorporation of iodine into thyroid hormone precursors and inhibiting thyroxine conversion	• Agranulocytosis is rare, but is a potentially life-threatening adverse effect. • Hepatoxicity • Must be discontinued 3–4 days before beginning radioactive iodine therapy

(continued)

TABLE 9.1 Medications for Various Medical Emergencies *(continued)*

INDICATIONS	MECHANISM OF ACTION	CONTRAINDICATIONS, PRECAUTIONS, AND ADVERSE EFFECTS
Alpha-/beta-adrenergic agonists (e.g., epinephrine)		
• Hypersensitivity/anaphylaxis (IM) • Hypotension secondary to septic shock (IV) • Cardiac arrest	• Act as a nonselective alpha- and beta-adrenergic agonist to promote vasoconstriction, improve ventricular contraction, increase heart rate, and relax bronchial smooth muscle	• Concentrations of epinephrine vary depending on indication: 1:1,000 concentration is used for anaphylaxis, and 1:10,000 concentration used for cardiac indications. • Immediate IM injection of epinephrine 1 mg/mL concentration is indicated for first-line treatment of anaphylaxis; additional doses may be required. • Ensure patient is sufficiently educated regarding proper use of the epinephrine auto-injector; advise patients to always seek emergent care after using epinephrine. • Tachycardia and hypertension may occur, as well as palpitations, tremors, anxiety, and headache. • See Chapter 2 for more information regarding cardiac arrest and indications for epinephrine.
Potassium binders (e.g., kayexalate)		
• Treatment of hyperkalemia	• Bind to potassium in the GI tract to facilitate fecal elimination of excess potassium	• May alter GI drug absorption; must be administered 3 hours before or 3 hours after any other medications. • Elimination of potassium may take several hours; not an appropriate treatment of life-threatening hyperkalemia. • Use with caution in patients with hypocalcemia. • Contraindicated for patients with abnormal bowel function; will cause loose stools.
Short-acting human insulins and analogs (e.g., Humulin R)		
• Type 1 DM • Type 2 DM	• Act as endogenous insulin • Insulin stops breakdown of, and allows storage of, glucose, fat, and amino acids	• Monitor blood glucose; may cause hypoglycemia

(continued)

TABLE 9.1	Medications for Various Medical Emergencies *(continued)*	
INDICATIONS	**MECHANISM OF ACTION**	**CONTRAINDICATIONS, PRECAUTIONS, AND ADVERSE EFFECTS**
Thyroid agents (e.g., levothyroxine)		
• Hypothyroidism	• Thyroid hormone replacement acts the same as endogenous thyroid hormone	• Contraindicated in adrenal insufficiency • Use caution in patients with diabetes, hypopituitarism, and cardiac disease. • Adverse effects include anxiety, angina, tachycardia, and palpitations. • May cause alopecia.

GI, gastrointestinal; CNS, central nervous system; COPD, chronic obstructive pulmonary disease; DM, diabetes mellitus; IM, intramuscular; IV, intravenous.

Nursing Interventions *(continued)*

- Provide mechanical ventilation for patients with decreased level of consciousness (LOC) who are unable to maintain airway until condition improves; assist with endotracheal intubation and respiratory management, if needed.
- Establish intravenous (IV) access and draw blood for lab tests as ordered. Repeat laboratory draws as ordered to trend CMP.
- Administer medications, such as steroids, as ordered.
- Initiate fluid resuscitation to achieve mean arterial pressure (MAP) greater than 65 mmHg.
- Administer vasopressors if the patient remains hypotensive after fluid resuscitation.
- Prepare for central line placement.
- Monitor intake and output (I/O). Assist with 24-hour urine collection, if ordered.
- Prepare patient for admission.

Patient Education

- If diagnosed with primary adrenal insufficiency, understand the disease process and the importance of taking steroid medication as prescribed to prevent adrenal crisis. Consider wearing a medical alert bracelet or necklace after diagnosis and carry an emergency card with medications, dosages, and contact information in wallet or purse. Learn to identify triggers for addisonian crisis, recognize symptoms, and keep a hydrocortisone injection kit available in case of emergency. Seek emergency care if symptoms persist after administration of steroid injection.
- If instructed to discontinue steroid medication for the treatment of Cushing syndrome, follow medication taper instructions to limit steroid withdrawal complications.
- Monitor for signs of abnormal blood glucose levels if adrenal dysfunction is present. Demonstrate use of glucose meter for blood sugar checks, if prescribed.
- If discharged home with plans for later surgical intervention (adrenalectomy for pheochromocytoma or pituitary tumor excision for Cushing disease), monitor symptoms and follow up with specialists as instructed.
- Seek emergent care for symptoms, such as chest pain, palpitations, shortness of breath, severe headache, weakness, altered mental status, or loss of consciousness.

DIABETES MELLITUS

Overview

- *Diabetes mellitus (DM)* is a metabolic disease characterized by the inability of the body to produce and/or use insulin, resulting in inappropriate hyperglycemia and impaired glucose tolerance. *Type 1 diabetes* is caused by an autoimmune response in which the body attacks and destroys pancreatic cells that produce insulin, causing hyperglycemia. *Type 2 diabetes* occurs when the cells in the body become resistant to insulin and the pancreas cannot make enough insulin to meet the body's demands, leading to an accumulation of glucose. Blood glucose regulation is vital in maintaining homeostasis; glucose levels are expected to fluctuate within a narrow range, with normal fasting blood glucose between 70 and 110 mg/dL.

[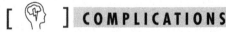] **COMPLICATIONS**

Complications of hypo- and hyperglycemia include altered mental status, decreased LOC, cerebral edema, arrhythmias, seizures, coma, and death.

[ ] **ALERT!**

Abnormal blood sugar may be the result of infection, liver disease, administration of medications such as insulin or corticosteroids, changes in diet, increased physiologic or psychological stress, pregnancy, or alcohol ingestion.

- Diabetic ketoacidosis (DKA) is a life-threatening complication of diabetes that occurs when the body produces excessive ketones secondary to the breakdown of fat in the absence of insulin needed for carbohydrate metabolism, leading to a state of intracellular dehydration. DKA can occur over hours to days and is characterized by an elevated blood glucose level (greater than 250 mg/dL), acidosis (pH less than 7.3 and serum bicarbonate less than 18 mEq/L), and ketonemia and/or ketonuria; DKA most commonly occurs in type 1 diabetes but may occur in type 2.

- Hyperosmolar hyperglycemic state (HHS) is a complication that typically occurs in patients with type 2 DM and may be defined as an extreme elevation in blood glucose (greater than 600 mg/dL) without ketosis. HHS occurs gradually over the course of several days, and patients typically experience polydipsia, polyuria, and dehydration as the body attempts to eliminate excess glucose in the urine. Table 9.2 compares presentations of HHS and DKA.

TABLE 9.2   DKA and HHS Signs and Symptoms

	HHS	DKA
Blood glucose	Greater than 600 mg/dL	• Greater than 250 mg/dL
Acidosis	• No	• Yes • Fruit-scented breath
Ketones	• Small ketonuria • Low to no ketonemia	• Positive
Respirations	• Tachypnea	• Kussmaul respirations
Onset of symptoms	• Gradual (over the course of several days)	• Rapid (over the course of hours to days)

DKA, diabetic ketoacidosis; HHS, hyperosmolar hyperglycemic state.

Signs and Symptoms

- Hypoglycemia: altered mental status/confusion; anxiety; decreased LOC/coma; diaphoresis (cool, clammy skin); headache; hunger; palpitations; tremor
- Hyperglycemia: altered mental status/confusion; blurred vision; decreased LOC/lethargy; polydipsia; polyphagia; polyuria; warm, dry skin; weight loss

Diagnosis

Labs

- Arterial blood gases (ABGs) and venous blood gases (VBGs): mild DKA—pH of 7.25 to 7.3 and serum bicarbonate of 15 to 18 mEq/L; moderate DKA—pH of 7.0 to 7.24 and serum bicarbonate of 10 to less than 15 mEq/L; severe DKA—pH of less than 7.0 and serum bicarbonate of less than 10 mEq/L
- Diagnostic criteria for DM: fasting blood glucose—nothing by mouth for at least 8 hours before the test; normal—less than 100 mg/dL; prediabetes—100 to 125 mg/dL; diabetes—126 mg/dL or higher
- Hemoglobin A1c (HbA1c) to measure average blood sugar for the past 2 to 3 months: normal—less than 5.7%; prediabetes—5.7% to 6.5%; diabetes—6.5% or higher
- Fingerstick glucose level: hypoglycemia—blood glucose of less than 70 mg/dL; hyperglycemia—blood glucose of greater than 125 mg/dL when fasting or greater than 180 mg/dL if postprandial
- Beta-hydroxybutyrate: greater than 3.8 mmol/L diagnostic for DKA in known diabetic patients
- Blood osmolality: greater than 320 mOsm/kg with severe hyperglycemia and without ketoacidosis diagnostic for HHS
- Comprehensive metabolic panel (CMP): anion gap greater than 10 mEq/L significant for acidosis
- UA: ketones and glucose found in the urine of patients with DKA
- Urine culture: patients with diabetes at increased risk for urinary tract infection due to excessive glucose in the urine

Diagnostic Testing

There are no tests specific to diagnosing abnormal blood glucose. However, the following may be helpful for differential diagnostic values:

- Head CT scan for altered mental status
- EKG if presenting with abnormal electrolyte values

Treatment

- Treat blood sugar below 70 mg/dL with the following: If the patient is alert and able to drink fluids, provide orange juice (10–15 g of simple carbohydrates). If the patient is altered and oral (PO) intake is contraindicated, give 1 amp dextrose IV (20–50 g of 50% IV dextrose solution).
- Treat elevated blood sugar (without DKA) with the following: normal saline to restore fluid balance; insulin IV or subcutaneous (SC). After a thorough examination with assessment/treatment of underlying causes, the patient may be discharged when blood sugar falls below 250 to 350 mg/dL. ▶

[ ] **NURSING PEARL**

Kussmaul respirations are a pattern of labored breathing that occurs secondary to acidosis in DKA. The nurse may observe the patient breathing deeply and rapidly, and the breath often takes on a sweet, fruity odor.

[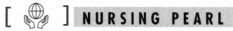] **NURSING PEARL**

Anion gap is calculated by subtracting the sum of chloride and bicarbonate from the serum sodium level. A level greater than 20 is indicative of DKA.

Treatment *(continued)*

- HHS treatment recommendations are as follows: Maintain SpO_2 greater than 96%. Monitor airway; do not use succinylcholine for intubation without first obtaining serum potassium level. Administer fluid resuscitation to maintain systolic blood pressure above 90 mmHg. Administer insulin after potassium level is corrected. Administer IV insulin because IM and SC administration is not consistently absorbed; IV insulin drip may be started.
- DKA treatment is as follows: Maintain SpO_2 greater than 96%. Administer fluid resuscitation (for adult patients, typically 10 mL/kg normal saline [NS] over 1 to 2 hours); if a severe hemodynamic compromise occurs, initiate vasopressors. Assess and correct potassium prior to insulin administration. Administer insulin (lispro SC or regular insulin IV drip). Administer bicarbonate if pH less than 7.1.
- Reassess blood sugar frequently (every half hour or per protocol).
- Assess and treat underlying causes.
- Administer dextrose-containing IV fluid once serum glucose is between 200 and 250 mg/dL.
- Admit patient if blood sugar is not controlled or if continued treatment of the underlying cause is needed.

Nursing Interventions

- Place patient on continuous pulse oximetry and cardiac monitoring; alert emergency provider to changes in vital signs or cardiac rhythm. Assist to quickly obtain an EKG for interpretation by the emergency provider.
- Perform head-to-toe assessment. Immediately assess blood glucose if the patient presents with altered mental status or decreased LOC; if patient is hypoglycemic, alert provider and immediately proceed with interventions to correct blood sugar. Review prescribed medications and discuss recent oral intake and dietary changes. If the patient is diabetic, inquire regarding any prescribed oral therapies or insulin management and inspect for an insulin pump, noting settings if present. Conduct respiratory assessment, noting any abnormal breathing pattern (such as Kussmaul respirations). Perform careful skin assessment for all patients with diabetes, noting temperature and moisture and examining for wounds/ulcerations to feet and pressure points, if applicable.
- Establish IV access and draw blood for lab tests as ordered. Patients often require additional peripheral IV access if the need for insulin infusion is anticipated. Additional serum samples should be obtained as needed to reassess CMP after interventions.
- Administer medications as prescribed. IV fluids should be administered at a controlled rate using a medication pump to prevent complications such as fluid overload, hypoglycemia, and cerebral edema. The patient should be monitored closely during insulin infusion, frequently reassessing blood glucose as ordered.
- Monitor I/O.
- Assist with transfer to critical care unit, if needed, for continued blood sugar management and close monitoring.

Patient Education

- Monitor blood glucose daily before meals, at bedtime, and when feeling symptomatic using a home blood glucose monitoring device. ▶

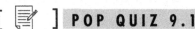 **POP QUIZ 9.1**

A patient with a history of poorly controlled diabetes arrives with Kussmaul breathing, blood sugar greater than 600 mg/dL, and decreased mental status. What does the nurse suspect this patient is suffering from?

Patient Education *(continued)*

- Know that early hypoglycemic symptoms include behavioral changes (anxiety and irritability), diaphoresis, fatigue, hunger, palpitations, and tachycardia. Late hypoglycemic symptoms include confusion, lethargy, slurred speech, seizures, and coma. Treat with 15 to 20 g of fast-acting carbohydrates (e.g., soda, fruit juice, glucose gel, or tablet) and recheck blood glucose 15 minutes later. If blood glucose values after rechecking remain below 70 mg/dL, repeat the preceding steps until blood glucose is higher than 70 mg/dL. If unable to take food or drink by mouth, use the emergency glucagon kit. Make sure family and friends know how to use the kit or know to call 911 for assistance.
- Know that hyperglycemic symptoms may manifest as altered mental status, abdominal pain, fatigue and lethargy, frequent urination, thirst, and vomiting. Treat elevated blood glucose values with a prescribed diabetes management plan. This may include increasing short-acting insulin dose or adjusting diet to manage hyperglycemia. Count carbohydrate grams and follow the recommended low-carbohydrate diet. Rotate insulin injection sites: abdomen, upper arm, thigh, lower back, hips, or buttocks. Conduct daily skin assessments at home. Engage in exercise as instructed by the provider.
- Be aware of triggers for abnormal blood sugar, such as alcohol use, steroid use, illness, or injury.
- Follow up with endocrinology as instructed for ongoing disease management.

THYROID DISORDERS

Overview

- The thyroid plays a vital role in regulating metabolism; dysfunction of the thyroid gland may be due to pituitary dysfunction, autoimmune causes, or changes in iodine intake.
- *Hyperthyroidism* (overactive thyroid) occurs when the thyroid produces abnormally low amounts of thyroid-stimulating hormone (TSH) and high amounts of thyroxine (T4). Overproduction of ▶

[ ] **COMPLICATIONS**

Complications of thyroid disorders include myxedema coma (hypothyroidism) and thyroid storm (hyperthyroidism), which may be fatal if untreated. Table 9.3 shows more information regarding signs and symptoms of myxedema coma and thyroid storm.

TABLE 9.3 Comparison of Signs and Symptoms of Myxedema Coma and Thyroid Storm

MYXEDEMA COMA	THYROID STORM
Acute psychosis	Altered mental status
Altered mental status	Arrhythmias
Arrhythmias	Coma
Bradycardia	Hyperthermia, maybe extreme
Fatigue	Nausea, vomiting, and diarrhea
Hypotension	Restless
Hypothermia	Tachycardia
Multiorgan complications	Tremors
Tongue swelling	
Weak respiratory function	

Overview (continued)

T4 results in increased metabolism and systemic vascular resistance. The most common cause of hyperthyroidism is Graves disease, an autoimmune disorder. Untreated hyperthyroidism can result in a thyroid storm, which is a hypermetabolic state causing tachycardia, increased gastrointestinal (GI) motility, diaphoresis, anxiety, and fever. Failure to identify and treat thyroid storm can result in death.

- *Hypothyroidism* (underactive thyroid) occurs when the thyroid produces abnormally low amounts of T4 and high amounts of TSH. Hypothyroidism can cause decreased cardiovascular response and metabolism and increased vascular resistance. The most common cause of hypothyroidism is an autoimmune disorder known as Hashimoto's thyroiditis. Untreated hypothyroidism (often with a precipitating stressor, such as an infection or cold exposure) can result in myxedema coma, a rare presentation of severe hypothyroidism. Patients may experience encephalopathy, fluid retention, seizures, hyponatremia, hypoglycemia, arrhythmias, cardiogenic shock, and respiratory failure.
- Female patients are at significantly higher risk for thyroid disorders. Patients are also at increased risk for thyroid disease if older than 60 years or if diagnosed with other autoimmune conditions.

Signs and Symptoms

- Hypothyroidism: bradycardia; brittle nails; cold intolerance; constipation; cognitive impairment; depression; decreased sweating; dry skin and hair; edema of the hands and face; enlarged thyroid gland; fatigue; hair loss; joint and muscle pain/cramps; lethargy; memory loss; muscle fatigue; slowed heart rate; sleep disturbances; weakness; weight gain
- Hyperthyroidism: anxiety; diarrhea; dyspnea; fatigue; fine tremors; exophthalmos; hair loss; heat intolerance; increased sweating; increased incidence of atrial fibrillation; insomnia; irritability; nervousness; palpitations; tachycardia; tremors; weight loss despite increased appetite; weakness

Diagnosis

Labs

- ABG: specific to myxedema coma to assess hypoxia and hypercapnia
- CMP: patients with hypothyroidism may experience electrolyte abnormalities such as hyponatremia and hypoglycemia
- CBC: patients with hypothyroidism may be anemic
- Thyroid blood tests (normal ranges may vary among laboratories): Hypothyroidism typically presents with high TSH, low triiodothyronine (T3), and low T4. Hyperthyroidism usually presents with low TSH, high T3, and high T4.
- UA: to rule out infection
- Urine or serum human chorionic gonadotropin (hCG) before administering medications

Diagnostic Testing

The following radiographic imaging may be used in the ED to diagnose possible causes of thyroid dysfunction:

- Chest x-ray to rule out infection
- EKG
- MRI of brain and/or orbits to assess pituitary gland and visualize Graves ophthalmopathy
- Thyroid radioactive iodine uptake and scan to establish etiology of hyperthyroidism. A high iodine uptake is consistent with Graves disease; a low uptake is consistent with subacute thyroiditis.
- Thyroid ultrasound to assess size and vasculature of thyroid

Treatment

- The following therapies may be used to treat hyperthyroidism: Beta-blockers, often propranolol, are used to manage symptoms of palpitations, anxiety, and/or tremors associated with hyperthyroidism. Radioactive iodine may be used to destroy the thyroid gland in patients with a benign or malignant overactive thyroid. If applicable, obtain a negative pregnancy test before administration. Thiourea drugs, such as propylthiouracil and methimazole (see Table 9.1), may be used to inhibit the production of thyroid hormone. Radioactive iodine-131 may be used to destroy thyroid cells. Patients may require surgical intervention for subtotal thyroidectomy.

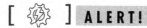

[ ] ALERT!

Aspirin is contraindicated in thyroid storm because it may increase free thyroid hormone.

- Patients in thyroid storm require supportive care and fluid resuscitation; treatment with beta-blockers (such as propranolol), antithyroid agents (such as propylthiouracil), and glucocorticoids (such as dexamethasone or hydrocortisone); and infusion of iodide Lugol's solution and sodium iodide to assist in blocking thyroid hormone production.
- Patients with hypothyroidism can be medically managed with levothyroxine (see Table 9.1), a synthetic form of T4.
- Patients presenting with signs and symptoms of myxedema coma require emergent IV administration of hydrocortisone and levothyroxine, as well as supportive measures, including intubation and mechanical ventilation (due to tongue swelling and respiratory compromise); cautious fluid resuscitation as needed; administration of vasopressors if hypotension does not improve with fluids; gradual rewarming measures (such as applying warm blankets and increasing ambient temperature).

Nursing Interventions

- Perform continuous pulse oximetry and cardiac monitoring in patients with suspected thyroid storm to alert the emergency provider to changes in vital signs or cardiac rhythm. Reassess blood pressure frequently, assisting to place the arterial line for continuous blood pressure monitoring, if needed. Assist to quickly obtain an EKG for interpretation by the emergency provider.
- Perform head-to-toe assessment. Inspect the neck, noting any thyroid gland enlargement (goiter) or thyroidectomy scar.
- Administer supplemental oxygen to maintain Spo$_2$ greater than 94%. Critically ill patients may require advanced airway; assist with placement of endotracheal tube (ETT) or manage noninvasive ventilation if needed.
- Establish IV access and draw blood for lab tests as ordered. Assist provider with central line placement if indicated; monitor site and dressing.
- Administer medications and IV fluids as prescribed.
- Titrate vasopressors, if ordered, to maintain a target MAP of 65 mmHg.
- Monitor I/O. If indicated, place a urinary catheter.
- Assist to optimize nutrition; the addition of glucose, multivitamins, thiamine, and folate may be considered to correct deficits secondary to hypermetabolism.

Patient Education

- Learn to recognize symptoms of hyperthyroidism and hypothyroidism.
- If diagnosed with hyperthyroidism, seek emergent care for signs of thyroid storm, including shortness of breath, worsening fatigue, palpitations, and tremors.
- If prescribed radioactive iodine, take special precautions during the first week to reduce radiation exposure to others. Arrange to have others take care of any small children who reside in the home. Avoid physical contact with others and maintain a distance of at least 3 feet from people younger than 18 years and people who are pregnant. Avoid sharing dishware or eating utensils with anyone in the household. Wash items immediately after use. Avoid sharing towels or washcloths with others. Flush the toilet twice after use. Rinse sinks and tubs out after use. Sleep alone. Wash towels, bed linens, and any clothing that may contact urine or sweat.
- If diagnosed with hypothyroidism, seek emergent care for symptoms of impending myxedema crisis, such as altered mental status, lethargy, or periorbital edema.
- If prescribed levothyroxine, adhere to medication instructions as prescribed: Take on an empty stomach; take at the same time every day; swallow the pill whole; do not crush it; take with 8 ounces of water.

IMMUNOLOGIC AND HEMATOLOGIC EMERGENCIES

ANEMIA

Overview

- *Anemia* indicates a reduction in the number or volume of red blood cells (RBCs) or a reduction in hemoglobin and hematocrit circulating throughout the body.
- Anemia causes a reduction in the blood's oxygen-carrying capacity, resulting in hypoxia.
- *Sickle cell anemia* is a common inherited form of anemia. Hallmark findings include crescent- or sickle-shaped RBCs that have decreased oxygen-carrying capacity and can obstruct blood flow to other areas of the body.
- Timely recognition and intervention are key to preventing severe complications.
- The three causes of anemia are shown in Table 9.4.

[🧠] **COMPLICATIONS**

Severe untreated anemia can affect patients of different age groups differently. In younger populations, impaired neurologic development may occur. In pregnancy, severe anemia can lead to early labor and premature birth. Complications for severe anemia, such as multiorgan failure or death, are most common in the older adult population due to preexisting comorbidities in this population.

TABLE 9.4 Conditions That Cause Anemia		
BLOOD LOSS	**INCREASED RBC DESTRUCTION**	**REDUCED RBC PRODUCTION**
• Acute • Chronic • May be related to coagulopathies, frequent phlebotomy, surgery, and trauma	• Damage by artificial valves • Immune destruction (e.g., hemolytic transfusion reaction) • Inherited disorders (e.g., sickle cell) • RBC membrane defects • Splenic destruction	• Aplastic anemia • Bone marrow malignancies • Chemotherapy or radiation • Chronic inflammatory conditions • Chronic kidney disease • Nutritional deficiencies • Vitamin B$_{12}$ • Folate • Iron • Stem cell transplant

RBC, red blood cell.

Signs and Symptoms

Mild anemia may be asymptomatic. Severe anemia symptoms include:

- Altered mental status
- Brittle nails
- Chest pain
- Decreased exertional tolerance
- Delayed growth
- Dizziness
- Dyspnea, especially on exertion
- Fatigue, weakness, and lethargy
- Hair loss
- Headache
- Hypotension
- Jaundice
- Koilonychia (spooning nails)
- Pallor
- Petechiae
- Pica
- Splenomegaly or hepatomegaly
- Tachycardia

Sickle cell symptoms include:

- Acute and/or chronic pain
- Dactylitis (swelling of hands and feet)
- Infections and fever
- Priapism
- Vision problems

[🤲] **NURSING PEARL**

The preparation for a stem cell transplant causes anemia, but low RBCs persist following the transplant until the new bone marrow is able to produce the appropriate number of RBCs.

[⚡] **ALERT!**

Patients with sickle cell anemia may present to the ED with sickle cell crisis triggered by infection, hypoxia, acidosis, and dehydration, among other stressors. Sickle cell crises are classified in one of three categories (Table 9.5). Identification of the appropriate phase of crisis can help guide treatment.

TABLE 9.5 Manifestations of Sickle Cell Crisis	
Hematologic aplastic crisis	• Exacerbation of anemia with a significant drop in hemoglobin • Sickled cells: have a 10–20-day half-life • Sickled cells frequently sequestered by spleen • Symptomatic anemia
Infectious crisis	• Elevated risk of secondary infections (e.g., pneumonia, bloodstream infections, meningitis, and osteomyelitis) • Sickle cell occlusions in the spleen reducing immunologic function
Vaso-occlusive crisis	• Microvascular occlusions caused by sickled red blood cells • Severe pain possible in abdomen, chest, bones, and joints • Tissue and organ ischemia

Diagnosis

Labs

- Vitamin B$_{12}$: less than 180 ng/L
- Blood films/smears: may show abnormally sized RBCs
- Bilirubin: may be greater than 1.2 mg/dL in hemolytic anemia
- CBC: hemoglobin—may be less than 13 g/dL in men and less than 12 g/dL in women; hematocrit—less than 38% in men and less than 35% in women
- Coombs test: may be positive
- Iron/ferritin: less than 30 ng/mL
- Folate: less than 2.7 ng/mL
- High-performance liquid chromatography (for sickle cell anemia)
- Reticulocyte count: less than 0.5%
- Serum iron: may be less than 60 μg/dL
- Stool, guaiac test: may be positive
- Total iron-binding capacity

Diagnostic Testing

- Chest x-ray
- CT scan
- Upper GI endoscopy (if suspected GI hemorrhage)
- Pelvic ultrasound

[🔆] **ALERT!**

If severe anemia results in angina, myocardial infarction, heart failure, or arrhythmias, cardiology should be consulted immediately for evaluation.

Treatment

- Dependent on etiology
- Aplastic anemia: bone marrow transplant
- Vitamin B$_{12}$, iron, or folate deficiency: PO or IV replacement of vitamin B$_{12}$, folate, or iron and blood transfusion
- Chronic anemia: renal failure: erythropoietin; autoimmune or rheumatologic condition: management of causative disease
- RBC destruction (hemolytic anemia): sickle cell—blood transfusions, exchange transfusions, antibiotics, opioids, hydroxyurea, IV hydration, oxygen therapy, stem cell/bone marrow transplant; medication mediated—discontinue medication immediately, if possible; disseminated intravascular coagulation (DIC)—antifibrinolytic agents; faulty mechanical valves—valve replacement treatment; persistent despite treatment—splenectomy as indicated

Nursing Interventions

- Administer oxygen, medications, IV hydration, and blood products as ordered.
- Assess airway, breathing, and circulation.
- Assess for signs of hemorrhage and occult bleeding.
- Assess for signs of infection.
- Assess for signs of respiratory distress or hypoperfusion.
- Assess for worsening signs of fatigue, weakness, and lethargy.
- Draw and monitor serial CBCs to assess RBCs, hemoglobin, and hematocrit.
- Elevate extremities to prevent swelling.
- Monitor electrolyte and blood levels after transfusion of blood products. ▶

Nursing Interventions *(continued)*

- Monitor perfusion and oxygenation.
- Position patient with head of bed (HOB) at 30 degrees or higher to improve oxygenation and perfusion.
- Prepare patient for administration of blood transfusion for severe anemia.
- Promote appropriate diet choices for deficiency anemias.
- Provide therapeutic communication and support: discuss conditions specific to anemia diagnosis and assess willingness to accept blood transfusions.

Patient Education

- After discharge, avoid extreme temperatures and changes in altitude that could cause a vaso-occlusive crisis.
- Avoid drug or drug class if hemolytic anemia is a result of medication therapy.
- Avoid smoking due to nicotine's ability to attach to hemoglobin and cause decreased oxygen delivery.
- Follow-up regularly with a hematologist (sickle cell anemia, phenylketonuria, glucose-6-phosphate dehydrogenase deficiency) for monitoring.
- If the spleen is compromised, follow infection prevention techniques: handwashing; staying up to date on vaccinations; taking prophylactic antibiotics as prescribed
- Increase iron-rich foods (e.g., legumes, red meat, seafood, and dark green leafy vegetables) in diet (for iron deficiency anemia).
- Incorporate vitamin C–containing foods (e.g., citrus fruits, and broccoli) to enhance iron absorption (for iron deficiency anemia).
- Recognize that black tarry stools and constipation may occur with iron replacement therapy.
- Recognize that fortified foods are necessary to treat vitamin B$_{12}$ deficiency.
- Self-monitor for symptoms of worsening anemia.
- Take medications and iron or vitamin supplements as indicated by the provider.

COAGULOPATHIES

Overview

- *Coagulopathy* is any alteration in baseline hematologic function, that results in impaired clot formation
- Coagulopathies can be acquired or genetic.

Signs and Symptoms

- Cyanosis
- End organ damage
- Excessive or unexplained bleeding or bruising

 COMPLICATIONS

Massive blood transfusion may cause hypothermia, acidosis, and coagulopathy, as well as a variety of electrolyte abnormalities. Be sure to monitor electrolyte levels after administration of blood products and replace electrolytes as needed. Citrate toxicity may also occur with rapid transfusion, resulting in hypocalcemia due to citrate binding to serum calcium.

[🌐] **NURSING PEARL**

Megaloblastic anemia is caused by folate deficiency, and pernicious anemia is caused by vitamin B$_{12}$ deficiency.

[🧠] **COMPLICATIONS**

Coagulopathies can result in hemorrhage or vaso-occlusive manifestations. Hemorrhagic complications range from mild bruising to stroke, hemorrhagic shock, and death. Vaso-occlusive manifestations include severe conditions such as end organ ischemia, renal dysfunction, stroke, pulmonary embolism, myocardial infarction, and death.

 COMPLICATIONS

Onset of heparin-induced thrombocytopenia (HIT) is typically 5 to 10 days after initiation of therapy; however, symptoms can begin in less than 24 hours if the patient has antibodies due to previous heparin exposure.

- Fatigue
- Jaundice
- Petechiae
- Purpura

Diagnosis
Labs
- Basic metabolic panel (BMP)
- CBC
- Coagulation studies; D-dimer; fibrinogen; prothrombin time (PT) and international normalized ratio (INR); partial thromboplastin time (PTT)
- HIV and/or hepatitis C virus tests
- Peripheral blood smear

Diagnostic Testing
- Bone marrow biopsy
- Imaging to identify potential hemorrhage, bleeding, or thrombosis: CT scan; MRI; ultrasound
- Ultrasonography of the spleen

Treatment
- Treatment is dependent on condition and severity and may include the following: blood product administration and/or clotting factor replacement; oxygen and ventilatory support; two large-bore IV lines and/or central line access; management of condition precipitating coagulopathies (if known); medications (see Table 9.1); splenectomy for certain coagulopathies
- Treatment of medication-induced coagulopathy varies by etiology (Table 9.6). Vitamin K is used for warfarin-induced coagulopathy. Treatment of HIT involves discontinuation of heparin administration and heparin-dosed agents. There is no specific antidote for platelet inhibitor-induced coagulopathy; it is treated symptomatically.

[⚡] **ALERT!**

Platelet administration for thrombotic thrombocytopenic purpura (TTP) is typically contraindicated in the absence of severe hemorrhage. In TTP, large circulating multimers of von Willebrand factor cause platelets to adhere to vessel endothelium. Due to this pathophysiology, platelet administration can lead to vaso-occlusive crisis and end organ ischemia.

TABLE 9.6 Medication-Induced Acquired Coagulopathies	
PLATELET INHIBITORS	**HEPARIN-INDUCED THROMBOCYTOPENIA**
• Agranulocytosis	• Chest pain
• Angioedema	• Chills
• Aplastic anemia	• Development of new blood clot
• Bronchospasm	• Dyspnea
• Erythema multiforme	• Ecchymosis
• Hepatic failure	• Enlargement or extension of blood clot
• Pancreatitis	• Fever
• Pancytopenia	• Hypertension
• Peptic ulcer	• Rash or sore around the injection site
• Stevens-Johnson syndrome	• Sudden onset of pain, redness, and swelling of an arm or leg
• Thrombotic thrombocytopenic purpura	• Tachycardia
	• Weakness, numbness, painful extremity movement

Nursing Interventions

- Apply supplemental oxygen if indicated.
- Assess abdomen for potential signs of retroperitoneal bleeding, such as abdominal or back pain or bruising to flanks.
- Assess airway, breathing, and circulation.
- Assess for coffee-ground emesis or black stool.
- Assess neurologic status for potential change, possibly indicative of intracranial bleed.
- Draw and monitor CBC and clotting factor laboratory trends.
- Maintain activity precautions until coagulopathy is reversed.
- Monitor for hypothermia and provide warming as indicated.
- Monitor perfusion and oxygenation.
- Monitor vital signs for changes related to hypovolemia or excessive bleeding (tachycardia, hypotension).
- Position patient with HOB at 30 degrees or higher to assist with improved oxygenation and perfusion.
- Provide therapeutic communication and support.

[ ] **NURSING PEARL**

Hypothermia in patients with coagulopathies should be monitored and treated. Warming measures should be provided as needed, such as increasing ambient temperature and applying warm blankets. Hypothermia can worsen the clinical effect of coagulopathies and increase mortality risk.

Patient Education

- Adhere to fall safety precautions by removing tripping hazards. Consider installing handrails or ramps as needed.
- Adhere to follow-up visit schedule.
- Adhere to schedule of serial blood tests to monitor coagulation levels.
- Contact provider or go to ED for severe headache, weakness, numbness, confusion, coughing or vomiting up large amounts of blood; bleeding that will not stop after 10 minutes of firm pressure or uncontrolled bleeding; bright red blood in stool; signs of occult bleeding such as black tarry stools; fall; or head injury.
- Follow activity orders based on coagulopathy levels.
- For minor bleeding wounds, hold firm pressure for 10 minutes.
- Take all medications as prescribed.

FEVER

Overview

- Fevers are a common complaint in the ED. Normal body temperature is 98.6°F (37°C); typically, patients are considered febrile if their body temperature reaches 100.4°F.
- Infection is the most likely source of fever, but noninfectious causes, such as thyroid dysfunction and drug ingestion, may also impact thermoregulatory mechanisms and lead to the development of fever.
- In certain populations, such as neutropenic patients and young children, fever may be the only sign of infection.
- Risk factors for developing a fever include infections, inflammatory conditions such as autoimmune diseases, head injuries (neurogenic fever), heat exposure, malignancies, and anything that may prompt an immune response, such as receiving immunizations (e.g., DTaP).

Signs and Symptoms

- Chills
- Dehydration
- Elevated temperature

- Flushed skin
- Headache
- Muscles aches
- Sweating
- Weakness

Diagnosis

Labs

- Blood cultures
- Cultures of CSF, wounds, urine and stool, throat, peritoneal fluid, and pleural fluid
- CBC
- CMP
- UA

Diagnostic Testing

The following imaging may be used in the ED to investigate potential sources of fever:

- X-ray
- CT
- Ultrasound

Treatment

- Antipyretics should be administered (see Table A.2).
- Antibiotics may be prescribed for suspected bacterial infections (see Table A.1).
- Neutropenic patients should be isolated and placed on neutropenic precautions to reduce the risk for infection (including using personal protective equipment and positive-pressure rooms, enforcing visitor restrictions, maintaining a clean environment, and implementing diet modifications such as eliminating fresh fruits and vegetables).
- Fluid resuscitation may be indicated. Increasing oral fluid intake may be appropriate.
- Lumbar puncture, paracentesis, or thoracentesis may be indicated to obtain cultures to investigate possible infection sources.

Nursing Interventions

- Assess vital signs, including temperature, and alert provider if fever or signs of infection are present.
- Perform head-to-toe assessment, observing for possible sources of infection. Auscultate heart and lung sounds, noting any abnormalities such as adventitious lung sounds. Inspect skin, evaluate for breakdown, and inspect wounds for drainage or erythema. Conduct GI and genitourinary (GU) assessments, noting complaints such as pain, vomiting, or changes in bowel or bladder habits to assist in identifying the cause of fever. For pediatric patients, obtain the history of present illness from caregivers and obtain an accurate weight to accurately administer weight-based antipyretic medications.
- If needed, establish IV access and draw blood for lab tests as ordered. Collect blood cultures as ordered per institutional protocol (typically, drawn from two separate sites, at least 10 minutes apart, before initiating antibiotic treatment).
- Administer medications as prescribed. Continue to reassess fever to determine the need for additional antipyretic therapy.
- If ordered, place a temperature-sensing urinary catheter to obtain a sterile urine sample and facilitate core temperature monitoring.
- Monitor for signs of worsening fever and infection, reassessing frequently for signs of sepsis and septic shock.

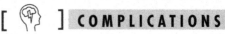

COMPLICATIONS

Febrile seizures may occur in young children (usually ages 6 months to 5 years) in response to an elevated temperature. These seizures are often tonic-clonic and typically last less than 15 minutes. Most patients suffer no long-term neurologic damage.

Patient Education

- Identify signs and symptoms of fever and learn to assess fever accurately using an oral, temporal, axillary, or rectal thermometer.
- Monitor temperature and identify appropriate pharmacologic and nonpharmacologic methods to reduce fever, including removing excess clothing and blankets and taking antipyretic medications as directed.
- Know that aspirin should not be used as an antipyretic for children due to the risk for Reye syndrome, a potentially lethal neurologic condition.
- Seek immediate care if a child younger than 3 months develops a temperature of 100.4°F (38°C) or greater. Know that the most accurate temperature assessment is obtained with a rectal thermometer.
- If neutropenic, seek immediate evaluation if fever or signs of infection occur.
- If prescribed antibiotics, finish the entire course of medications as prescribed, even if symptoms resolve.
- Return for evaluation if fever worsens or signs of worsening infection occur.

IMMUNE DEFICIENCIES

Overview

- *Immunodeficiency* is defined as an impairment in the regular function of the immune system resulting from lymphocyte, phagocyte, or system abnormalities.
- Immunodeficiency can be classified as acquired or genetic.
- Acquired immunodeficiencies: cancers (leukemia, multiple myeloma); chemotherapy and radiation; DM; graft-versus-host disease (Table 9.7); HIV and AIDS (Table 9.8); malnutrition; severe burns; steroid use; viral hepatitis
- Genetic immunodeficiencies: chronic granulomatous disease; chronic mucocutaneous candidiasis; congenital thymic aplasia (DiGeorge syndrome); hereditary angioedema; hyper-IgM syndrome; ►

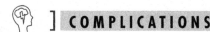

[🧠] COMPLICATIONS

Immunodeficiencies, such as HIV, leave a patient susceptible to bacterial, viral, and fungal infections. In the context of the immunocompromised patient, any infections may require emergent stabilizing care and admission to critical care to prevent multiorgan dysfunction and death.

TABLE 9.7 Types and Mechanisms of Transplant Rejection

Hyperacute rejection	• Antigen-antibody reaction within vessels of the organ • Immediate rejection in surgery or shortly thereafter • Ultimate vaso-occlusion and ischemia
Acute cellular rejection	• Occurs weeks to months after transplant • Sensitized cytotoxic T lymphocytes attack allograft • Typically reversible with immunosuppression
Chronic rejection	• May lead to organ failure and necessitate retransplantation • Not well managed with immunosuppressive medications • Slow immune-mediated response
Graft-versus-host disease	• Occurs within the first few months post transplant • Occurs when donor cells recognize host tissue as foreign • Managed with steroids and/or immunosuppressant medications

TABLE 9.8	World Health Organization Clinical Categories of HIV/AIDS
Stage 1	Asymptomatic or generalized lymphadenopathy
Stage 2	Weight loss, recurrent respiratory infections, oral lesions, fungal nail infections
Stage 3	AIDS-defining illnesses (e.g., *Pneumocystitis jiroveci* pneumonia, *Mycobacterium tuberculosis*, esophageal candidiasis) and malignancies (e.g., Kaposi sarcoma)

Overview *(continued)*

immunodeficiency with ataxia-telangiectasia; interleukin-12 receptor deficiency; leukocyte adhesion deficiency syndrome; major histocompatibility complex (MHC) deficiency (bare leukocyte syndrome); selective IgA deficiencies; severe combined immunodeficiency disease; X-linked agammaglobulinemia (Bruton disease); Wiskott-Aldrich syndrome

Signs and Symptoms

- Cough
- Diarrhea
- Fever
- Hepatomegaly
- Impaired wound healing
- Malaise and fatigue
- Opportunistic infections
- Oral lesions
- Signs of infection (may be recurrent): intrauterine infections; meningitis; otitis media; pneumonia or infections of the lung; recurrent staphylococcal infection; septicemia or bacteremia; sinus infections
- Sore throat
- Splenomegaly
- Transplant rejection: chills; dyspnea; fatigue; headache; malaise; night sweats; sore throat; pain with swallowing, voiding, or bowel movements
- Unexplained weight loss

Diagnosis

Labs

- Antibody activity: IgG antibodies: post antibody or post exposure; isohemagglutinins (IgM)
- Autoimmune studies: antinuclear antibodies; detection of anti-RBC, antiplatelet, and antineutrophil antibodies; organ-specific autoimmune antibodies
- Blood cultures to identify opportunistic infections
- Blood lymphocyte counts: total lymphocyte count; T lymphocyte counts: CD3, CD4, and CD8; B lymphocyte counts: CD19 and CD20; CD4/CD8 ratio
- BMP
- CBC with differential ▶

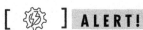 **ALERT!**

Presentation of HIV symptoms varies with stages of viral replication:

- ARS often presents with symptoms 2 to 4 weeks post exposure. Although patients may be highly infectious and likely to transmit the virus at this time, symptoms may be mild, and patients may associate symptoms with flu-like illness (fever, sore throat, headache, fatigue, muscle pain).

- About 3 to 12 weeks after contracting HIV, seroconversion is complete and serum antibodies become detectable; many patients are asymptomatic during this stage.

- Patients may remain asymptomatic for years even without treatment (period of clinical latency), although the virus continues to replicate and weaken the immune system over time; treatment with antiretroviral therapy at this time is highly effective in managing disease and decreasing likelihood of transmission.

- AIDS is the last stage of HIV infection and is marked by the development of certain illnesses associated with the immunocompromised state, such as opportunistic infection (pneumonia, tuberculosis) and certain cancers.

Labs (continued)

- Coagulation studies: factor V; fibrinogen; PT/INR
- Tumor markers
- QuantiFERON gold test

Diagnostic Testing

- Chest x-ray
- Additional radiographic imaging, such as CT and MRI, may be required to further evaluate immunocompromised patients for opportunistic infections, masses/malignancy, or other complications.

[ ] **NURSING PEARL**

CDC Categories of HIV Infection Based on CD4+

- Category 1: Greater than 500 cells/μL
- Category 2: 200 to 400 cells/μL
- Category 3: Less than 200 cells/μL

Treatment

- Bone marrow transplant
- Immunoglobulin therapy
- Management of immunosuppressive and chemotherapy agents
- Medications (see Table 9.1): antibiotics, antifungals, antivirals, immunosuppressors
- Nutritional supplements
- Treatment of secondary infections

Nursing Interventions

- Assess for signs of infection, including sepsis, hemodynamic instability, and shock.
- Place patient on neutropenic precautions. Place the patient in a private room, preferably with high-energy particular air (HEPA) filtration. Do not allow visitors or staff who exhibit signs of illness to enter. Obtain single-use equipment to use with the patient that will not be shared with other patients (e.g., stethoscopes, thermometers). All visitors and staff must perform hand hygiene and wear a surgical mask, gown, and gloves while in the room. Neutropenic precaution guidelines may vary slightly across healthcare facilities; refer to institutional guidelines.

Patient Education

- Adhere to instructions regarding ongoing disease maintenance, including following-up with specialists as needed.
- Implement neutropenic precautions as recommended by the provider. This may include frequent hand-washing, avoidance of large crowds, wearing a mask in certain public settings, and avoidance of certain raw or undercooked foods.
- Patients who have undergone transplant must maintain follow-up with their transplant team regarding long-term management, including antirejection therapy.
- If diagnosed with HIV, understand the importance of adhering to treatment plans, including methods of reducing HIV transmission and notification of HIV status to sexual partners.
- Monitor for signs of infection and seek care if symptoms, such as fever, chills, and flu-like symptoms, occur.
- Take all medications as prescribed. In addition to routine medications, some patients may be prescribed prophylactic antibiotics before certain procedures, such as dental work.

RENAL EMERGENCIES

ELECTROLYTE AND FLUID IMBALANCE

Overview

- Proper fluid and electrolyte balance is vital in maintaining homeostasis. Table 9.9 outlines potential causes of electrolyte imbalances: Conditions such as diabetes insipidus (DI) and syndrome of inappropriate antidiuretic hormone secretion (SIADH) lead to dysregulated fluid balance. DI may be classified as central or nephrogenic; central DI is caused by a decrease in the production of antidiuretic hormone (ADH), while nephrogenic DI is due to a defect in the renal tubules resulting in renal insensitivity to ADH. Patients with DI produce an excessive amount of dilute urine, leading to hypovolemia and electrolyte disturbance. SIADH is caused by excess secretion of ADH, which causes inappropriate fluid retention.
- Patients at increased risk for fluid and electrolyte imbalances include infants and young children; older adults; those with chronic conditions such as diabetes, Addison's disease, parathyroid dysfunction, and alcohol dependency; and those who take supplements (OTC or prescribed).
- Risk for electrolyte disturbance increases with any excessive GI or GU losses due to vomiting and diarrhea or increased urination due to diuretic use or renal disease.

Signs and Symptoms

- Variable and dependent on specific electrolyte abnormality (see Table 9.9)

Diagnosis

Labs

- CBC: hemoglobin and hematocrit typically elevated in dehydrated states
- CMP
- Magnesium
- Phosphorus
- UA
- Urine osmolality
- Urine sodium

Diagnostic Testing

- EKG
- Radiographic imaging, such as chest x-ray: may be indicated to assess for complications of fluid and electrolyte imbalances

 COMPLICATIONS

Complications of electrolyte and fluid imbalances include dysrhythmias, coma, and death.

 POP QUIZ 9.2

A patient presents to the ED complaining of heart palpitations, nausea, and vomiting. An EKG is obtained and is being reviewed by the provider. While listening to the report, the emergency nurse overhears that the patient started spironolactone recently after switching from furosemide. What potential electrolyte imbalance does the nurse suspect may be causing the patient's symptoms?

Treatment

- Patients with electrolyte abnormalities should be placed on continuous cardiac monitoring due to increased risk for arrythmias.
- Hypovolemia may be corrected with administration of IV fluids. Increased oral fluid intake may also be indicated.
- Patients may require diuretic medications for fluid overload.
- Fluid and electrolyte shifts caused by acute GI losses due to vomiting and diarrhea may require treatment with antiemetic and/or antidiarrheal medications, in addition to fluid volume replacement. ▶

Treatment *(continued)*

- Electrolyte abnormalities related to medications, such as diuretics, may require change in prescribed therapies if issues persist.
- Underlying chronic disease, such as congestive heart failure and chronic kidney disease, requires ongoing disease management to manage fluid balance and limit electrolyte disturbance.
- Trending of electrolytes is often indicated to evaluate response to treatment.

Nursing Interventions

- Place patient on continuous pulse oximetry and cardiac monitoring, alerting emergency provider to changes in vital signs or cardiac rhythm. Assist to quickly obtain an EKG for interpretation by the emergency provider.
- Perform head-to-toe assessment. Observe signs of fluid retention as evidenced by anasarca or peripheral edema. Perform respiratory assessment, noting any adventitious lung sounds (crackles) and orthopnea in patients with fluid overload. Note skin quality/turgor and observe mucous membranes for signs of dehydration. Evaluate for specific signs associated with electrolyte abnormalities, such as Trousseau and Chvostek signs. Conduct GI and GU assessments, noting complaints such as vomiting, diarrhea, or polyuria, which may contribute to electrolyte imbalance.
- Establish IV access and draw blood for lab tests as ordered. Repeat laboratory testing is often indicated to reassess electrolytes after treatment.
- Administer medications as prescribed. Conduct appropriate monitoring for prescribed fluid and electrolyte repletion (e.g., assessing deep tendon reflexes during magnesium infusion or monitoring for pain to IV site with potassium chloride infusion).
- Review prescribed medications and supplements with patient to ensure they are being taken appropriately.
- Discuss dietary habits and oral fluid intake to determine risk for nutritional electrolyte deficiencies.

[⚡] **ALERT!**

Patients who require treatment for abnormal sodium levels are at risk for serious complications. Central pontine myelinolysis may occur because of rapid sodium replacement in hyponatremia, and rapid overcorrection of hypernatremia may cause cerebral edema and seizures. Fluid administration, especially administration of hypotonic and hypertonic solutions, should be carefully monitored and administered using an IV pump.

Patient Education

- Discuss medications and supplements (both prescribed and OTC) with the provider prior to discharge and be aware of any associated risk for electrolyte abnormalities, dehydration, and fluid overload as applicable.
- Discuss ideal fluid intake with the provider prior to discharge and adhere to fluid restrictions as prescribed.
- Adhere to dietary changes as prescribed (e.g., increasing dietary calcium and vitamin D intake for hypocalcemia).
- Follow up as instructed for ongoing management as needed.

[📝] **POP QUIZ 9.3**

A patient arrives to the ED with multiple stab wounds. In the ED, massive transfusion protocol is initiated, and the patient receives 11 units of packed RBCs. What electrolyte imbalance may the patient experience after mass transfusion?

TABLE 9.9	Electrolyte Imbalances		
ELECTROLYTE	**CAUSES**	**SIGNS AND SYMPTOMS**	**TREATMENT**
Calcium (normal value: 8.5–10.5 mmol/L)			
Hypercalcemia	• Cancer • Hyperparathyroidism	• Arrythmias • Bone pain and fractures • Coma • Confusion • Depressed reflexes • Dehydration and polyuria • EKG changes including shortened ST and QT segments/intervals • Fatigue • Heart blocks • Hypotonicity • Lethargy • Neurologic changes including confusion, psychosis, personality changes, memory issues, stupor and coma, and nephrolithiasis • Seizures • Ventricular dysrhythmias • Weakness	• Furosemide to promote diuresis • Calcitonin • Hemodialysis if patient cannot tolerate additional fluids • High-rate IVF (0.9% NS)
Hypocalcemia	• Fluoride poisoning • Hypomagnesemia • Hypoparathyroidism • Mass transfusion of packed RBCs • Pancreatitis • Thyroid surgery • Toxic shock syndrome • Tumor lysis syndrome	• EKG changes: prolonged ST and QT segment and ventricular tachycardia • Facial paralysis • Hyperreflexia • Laryngeal spasm • Muscle cramps • Neurologic changes including anxiety, depression, or confusion • Numbness and tingling of the extremities and around the mouth • Positive Chvostek and Trousseau signs • Seizures • Tetany	Replacement with either calcium gluconate or chloride • Magnesium replacement • Vitamin D supplementation

(continued)

TABLE 9.9	Electrolyte Imbalances *(continued)*		
ELECTROLYTE	**CAUSES**	**SIGNS AND SYMPTOMS**	**TREATMENT**
Magnesium (normal value: 1.5-2.2 mg/dL)			
Hypermagnesemia	• Increased use of magnesium-containing medications such as laxatives and antacids • Renal failure	• Ataxia • Absent deep tendon reflexes • Bradyarrythmias • Cardiac arrest • Confusion • Drowsiness • Fatigue • Flushing • Muscular weakness • Paralysis • Respiratory depression/ arrest • Somnolence	• Ca^+ administration, which binds to and removes excessive Mg^+ • Dialysis • Diuresis with IVF 0.9% NS or furosemide
Hypomagnesemia	• Alcoholism • DKA, HHS • GI abnormalities • Malnutrition • Thyroid dysfunction	• Altered mental state • Cardiac arrythmias • Coma • Concurrent electrolyte/ hormonal abnormalities (hypocalcemia, hypoparathyroidism, hypokalemia) • Delirium • EKG changes, including widening QRS complex, peaked T wave, prolonged PR interval • Hyperreflexia • Muscle tremors • Ocular nystagmus • Positive Chvostek and Trousseau signs • Seizures • Tetany/tremors • Torsades de pointes	• IV magnesium sulfate max 1 g/min
Phosphate (normal value: 3–4.5 mg/dL)			
Hyperphosphatemia	• Renal failure	• Anxiety • Concurrent hypocalcemia • Deposition of calcium phosphate precipitates in skin, viscera, and blood vessels • Facial twitching • Irritability • Muscle dysfunction: tetany	• Aluminum hydroxide gel • Hypocalcemia treatments

(continued)

TABLE 9.9 Electrolyte Imbalances *(continued)*

ELECTROLYTE	CAUSES	SIGNS AND SYMPTOMS	TREATMENT
Hypophosphatemia	• Alcoholism • TPN	• CNS depression, including confusion and coma • Decreased stroke volume • Dysrhythmias • Fatigue • Lethargy • Muscle weakness, including decreased respiratory drive • Osteomalacia • Rhabdomyolysis	• Replacement with IV or PO sodium phosphate or potassium phosphate
Potassium (normal value: 3.5–5 mmol/L)			
Hyperkalemia	• Adrenal cortical insufficiency • Blood administration • Crush injuries • DKA • Potassium-sparing diuretic use • Renal failure • Rhabdomyolysis	• Bradycardia • Cardiac arrest • EKG abnormalities, including flattening or missing P waves, widening QRS complex, shortened QT interval, peaked T waves • Leg cramps • Paralysis of skeletal muscle • Respiratory failure • Weakness	• Calcium chloride, sodium bicarbonate, insulin, and glucose administration • Correction of acidosis • Dialysis • Elimination of drugs that may be the cause • Furosemide • Kayexalate
Hypokalemia	• GI loss • Malnutrition • Renal failure	• Arrythmias • Cardiac arrest • Decreased GI motility • EKG findings, including flattened T waves, emergence of the U wave, peaked P waves with increased amplitude • Fatigue • Hyperglycemia • Ileus • Muscle cramping • Paralysis • Respiratory failure • Weakness	• PO or IV potassium chloride replacement
Sodium (normal value: 135–145 mEq/L)			
Hypernatremia	• Water loss • Cushing syndrome • Hyperaldosteronism	• Altered mental status • Agitation • Coma	• Free water replacement via PO or through NG tube if tolerated enterally

(continued)

TABLE 9.9	Electrolyte Imbalances *(continued)*		
ELECTROLYTE	**CAUSES**	**SIGNS AND SYMPTOMS**	**TREATMENT**
Hypernatremia	• GI loss • DI • DKA • HHS	• Dehydration • Irritability • Lethargy • Seizures • Weakness	• IV fluid replacement with D5W or D5 ½NS if unable to tolerate orally • Slow correction to prevent cerebral edema or neurologic complications
Hyponatremia	• Fluid overload • Thiazide diuretics • SIADH • Renal failure • CHF • Cirrhosis with ascites • Hypothyroidism • Excess water intake	• Coma • Confusion • Headache • Irritability • Lethargy • Nausea • Seizures • Vomiting	• 3% NS IV • Gradual correction to prevent cerebral edema and osmotic demyelination • Sodium tablet administration and free water restriction

CHF, congestive heart failure; DI, diabetes insipidus; DKA, diabetic ketoacidosis; D5 ½NS, dextrose 5% in ½ normal saline solution; D5W, dextrose 5% in water; GI, gastrointestinal; HHS, hyperosmolar hyperglycemic state; IV, intravenous; IVF, intravenous fluid; NG, nasogastric; NS, normal saline; PO, orally; RBCs, red blood cells; SIADH, syndrome of inappropriate antidiuretic hormone secretion; TPN, total parenteral nutrition.

RENAL FAILURE

Overview

- Acute renal failure (ARF), also called acute kidney injury (AKI), is a sudden decline in glomerular filtration rate (GFR) and is typically reversible. Causes may be classified as prerenal (hypovolemia), intrarenal (nephrotoxic medications), or postrenal (strictures).

- Chronic renal failure (CRF), or chronic kidney disease (CKD), is the result of prolonged kidney damage and is irreversible. CRF leads to end-stage renal disease (ESRD), which may require peritoneal dialysis or hemodialysis.

- Complaints related to issues with dialysis access are common in the ED. Patients may present for evaluation of infection, bleeding, or clotted vascular access. Patients may also require emergent care for fluid and electrolyte abnormalities after a missed dialysis appointment. Bleeding from a fistula or graft requires direct pressure for 5 to 10 minutes; patients may seek emergency care if bleeding persists.

- Risk factors for renal disease can include hypovolemia, medications, calculi, hypertension, chronic kidney damage, DM, and infections of the kidney.

Signs and Symptoms

Renal failure affects every body system and has many symptoms of varying severity depending on the stage of disease, including:

- Altered mental status/decreased LOC
- Anemia
- Asterixis

[ ]   **ALERT!**

Chvostek sign is a twitching of the facial muscles that occurs with tapping on the facial anterior nerve. *Trousseau sign* is a carpopedal spasm that occurs while inflating a blood pressure cuff on the arm. Both signs are abnormal and may be indicative of hypocalcemia.

[ ]   **COMPLICATIONS**

Complications of renal failure can include hospitalization, electrolyte imbalances (e.g., hyperkalemia, hyperphosphatemia), rhabdomyolysis, seizures, coma, and death.

Signs and Symptoms *(continued)*

- Arrythmias
- Edema
- Ecchymosis
- Electrolyte imbalances
- Encephalopathy
- Hypertension
- Metabolic acidosis
- Nausea and vomiting
- Oliguria or anuria
- Peripheral neuropathy
- Pruritus
- Seizures
- Volume deficit or overload
- Weakness

Diagnosis

Labs

- Albumin
- Blood cultures (if infection is suspected)
- CBC
- CMP
- Creatinine clearance
- Creatine phosphokinase (CPK)
- Lactic dehydrogenase (LDH)
- Peritoneal fluid culture (if peritonitis is suspected)
- UA (if possible, to collect sample; anuria may occur in patients with renal failure)

Diagnostic Testing

- EKG
- X-ray: chest; kidneys, ureters, bladder
- Renal ultrasound
- CT scan: abdomen and pelvis; interventions may be required to prevent further renal damage if contrast must be used in emergent situations. Emergent dialysis may be indicated.

Treatment

- Identification and treatment of the underlying cause is vital in correcting renal failure.
- Early initiation of dialysis is recommended for acute and chronic renal failure. This may include hemodialysis, peritoneal dialysis, or continuous renal replacement therapy.
- Nephrotoxic agents should be avoided if possible, and medications should be dosed appropriately for patients with renal disease.
- Kidney transplant may be recommended depending on disease etiology.
- Medications should be administered. Patients may require medications to manage complications of ESRD; for example, a combination of IV sodium bicarbonate, glucose, and insulin may be used to treat hyperkalemia emergently. Blood transfusion may be necessary for anemia secondary to renal disease.
- Critically ill patients may require placement of invasive monitoring devices. ▶

[ ] **ALERT!**

AKI is diagnosed when creatinine increases by greater than or equal to 0.3 mg/dL (27 μmol/L) relative to a known baseline value within 48 hours or increases to greater than or equal to 1.5 times the known or presumed baseline value within 7 days. CKD is defined as the presence of kidney damage or decreased kidney function, as evidenced by an estimated GFR of less than 60 mL/min/1.73 m² for 3 or more months, irrespective of the cause.

[ ] **NURSING PEARL**

Stages of CKD

- Stage 1: Kidney damage with normal or slightly increased GFR (greater than 90 mL/min/1.73 m²)
- Stage 2: Mild loss in GFR (60–89 mL/min/1.73 m²)
- Stage 3: Moderate loss in GFR (30–59 mL/min/1.73 m²)
- Stage 4: Severe loss in GFR (15–29 mL/min/1.73 m²)
- Stage 5: Kidney failure (ESRD) requiring dialysis (GFR less than 15 mL/min/1.73 m²)

Treatment *(continued)*

- IV fluid resuscitation should be administered for hypovolemia.
- Urine output should be monitored.
- Nutrition should be optimized to reduce renal strain. This may include low-protein diet (0.6 to 0.8 g/kg/day); reduced sodium, potassium, and phosphate diet; and fluid restriction.

Nursing Interventions

- Obtain vital signs and place patient on continuous cardiac monitoring. Alert emergency provider to any abnormal vital signs or changes in cardiac rhythm. Assist with placement and monitoring of any invasive monitoring measures, such as an arterial line.
- Perform head-to-toe assessment, including obtaining GU history and noting dialysis schedule.
- Inspect dialysis access sites for signs of infection or bleeding. In patients receiving peritoneal dialysis, monitor for signs of peritonitis. Apply direct pressure if bleeding occurs from a vascular access site. Avoid using blood pressure cuff or tourniquet on same extremity as the dialysis access site.
- Assess arteriovenous fistula, if applicable. Auscultate for bruit and palpate for thrill. Assess skin color, pulse, and capillary refill of distal extremity.
- Monitor I/O. Place a urinary catheter, if indicated, for strict I/O.

Patient Education

- Be aware of the importance of adhering to treatment plans as prescribed. Ensure that all dialysis appointments are completed as ordered. Seek care if dialysis appointment is not completed.
- Adhere to dietary restrictions and fluid restrictions as prescribed.
- Take all medications as prescribed.
- Seek emergent evaluation if symptoms such as chest pain, shortness of breath, fluid retention (edema), or urinary retention occur.
- Avoid nephrotoxic agents (such as certain antibiotics, diuretics, contrast dye, statins, antihypertensives, benzodiazepines, and nonsteroidal anti-inflammatory drugs) unless directed by provider.
- Maintain blood sugars within target range if diabetes is present.
- Follow up with scheduled outpatient appointments, dialysis sessions, and blood draws.
- Learn about renal diet modifications, including any diet requirements with fluid restrictions, high protein, or low potassium, phosphate, and sodium.
- Self-monitor for signs of fluid overload (such as swelling in feet and ankles), worsening dyspnea, palpitations, or chest pain. Call for help if indicated.

SHOCK STATES

ANAPHYLACTIC SHOCK

Overview

- *Anaphylactic shock* is a subset of distributive shock, a state in which perfusion is compromised by a systemic vasodilatory response; other classifications of distributive shock include septic shock (see following section) and neurogenic shock (see Chapter 4).
- An *allergic reaction* is an abnormal hypersensitive response to a substance that usually does not cause harm; anaphylaxis is the most severe form of allergic reaction and can be life-threatening. Anaphylactic response involves the pulmonary, circulatory, integumentary, and central nervous systems, and symptoms may progress rapidly, causing respiratory failure and cardiac arrest.   ▶

Overview *(continued)*

- Risk factors for an allergic reaction or anaphylaxis include exposure to an allergen, a previous anaphylactic reaction, or asthma. Common causes of allergic reactions are environmental irritants such as pollen, foods such as nuts and eggs, insect bites and stings, and medications.

Signs and Symptoms

- Hives
- Difficulty swallowing
- Dyspnea
- Nausea, vomiting, and diarrhea
- Sense of impending doom
- Swollen throat
- Pale or flushed face
- Wheezing

Diagnosis

Labs

There are no laboratory tests specific to diagnosing acute allergic reaction or anaphylaxis; however, the following tests may be helpful in assessing patients with anaphylaxis:

- ABG
- CBC
- CMP

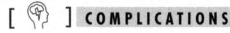 **COMPLICATIONS**

Complications of anaphylaxis include airway compromise, respiratory failure, circulatory collapse, and death.

Diagnostic Testing

There are no tests specific to diagnosing anaphylaxis and allergic reactions; however, imaging such as chest x-ray may be valuable in evaluating patients with respiratory distress or failure.

Treatment

- Continuous cardiac monitoring and pulse oximetry should be applied for all patients presenting with allergic reactions.
- Supplemental oxygen should be applied to maintain SpO_2 greater than 94%.
- Mild allergic reactions may be treated with oral or IV antihistamine medication, such as diphenhydramine (see Table 9.1). Glucocorticoids (see Table A.4) may also be used to reduce inflammation and control symptoms. Patients should be monitored for progression of symptoms, and additional medications may be required if signs of worsening reaction occur, such as facial or tongue swelling, throat or chest tightness, or airway edema.
- Patients with a history of severe allergic reactions or signs of anaphylaxis require immediate treatment with epinephrine injection to prevent respiratory compromise and anaphylactic shock. A dose of 0.01 mg/kg of epinephrine should be administered intramuscularly as soon as anaphylaxis is identified; patients should be closely monitored because an additional one to two doses may be required at 5- to 15-minute intervals to control symptoms. Administration of isotonic crystalloids is often required to support blood pressure and maintain perfusion. An infusion of IV epinephrine (typically a concentration of 1 µg/mL) may be required if symptoms are not controlled with fluids and repeated doses of IM epinephrine. Antihistamines and glucocorticoids are also indicated for management of severe allergic reactions. ▶

Treatment *(continued)*

- Patients experiencing anaphylaxis may require interventions to maintain airway if symptoms are not immediately controlled with medications. Intubation and mechanical ventilation may be indicated. If upper airway edema is severe, bedside cricothyroidotomy may be required to permit ventilation. Patients may experience refractory hypotension requiring vasopressors to maintain perfusion.

Nursing Interventions

- Immediately assess for airway patency and signs of respiratory distress. Alert emergency provider and proceed with emergent interventions if airway edema or signs of respiratory compromise are present. Administration of IM epinephrine should be prioritized for patients experiencing signs of anaphylaxis.
- Place patient on continuous cardiac monitoring and pulse oximetry and frequently reassess vital signs. Assist with placement of arterial line for continuous blood pressure monitoring, if indicated.
- Perform head-to-toe assessment with focused cardiovascular and respiratory assessments, noting any abnormal lung sound, such as stridor or wheezing.
- Apply supplemental oxygen to maintain SpO_2 greater than 94%.
- Establish IV access and administer medications as ordered.
- Continually reassess symptoms and monitor response to medications, alerting provider to any change in condition and titrating medications, such as vasopressors, as ordered.

Patient Education

- Avoid known allergens, if possible.
- Follow up with allergy specialist if referral was provided. Learn how and when to use epinephrine auto-injector. Always carry two injector epinephrine pens in case one fails to inject or if a second dose is required. Seek emergency care after injecting epinephrine.

SEPSIS AND SEPTIC SHOCK

Overview

- *Sepsis* is a systemic immune response to severe infection; this condition is associated with very high mortality rate and must be treated promptly to optimize outcomes.
- Sepsis usually occurs secondary to a bacterial infection, although more rarely the source may be viral or fungal.
- Many cases of sepsis are the result of healthcare-acquired infections.
- In 2016, the Society of Critical Care Medicine and the European Society of Intensive Care Medicine called sepsis "life-threatening organ dysfunction caused by a dysregulated host response to infection." Other changes proposed at this time included the elimination of SIRS (systemic inflammatory response syndrome) criteria for diagnosis of sepsis, elimination of the term "severe sepsis," and changes to best practice guidelines for resuscitation and antimicrobial management. SIRS criteria may still be used clinically. Criteria are as follows: temperature of less than 98.6°F (36°C) or greater than 100.4°F (38°C), heart rate greater than 90 bpm, respiration rate greater than 20 breaths/min, $PaCO_2$ less than 32 mmHg, and abnormal white blood cell (WBC) count.
- The Quick Sequential Organ Failure Assessment (qSOFA) has been recommended as a screening tool for prompt identification of sepsis. This tool quickly assigns patients a total score between 0 and 3, with a score of 2 or greater associated with high probability of extended hospitalization and death. One point is assigned for each of the following criteria: mentation (Glasgow Coma Scale score less than or equal to 14), tachypnea (greater than or equal to 22 breaths/min), and hypotension (systolic blood pressure less than 100 mmHg). ▶

Overview *(continued)*

- Patients are considered to be in septic shock if they are unable to maintain perfusion with MAP greater than 65 mmHg and lactic acid level remaining over 2 mmol/L despite adequate fluid resuscitation.
- Risk factors include age (younger than 1 year or older than 65 years), medication use (recent antibiotic use or long-term steroid administration), medical equipment use (e.g., urinary catheters, IV access devices, or surgically implanted devices), and presence of comorbid conditions, such as chronic obstructive pulmonary disease (COPD), DM, or CKD.

Signs and Symptoms

Patients may have variable symptoms depending on the source of infection and progression of disease. General symptoms that are likely to occur as sepsis progresses include the following:

- Altered mental status
- Delirium
- Delayed capillary refill (poor perfusion)
- Dyspnea
- Fever or hypothermia (temperature above 100.4°F [38°C] or below 96.8°F [36°C])
- Hypotension
- Skin changes: cold, clammy, mottled
- Tachypnea
- Tachycardia

[ ] **COMPLICATIONS**

Complications of sepsis include septic shock, multiple organ dysfunction syndrome (MODS), and death. MODS is associated with very high mortality rate and is diagnosed when organ dysfunction and/or ischemia is present in at least two organs.

Diagnosis

Labs

- ABG/VBG: PaO_2 greater than 300 mmHg significant for arterial hypoxemia.
- CBC: leukocytosis (WBC count over 12,000/μL) or leukopenia (WBC count under 4,000/μL); thrombocytopenia (platelet count less than 80,000/mm³ in critically ill septic patients).
- CMP: Hyperglycemia may occur, even in nondiabetic patients; serum creatinine typically increases by over 0.5 mg/dL in sepsis due to renal dysfunction in MODS; increased bilirubin (greater than 2–4 mg/dL) may occur due to hepatic dysfunction in MODS.
- Coagulation panel: Septic patients often develop changes in coagulation.
- Culture of suspected infection sources (blood, urine, wound, sputum, vascular access catheters).
- D-dimer: typically elevates in sepsis due to fibrinolysis.
- Lactic acid: In septic patients, lactic acid typically elevates; goal of resuscitation is often to decrease value to less than 2 mmol/L.
- Procalcitonin: Value greater than 0.5 ng/mL may be indicative of sepsis.

Diagnostic Testing

The primary diagnostic tool to screen for sepsis is careful assessment and laboratory analysis, although the following radiographic imaging may be valuable in discovering the infection source:

- CT scan of head, chest, or abdomen/pelvis (or any area of suspected infection)
- X-ray of chest or abdomen (or any area of suspected infection)
- EKG
- Ultrasound

Treatment

- The qSOFA scoring tool or institutional protocols should be used to identify patients at risk for developing sepsis.
- The Surviving Sepsis Campaign 2021 outlines interventions that should be performed once signs and symptoms of sepsis are identified. Interventions include: measurement of serum lactate level (obtain a second sample if over 2 mmol/L upon initial lab draw); obtaining blood cultures before initiating antibiotics; administration of broad-spectrum antibiotics (see Table A.1) immediately (ideally within 1 hour) if high clinical suspicion for sepsis or signs of shock are present; administration of 30 mL/kg balanced crystalloid fluids within first 3 hours of care for hypotensive patients or those with a serum lactate level of 4 mmol/L or greater; administration of vasopressors for persistent hypotension after fluid resuscitation, with a goal MAP of 65 mmHg or greater.
- Within the first 3 hours after signs of sepsis are identified, patients with signs of poor perfusion should receive at least 30 mL/kg of IV fluids (crystalloid solution such as Ringer's lactate solution recommended over NS for initial resuscitation).
- Norepinephrine is recommended as the first-line vasopressor.
- When possible, patients receiving broad-spectrum antibiotics should be transitioned to more targeted antimicrobial therapy once early culture results have been identified.
- Per guidelines, critically ill patients should be transferred to ICU within 6 hours to optimize outcomes.

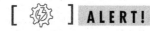

[⚡] ALERT!

Changes in coagulation that occur as sepsis progresses may lead to the development of DIC, which is often fatal.

Nursing Interventions

- Place patient on continuous pulse oximetry and cardiac monitoring, alerting emergency provider to changes in vital signs or cardiac rhythm. Reassess blood pressure frequently, assisting to place and monitor arterial line for continuous blood pressure monitoring if needed. Assist to quickly obtain an EKG for interpretation by the emergency provider.
- Perform head-to-toe assessment and assist in identifying possible sources of infection.
- Administer supplemental oxygen to maintain Spo_2 greater than 94%. Critically ill patients may require advanced airway; assist with placement of ETT or manage noninvasive ventilation if needed.
- Establish IV access and draw blood for laboratory tests as ordered. Prioritize obtaining blood cultures before administering medications. Patients with septic shock require placement of at least two large-bore peripheral IV lines initially. Administration of vasopressors up to a certain dosage should not be delayed until a central line is established. Assist provider with central line placement if indicated; monitor site and dressing.
- Administer medications and IV fluids as prescribed. Prioritize administration of antimicrobials within the first hour of care.
- Titrate vasopressors, if ordered, to maintain target MAP of 65 mmHg.
- Monitor I/O. If indicated, place urinary catheter to obtain urine sample and monitor output.
- Expedite transfer to critical care unit for continued treatment and monitoring.

Patient Education

- Recognize the signs and symptoms of sepsis. If immunocompromised, seek immediate care if signs of infection occur.
- If discharged home with vascular access devices in place, such as a peripherally inserted central catheter line or dialysis access port, adhere to instructions regarding skin care, cleansing, and dressing changes.
- Follow up as instructed for ongoing care and monitoring. Seek emergent care if signs of infection occur, such as fevers, localized erythema, or drainage from insertion site.
- Take all medications as prescribed, ensuring that any antibiotic regimen is completed as instructed to minimize antibiotic resistance.

RESOURCES

Alghamdi, M. A., Alzahrani, A. M., Alshams, H. A., Saif, M. H. A., Moafa, A. M., Alenzi, M. M., Seadawi, L. E., Ali, A. K. A., Al-Hufayyan, N. S., & Mujallid, M. F. (2021). Hyperosmolar hyperglycemic state management in the emergency department; Literature review. *Archives of Pharmacy Practice, 12*(1), 37–40. https://doi.org/10.51847/8gxTO9C75T

Almeida, S. L. (2020). Communicable diseases and organisms in the health care setting. In V. Sweet & A. Foley (Eds.), *Sheehy's emergency nursing: Principles and practice* (7th ed., pp. 186–187). Elsevier.

Atkins, R. C. (2005). The epidemiology of chronic kidney disease. *Kidney International. 67*(Suppl. 94), S14–S18. https://doi.org/10.1111/j.1523-1755.2005.09403.x

Barthel, A., Benker, G., Berens, K., Diederich, S., Manfras, B., Gruber, M., Kanczkowski, W., Kline, G., Kamvissi-Lorenz, V., Hahner, S., Beuschlein, F., Brennand, A., Boehm, B., Torpy, D., & Bornstein, S. (2019). An update on Addison's disease. *Experimental and Clinical Endocrinology & Diabetes, 127*(02/03), 165–175. https://doi.org/10.1055/a-0804-2715

Baugh, C. W., Faridi, M. K., Mueller, E. L., Camargo, C. A. Jr., & Pallin, D. J. (2019). Near-universal hospitalization of US emergency department patients with cancer and febrile neutropenia. *PloS One, 14*(5) Article, e0216835 https://doi.org/10.1371/journal.pone.0216835

Baxter, C. S. (2020). Renal and genitourinary emergencies. In V. Sweet & A. Foley (Eds.), *Sheehy's emergency nursing: Principles and practice* (7th ed., pp. 273–274). Elsevier.

Christ-Crain, M., Winzeler, B., & Refardt, J. (2021). Diagnosis and management of diabetes insipidus for the internist: An update. *Journal of Internal Medicine, 290*(1), 73–87. https://doi.org/10.1111/joim.13261

Desai, S., & Seidler, M. (2017). Metabolic and endocrine emergencies. In C. K. Stone & R. L. Humphries (Eds.), *CURRENT diagnosis & treatment: Emergency medicine* (8th ed, Chapter 43). McGraw Hill. https://accessemergencymedicine.mhmedical.com/content.aspx?bookid=2172&sectionid=165068628

Dodd, A., Hughes, A., Sargant, N., Whyte, A. F., Soar, J., & Turner, P. J. (2021). Evidence update for the treatment of anaphylaxis. *Resuscitation, 163*, 86–96. https://doi.org/10.1016/j.resuscitation.2021.04.010

Gunda, M., Bantu, S., Jakka, B., & Thudi, V. (2020, April–May). MON-LB041 Pheochromocytomal—Ilusive myriad of symptoms. *Journal of the Endocrine Society, 4*(Suppl. 1), A1023. https://doi.org/10.1210/jendso/bvaa046.2030

Gupta, A., & Moore, J. A. (2018). Tumor lysis syndrome. *JAMA Oncology, 4*(6), 895. https://doi.org/10.1001/jamaoncol.2018.0613

Kiernan, C. M., & Solórzano, C. C. (2020). Surgical approach to patients with hypercortisolism. *Gland Surgery, 9*(1), 59–68. https://doi.org/10.21037/gs.2019.12.13

Kuiper, B. (2020). Fluids, fluid replacement, electrolytes, and vascular access. In V. Sweet & A. Foley (Eds.), *Sheehy's emergency nursing: Principles and practice* (7th ed., pp. 198–201). Elsevier.

Lambert, M. P., & Gernsheimer, T. B. (2017). Clinical updates in adult immune thrombocytopenia. *Blood, 129*(21), 2829–2835.https://doi.org/10.1182/blood-2017-03-754119

Lee, S. M., & An, W. S. (2016). New clinical criteria for septic shock: Serum lactate level as new emerging vital sign. *Journal of Thoracic Disease, 8*(7), 1388–1390. https://doi.org/10.21037/jtd.2016.05.55

Levi, M. (2018). Pathogenesis and diagnosis of disseminated intravascular coagulation. *International Journal of Laboratory Hematology, 40*(Suppl. 1), 15–20. https://doi.org/10.1111/ijlh.12830

Levy, M. M., Evans, L. E., & Rhodes, A. (2018). The surviving sepsis campaign bundle: 2018 update. *Intensive Care Medicine, 44(6)*, 925–928. https://doi.org/10.1007/s00134-018-5085-0

Logee, K. (2020). Pediatric emergencies. In V. Sweet & A. Foley (Eds.), *Sheehy's emergency nursing: Principles and practice* (7th ed., pp. 570–571). Elsevier.

Mentrasti, G., Scortichini, L., Torniai, M., Giampieri, R., Morgese, F., Rinaldi, S., & Berardi, R. (2020). Syndrome of inappropriate antidiuretic hormone secretion (SIADH): Optimal management. *Therapeutics and Clinical Risk Management, 16*, 663–672. https://doi.org/10.2147/TCRM.S206066

Moore, B. J., & Torio, C. M. (2017). Acute renal failure hospitalizations, 2005–2014 [HCUP Statistical Brief #231]. Agency for Healthcare Research and Quality. https://www.hcup-us.ahrq.gov/reports/statbriefssb231-Acute-Renal-Failure-Hospitalizations.pdf

Mouri, M., & Badireddy, M. (2021). Hyperglycemia. In *StatPearls*. StatPearls Publishing. https://www.ncbi.nlm.nih.gov/books/NBK430900

Nasr, I. F. (2014). *Adrenal emergencies*. In S. C. Sherman, J. M. Weber, M. A. Schindlbeck, & R. G. Patwari (Eds.), *Clinical emergency medicine* (Chapter 69). McGraw-Hill. https://accessemergencymedicine.mhmedical.com/content.aspx?bookid=991&sectionid=55139185

Nieman, L. K. (2015). Cushing's syndrome: Update on signs, symptoms and biochemical screening. *European Journal of Endocrinology, 173*(4), M33–M38. https://doi.org/10.1530/EJE-15-0464

Pasquel, F. J., & Umpierrez, G. E. (2014). Hyperosmolar hyperglycemic state: A historic review of the clinical presentation, diagnosis, and treatment. *Diabetes Care, 37*(11), 3124–3131. https://doi.org/10.2337/dc14-0984

Peyvandi, F., Garagiola, I., & Biguzzi, E. (2016). Advances in the treatment of bleeding disorders. *Journal of Thrombosis and Haemostasis, 14*(11), 2095–2106. https://doi.org/10.1111/jth.13491

Prescribers' Digital Reference. (n.d.-a). *Adrenalin (epinephrine)* [Drug information]. https://www.pdr.net/drug-summary/Adrenalin-epinephrine-3036#10

Prescribers' Digital Reference. (n.d.-b). *Dexamethasone sodium phosphate* [Drug information]. https://www.pdr.net/drug-summary/Dexamethasone-Sodium-Phosphate-Injection--USP-10-mg-mL-dexamethasone-sodium-phosphate-1725#14

Prescribers' Drug Reference. (n.d.-c). *Humulin R (regular, human insulin (rDNA origin))* [Drug information]. https://www.pdr.net/drug-summary/Humulin-R-regular--human-insulin--rDNA-origin--2912#14

Prescribers' Drug Reference. (n.d.-d). *Hydrea (hydroxyurea)* [Drug information]. https://www.pdrnetdrug-summary/Hydrea-hydroxyurea-888#15

Prescribers' Digital Reference. (n.d.-e). *Levophed (norepinephrine bitartrate)* [Drug information]. https://www.pdr.net/drug-summary/Levophed-norepinephrine-bitartrate-868#7

Prescribers' Digital Reference. (n.d.-f). *Levothyroxine sodium* [Drug information]. https://www.pdr.netdrug-summary/Levothyroxine-Sodium-Injection-levothyroxine-sodium-3865#15

Prescribers' Digital Reference. (n.d.-g). *Propylthiouracil* [Drug information]. https://www.pdr.net/drug-summary/Propylthiouracil-propylthiouracil-787#14

Pritts, W. S. (2020). Hematologic and oncologic emergencies. In V. Sweet & A. Foley (Eds.), *Sheehy's emergency nursing: Principles and practice* (7th ed., pp. 314–318). Elsevier.

Recznik, C. T. (2020). Endocrine emergencies. In V. Sweet & A. Foley (Eds.), *Sheehy's emergency nursing: Principles and practice* (7th ed., pp. 299–308). Elsevier.

Rhodes, A., Evans, L. E., Alhazzani, W., Levy, M. M., Antonelli, M., Ferrer, R., Kumar, A., Sevransky, J. E., Sprung, C. L., Nunnally, M. E., Rochwerg, B., Rubenfeld, G. D., Angus, D. C., Annane, D., Beale, R. J., Bellinghan, G. J., Bernard, G. R., Chiche, J.-D., Coopersmith, C., . . . Dellinger, R. P. (2017). Surviving sepsis campaign: International guidelines for management of sepsis and septic shock. *Intensive Care Medicine, 43*, 304–377. https://doi.org/10.1007/s00134-017-4683-6

Shaker, M. S., Wallace, D. V., Golden, D., Oppenheimer, J., Bernstein, J. A., Campbell, R. L., Dinakar, C., Ellis, A., Greenhawt, M., Khan, D. A., Lang, D. M., Lang, E. S., Lieberman, J. A., Portnoy, J., Rank, M. A., Stukus, D. R., Wang, J., Riblet, N., Bobrownicki, A., . . . Wickham, A. (2020). Anaphylaxis—A 2020 practice parameter update, systematic review, and Grading of Recommendations, Assessment, Development and Evaluation (GRADE) analysis. *Journal of Allergy and Clinical Immunology, 145*(4), 1082–1123. https://doi.org/10.1016/j.jaci.2020.01.017

Sheikh-Ali, M., Karon, B. S., Basu, A., Kudva, Y. C., Muller, L. A., Xu, J., Schwenk, W. F., & Miles, J. M. (2008, April 1). *Can serum β-hydroxybutyrate be used to diagnose diabetic ketoacidosis? Diabetes Care, 31*(4), 643–647. https://doi.org/10.2337/dc07-1683

Simmons, J., & Pittet, J.-F. (2015, April). The coagulopathy of acute sepsis. *Current Opinion in Anaesthesiology, 28*(2), 227–236. https://doi.org/10.1097/ACO.0000000000000163

Singer, M., Deutschman, C.S., Seymour, C.W., Shankar-Hari, M., Annane, D., Bauer, M., Bellomo, R., Bernard, G. R., Chiche, J.-D., Coopersmith, C. M., Hotchkiss, R. S., Levy, M. M., Marshall, J. C., Martin, G. S., Opal, S. M., Rubenfeld, G. D., van der Poll, T., Vincent, J.-L., & Angus, D. C. (2016). The third international consensus definitions for sepsis and septic shock (sepsis-3). *Journal of the American Medical Association, 315*(8), 801–810. https://doi.org/10.1001/jama.2016.0287

Subekti, I., & Pramono, L. A. (2018, June 26). Current diagnosis and management of Graves' disease. *Acta Medica Indonesiana, 50*(2), 177–182.

Sundén-Cullberg, J., Rylance, R., Svefors, J., Norrby-Teglund, A., Björk, J., & Inghammar, M. (2017). Fever in the emergency department predicts survival of patients with severe sepsis and septic shock admitted to the ICU. *Critical Care Medicine, 45*(4), 591–599. https://doi.org/10.1097/CCM.0000000000002249

10 MAXILLOFACIAL EMERGENCIES

ACUTE VESTIBULAR DYSFUNCTION

Overview

- *Acute vestibular dysfunction* is the result of either peripheral or central disturbances that affect the body's balance system.
- An example of peripheral vestibular dysfunction, also called vestibular neuritis, is inflammation of the vestibulocochlear nerve inside the inner ear.
- An example of a central cause of vestibular dysfunction is ischemic stroke.
- *Ménière's disease* is a peripheral vestibular disorder caused by a collection of fluid to the inner ear that results in episodic vertigo, tinnitus, and hearing loss.

 COMPLICATIONS

Complications of acute vestibular dysfunction can include benign paroxysmal positional vertigo, persistent postural-perceptual dizziness, and falls.

Signs and Symptoms

- Anxiety
- Calcium deposits in the inner ear
- Disorientation
- Dizziness
- Falling
- Nausea and vomiting
- Nystagmus
- Tinnitus
- Vertigo

Diagnosis

Labs

- Complete blood count (CBC)
- Comprehensive metabolic panel (CMP)
- Urinalysis

Diagnostic Testing

- Head CT or MRI
- Physical examination, such as audiometric testing
- HINTS examination

 NURSING PEARL

HINTS examination refers to a head impulse test, evaluation of nystagmus, and a test of skew.

Treatment

- Benzodiazepines such as alprazolam, clonazepam, and lorazepam (see Table A.2)
- Medications to control symptoms: antiemetics such as metoclopramide and ondansetron
- Neurology and/or otolaryngology consult
- Physical therapy/occupational therapy consult for positional therapies such as Epley, Semont, and Foster maneuvers ▶

Treatment *(continued)*

- Ruling out of stroke
- Vestibular suppressants such as diphenhydramine and meclizine (see Table 10.1)

TABLE 10.1 Maxillofacial Common Medications		
INDICATIONS	**MECHANISM OF ACTION**	**CONTRAINDICATIONS, PRECAUTIONS, AND ADVERSE EFFECTS**
Anesthetics (let, topical cocaine hydrochloride)		
• Topical numbing	• Block the signals at the nerve endings in the skin	• Do not overuse. • Medication may cause blistering, dry skin, and hives.
Antibiotics (quinolone drops)		
• Middle ear infections	• Treat gram-negative organisms	• Medication may cause perforated eardrum, which could lead to hearing loss.
Antifibrotics (topical TXA)		
• Treatment of bleeding	• Inhibit plasminogen formation	• Medication is contraindicated in preexisting active thromboembolic disorder.
Antihistamines (diphenhydramine, meclizine)		
• Allergic rhinitis • Vertigo • Nystagmus	• Compete to bind at H1 receptor sites with free histamine	• Use caution in patients with asthma, as secretions can become thicker. • Avoid in closed-angle glaucoma and in patients with increased IOP.
Antivirals (acyclovir)		
• Treatment of herpes infections and shingles	• Inhibit viral replication	• Side effects are dizziness and drowsiness. • Medication is contraindicated for renal failure and immunocompromised patients.
Corticosteroids (fluticasone)		
• Decrease inflammation and swelling	• Bind and activate glucocorticoid receptors, decreasing activation of lipocortin	• Use caution, as the medication may weaken immune system, which may increase risk of infection.
Decongestants (oxymetazoline, pseudoephedrine)		
• Allergic rhinitis	• Cause vasoconstriction of the nasal mucosa and reduce nasal congestion	• Do not use in patients with uncontrolled hypertension, CAD, DM, closed-angle glaucoma, or hyperthyroidism.
Disease-specific immunoglobulins (HyperRAB)		
• Postexposure rabies prophylaxis	• Provide passive immunity	• Administer to infiltrate in and around wounds; remaining dose to be administered IM. • Do not administer via IV route. • Do not put the vaccine in the same arm as immunoglobulin.
Rabies vaccine (RabAvert)		
• Postexposure rabies prophylaxis	• Provides active immunity by using the rabies antigen to produce specific antibodies against rabies	• Use with caution in patients with bleeding disorders, as it is given IM. • Do not give via IV or SQ route. • Use caution in patients with egg or bovine hypersensitivity and neomycin hypersensitivity.

CAD, coronary artery disease; DM, diabetes mellitus; IM, intramuscular; IOP, intraocular pressure; IV, intravenous; LET, lidocaine/epinephrine/tetracaine; SQ, subcutaneous; TXA, tranexamic acid.

Nursing Interventions

- Administer medications to control symptoms.
- Conduct focused neurologic examination and assess stroke scale.
- Place patient on fall precautions and use standby assist.

Patient Education

- Dietary changes may help with Ménière's disease (e.g., limiting salt, caffeine, and alcohol).
- Follow up for possible vestibular rehabilitation therapy to maximize balance and central nervous system compensation for disequilibrium symptoms.
- Practice exercises to improve balance; follow up with physical therapy/occupational therapy if ordered.
- Use hearing amplification devices for hearing loss.
- Vertigo associated with stroke-like symptoms is a medical emergency; seek medical care immediately.

[ ] **POP QUIZ 10.1**

An older adult patient arrives to triage via emergency medical services with a chief complaint of a fall. The patient reports that they were walking when suddenly they felt a room-spinning sensation and fell. The patient is alert but appears disoriented. The patient is not on anticoagulation medication and did not hit their head. The patient does not have chest pain or shortness of breath. What other emergent condition should the nurse evaluate for during triage?

DENTAL CONDITIONS

Overview

- Dental pain, or odontalgia, is usually caused by dental caries.
- Children's teeth erupt from ages 6 months to 3 years.
- The Ellis classification is used to identify fractures of anterior teeth. Class I fractures involve only enamel, and teeth appear white; class II fractures go through enamel and reveal dentin; class III fractures are considered a dental emergency. They are injuries of the enamel, dentin, and pulp. Pain is significant because exposure of the nerve occurs.
- Tooth avulsion occurs when the tooth is completely removed from the socket.
- Pericoronitis occurs in erupting molars that are impacted or crowded.
- Gingivitis is a common factor in tooth loss and is a result of poor dental hygiene.
- *Ludwig's angina* is a bilateral infection of the submandibular space, which consists of two compartments in the floor of the mouth: the sublingual space and the submylohyoid (submaxillary) space. It is an aggressive, rapidly spreading dental-associated cellulitis that often arises from an infected mandibular molar tooth; this infection can be a medical emergency with the potential for airway obstruction, and it requires careful monitoring.

[ ] **COMPLICATIONS**

Complications from dental emergencies can include abscess, pulpitis, pulpal necrosis, sepsis, aspiration of teeth or tooth fragments, loss of teeth, malocclusion, facial swelling, and airway obstruction.

Signs and Symptoms

- Bleeding
- Cellulitis of the face and neck (dental abscess)
- Erythema
- Ludwig's angina: chills/fever; drooling; dysphasia; malaise; mouth pain; neck pain; swelling under the tongue; tender, "woody" induration
- Malodorous breath ▶

[⚡] **ALERT!**

A high fever in teething children should not be attributed to the erupting teeth. Other disease processes should be considered.

Signs and Symptoms (continued)

- Pain
- Purulent exudate
- Sensitivity to heat, cold, or air

Diagnosis

Labs

- Arterial blood gases (if concern for respiratory compromise)
- Blood cultures (if systemic infection is suspected)
- CBC
- Fluid culture if incision and drainage is performed

Diagnostic Testing

- Chest x-ray to assess for aspiration
- CT of the head and neck
- Maxillofacial CT
- X-ray of the neck

Treatment

- Avulsed teeth: submerged in an isotonic solution, warm milk, saline, or saliva (keeping tooth between gum and cheek); replaced within 30 minutes once exposed to air
- Incision and drainage for a dental abscess and Ludwig's angina
- Intubation or tracheostomy placement; mechanical ventilation possible for Ludwig's angina
- Medications: analgesia such as acetaminophen and nonsteroidal anti-inflammatory drugs (NSAIDs; see Table A.2); antibiotics (see Table A.1); antimicrobial mouthwash to prevent gingivitis; prophylactic tetanus shot
- Possible extraction for fractured teeth; dental consult
- Referral to dentist or oral surgeon
- Soft-food or liquid diet

Nursing Interventions

- Assess for signs of child abuse.
- Assess for signs of head trauma or other maxillofacial injuries.
- Elevate the head of the bed and suction excess secretions in patients with impaired swallowing or impaired management of oral secretions.
- Hold avulsed teeth by the crown; do not touch the bottom to avoid damaging the ligaments.
- Monitor airway patency.
- Place an avulsed tooth in milk, saline, or under the tongue of a patient who is awake and alert, if unable to reimplant immediately.

Patient Education

- Brush teeth twice daily with fluoride toothpaste to prevent tooth decay.
- Finish the entire course of oral antibiotics as prescribed.
- Floss teeth daily.
- Follow up with routine dental care.
- Wear protective mouth equipment when playing sports.

[ ] **POP QUIZ 10.2**

An adult patient arrives to the ED complaining of der pain. The patient has a history of methamphetamine and diabetes mellitus and reports not having been to dentist in years. During the assessment, the nurse reali that the patient is drooling and febrile, and the neck appe swollen on one side. What condition may this patient h and what is the priority management?

EPISTAXIS

Overview

- Bleeding in the nose can occur posteriorly or anteriorly. Anterior bleeds are the most common, are often self-limiting, and can be managed in the primary care setting. Posterior nosebleeds involve larger blood vessels (e.g., sphenopalatine artery), which can result in significant hemorrhage.
- Risk factors for epistaxis can include infections, trauma, foreign bodies, anticoagulant medication, tumors, dry air, colds, allergies, pregnancy, and clotting disorders.

[🧠] **COMPLICATIONS**

Complications of epistaxis can include excessive blood loss that requires a blood transfusion. Nausea, vomiting, and possible aspiration can also occur. If the patient is taking anticoagulant medication, reversal agents may be considered, if necessary.

Signs and Symptoms

- Blood oozing from one or both nares
- Frequent swallowing
- Hematochezia or melena from swallowed blood
- Tasting blood in the back of the mouth

Diagnosis

Labs

- CBC
- Prothrombin time (PT), partial thromboplastin time (PTT), international normalized ratio (INR)
- Type and screen

Diagnostic Testing

There are no diagnostic tests specific to diagnosing epistaxis; however, imaging may be required if epistaxis occurs secondary to trauma.

Treatment

- Adequate airway, breathing, and circulation
- Anterior bleeding source: cauterization with silver nitrate or electrocautery
- Blowing nose to remove excess blood/clots: Clinician sprays the nares with oxymetazoline to hasten hemostasis. Patient pinches the alae tightly against the septum and holds for 10 minutes.
- Consult for emergent otolaryngologic intervention
- Fluid resuscitation
- Lidocaine, epinephrine, tetracaine (LET) solution to numb gums/teeth (see Table 10.1)
- Medications and blood products, if indicated: oxymetazoline to stop bleeding in nares (see Table 10.1)
- Nasal packing to tamponade local bleeding
- Prophylactic antibiotics (see Table A.1)
- Patients with a posterior bleeding: packing with a specially developed nasal balloon catheter or a Foley catheter
- Surgical ligation of blood vessels (posterior)
- Topical cocaine hydrochloride as local anesthetic (see Table 10.1)
- Topical tranexamic acid for stopping hemorrhage (see Table 10.1)

Nursing Interventions

- Adhere to appropriate precautions (gloves, mask, eyewear, and gown) if significant hemorrhage is noted.
- Assist the patient to an upright position and tilt head forward and down.
- Encourage patient to clear secretions to reduce risk for emesis and aspiration.
- Establish intravenous (IV) access and draw blood for lab tests.
- Monitor airway patency, especially in a posterior nosebleed, and have suction accessible.
- Monitor amount of blood loss.
- Monitor for signs and symptoms of blood transfusion reaction, if indicated.
- Provide emesis basin to catch blood and expectorated clots.

Patient Education

- If nasal packing is present, monitor for signs and symptoms of toxic shock syndrome: high fever; low blood pressure; headache; rapid heartbeat; nausea and vomiting; malaise and confusion; rashes on the soles and palms; peeling of the skin.
- Remove packing for an anterior nosebleed in 48 hours.
- If a nosebleed is present, lean forward slightly and pinch the two nares together.
- Place an icepack on the bridge of the nose to create vasoconstriction in the vessels.
- Do not blow, pick, or rub the nose after a nosebleed is resolved.

FACIAL NERVE DISORDERS

Overview

- *Bell's palsy* is an acute dysfunction of the facial nerve that causes temporary paralysis on one side of the face.
- *Ramsay Hunt syndrome*, also known as herpes zoster oticus or geniculate ganglion herpes zoster, is a late complication of varicella-zoster virus infection, resulting in inflammation of the geniculate ganglion of cranial nerve VII.

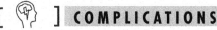 **COMPLICATIONS**

Complications of facial nerve disorders can incluc postherpetic neuralgia, eye damage, permanent heari loss, facial weakness, dry eyes, depression, and vertigo.

- Trigeminal neuralgia is characterized by recurrent brief episodes of unilateral electric shock–like pains in the distribution of one or more divisions of the fifth cranial (trigeminal) nerve that typically are triggered by innocuous stimuli. The attacks can last seconds to minutes; however, they can also cluster over a couple of hours.
- Facial nerve disorders can lead to depression related to facial pain and image changes.
- Risk factors for facial nerve disorders can include pregnancy, diabetes mellitus, upper respiratory infection, multiple sclerosis, and Lyme disease.

Signs and Symptoms

See Table 10.2.

Diagnosis

Labs

- CBC
- CMP
- Erythrocyte sedimentation rate
- Tick panel (Lyme antibody test)

TABLE 10.2 Signs and Symptoms of Facial Nerve Disorders

	BELL'S PALSY	RAMSAY HUNT SYNDROME	TRIGEMINAL NEURALGIA
Altered taste	X	X	
Burning or shocking facial pain			X
Drooling	X	X	
Facial paralysis (muscles of the upper face, forehead, and brow typically involved)	X	X	
Hearing loss		X	
Tearing	X	X	
Vesicular rash around one ear		X	

Diagnostic Testing

▪ There are no diagnostic tests specific to facial nerve disorders. However, testing is often indicated to rule out other causes.

Treatment

▪ Pain control for trigeminal neuralgia: carbamazepine; oxcarbazepine
▪ Ruling out a stroke diagnosis
▪ Surgical consult for uncontrolled cases
▪ Symptom control for Bell's palsy; corticosteroids to reduce nerve inflammation (see Table A.4); antivirals like acyclovir (see Table 10.1); artificial tears to prevent ocular trauma from dry eyes

Nursing Interventions

▪ Administer eye care (e.g., artificial tears, protective eye covering).
▪ Assess for depression.
▪ Assess for facial and oral injuries on affected side.
▪ Complete a neurologic examination.
▪ Ensure proper precautions for patients with Ramsay Hunt syndrome.
▪ Monitor for signs of aspiration.
▪ Provide aspiration precautions; use safe swallowing practices and keep patients from pocketing pills.
▪ Provide eye care.

Patient Education

▪ Follow up with provider about surgery for trigeminal neuralgia.
▪ Protect the eyes with goggles or glasses.
▪ Receive the varicella and shingles vaccines.
▪ Use an eye patch at night if there is inability to close the eye completely. Do not use tape, as it can scratch the cornea if it moves.
▪ Use artificial tears to prevent dry eyes and cornea complications.

[⚙] **ALERT!**

Ramsay Hunt syndrome is a complication of herpes zoster infection. Ensure that while the rash is present and the vesicles are not healed over into scabs, those caring for the patient are up to date on varicella vaccination. People who are pregnant, immunocompromised, or unvaccinated against varicella or who have never had varicella should not be near the patient while the open vesicles are present. Patients should not return to work until the shingles have crusted over.

FOREIGN BODIES

Overview

- Foreign bodies in the maxillofacial area can cause temporary or permanent damage.
- Caustic agents require prompt evaluation to minimize damage.

Signs and Symptoms

- Audio changes
- Edema to the nasal mucosa
- Epistaxis
- Feeling of "something moving" inside the ear or nose
- Pain
- Purulent and odorous ear and nasal discharge

[ ] COMPLICATIONS

Complications of foreign bodies in the maxillofacial area can include aspiration, infection, ruptured tympanic membrane, hearing loss, otitis media, epistaxis, sinusitis, and nasal septum perforation.

[ ] ALERT!

Button batteries and paired magnets in the nose are an emergency and require urgent removal to prevent serious damage.

Diagnosis

Labs

- CBC (if infection suspected)

Diagnostic Testing

- Otoscope examination
- X-ray if unable to visualize the object (e.g., button battery)

Treatment

- Dislodging nasal foreign bodies with caution, as they can become aspirated
- Evaluation for ruptured tympanic membrane
- Irrigation of ears, except if a ruptured tympanic membrane, soft material (e.g., cooked vegetable), button battery, or infection is suspected
- Medications (see Tables 10.1 and A.1): acetaminophen; antibiotics; local analgesia such as LET; NSAIDs.
- Positive pressure (administered by closing unaffected naris and administering positive pressure by mouth, often performed by caregiver) in attempt to dislodge the nasal foreign body
- Possible conscious sedation for extraction
- Termination of live insect using mineral oil or 2% lidocaine in the ear

Nursing Interventions

- Administer pain medications, if ordered.
- Assist in foreign body removal, if indicated.
- Monitor for aspiration.
- Monitor for signs and symptoms of infection.

Patient Education

- Do not blindly attempt to remove a foreign body.
- Do not insert foreign objects (e.g., cotton swabs) in the ears or nares.
- Keep small objects out of reach of children.

MAXILLOFACIAL INFECTIONS

Overview

- Rhinitis occurs when the mucous membranes in the nose become inflamed and swollen.
- Sinusitis occurs as a result of paranasal sinus secretions being blocked, causing inflammation of the mucosa.
- *Mastoiditis* is an infection of the mastoid bone, located just behind the ear.
- Otitis can occur externally or internally. Otitis externa (OE) involves the external ear canal and the outer ear and is also known as swimmer's ear; otitis media (OM) involves the middle ear and is usually caused by bacteria. It can cause mastoiditis.
- *Labyrinthitis* is inflammation of both branches of the vestibulocochlear nerve.

[🧠] **COMPLICATIONS**

Complications of maxillofacial infections can include orbital cellulitis, abscess, sepsis, meningitis, brain abscess, and osteomyelitis.

Signs and Symptoms

- Cough
- Difficulty smelling
- Headache
- Fatigue
- Sinus pressure
- Purulent ear drainage
- Purulent nasal drainage
- Swollen nasal mucosa
- Tinnitus (labyrinthitis)
- Vertigo (labyrinthitis)

Diagnosis

Labs

- Blood cultures
- CBC
- CMP

Diagnostic Testing

- CT scan of head and face

Treatment

- Mastoidectomy for mastoiditis
- Medications (see Tables 10.1, A.1, and A.2): antibiotics specific to infection; analgesia such as acetaminophen or NSAIDs; decongestants to assist with clearing sinusitis and rhinitis; meclizine (for labyrinthitis); topical or intranasal steroids such as fluticasone to decrease inflammation in nares or sinuses
- Warm and moist compresses for pain

Nursing Interventions

- Monitor for signs and symptoms of systemic infection.
- Obtain blood cultures prior to administering antibiotics.

Patient Education

- Do not use topical decongestants (e.g., Afrin) for more than 3 days to prevent rebound nasal congestion.
- Identify and avoid allergens that trigger allergic rhinitis.
- If chronic OM occurs, talk to the provider about myringotomy tube placement.
- Keep the ear dry if OE or OM is present.
- Use a humidifier.

PERITONSILLAR ABSCESS

Overview

- A *peritonsillar abscess* is a collection of pus located between the capsule of the palatine tonsil and the pharyngeal muscles.
- A peritonsillar abscess is often the result of untreated or chronic tonsillitis or pharyngitis and may compromise the upper airway or spread to the surrounding structures.

[🧠] **COMPLICATIONS**

Complications of a peritonsillar abscess can include aspiration, sepsis, and airway obstruction.

Signs and Symptoms

- Anxiety
- Drooling
- Dysphagia
- Fatigue
- Fever
- "Hot potato" voice (defect in voice resonance causing voice to have a muffled quality)
- Severe sore throat

Diagnosis

Labs

There are no lab tests specific to diagnosing peritonsillar abscess. However, the following may help gauge the level of illness and direct therapy:

- Blood cultures
- CBC
- CMP
- Gram stain, culture (aerobic and anerobic) of abscess fluid if a drainage procedure is performed

Diagnostic Testing

- CT soft tissue neck
- Intraoral or submandibular ultrasonography

Treatment

- Assessment of degree of upper airway obstruction
- IV fluid resuscitation
- Medications (see Tables A.1, A.2, and A.4): acetaminophen; antibiotics such as penicillin and clindamycin; NSAIDs for pain and fever control; steroids such as dexamethasone
- Needle aspiration for most patients
- Surgical consult for patients who have airway complications or are resistant to antibiotics; may require incision and drainage or abscess tonsillectomy

Nursing Interventions

- Administer medications as ordered.
- Establish IV access and draw laboratories.
- Maintain a patent airway.
- Monitor airway for swelling and upper respiratory complications, such as stridor and increasing inability to swallow.
- Monitor for signs and symptoms of airway compromise.
- Monitor for signs of sepsis.
- Perform continuous pulse oximetry.
- Place the patient in an upright position.
- Suction excess secretions.

Patient Education

- Finish the entire course of antibiotics as prescribed, even if feeling better.
- Follow a soft diet of foods like gelatin, yogurt, frozen juice pops, and ice cream.
- Maintain regular dental care.
- Seek immediate medical care if you are having difficulty breathing or swallowing.

RUPTURED TYMPANIC MEMBRANE

Overview

- A *ruptured tympanic membrane* is a tear or hole in the eardrum.
- Risk factors for a ruptured tympanic membrane can include OM, trauma, foreign body in the ear, and being a child.

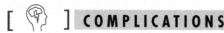 **COMPLICATIONS**

Complications of a ruptured tympanic membrane can include infection, hearing loss, and middle ear cyst.

Signs and Symptoms

- Cerebrospinal fluid (CSF) leak, possibly presenting as clear/colorless discharge from the ear (in basilar skull fractures)
- Hearing loss
- Nausea and vomiting
- Pain
- Sanguineous or purulent exudate
- Vertigo

Diagnosis

Labs

- Fluid culture

Diagnostic Testing

- Head CT and/or x-ray
- Otoscope examination
- Tuning fork evaluation

Treatment

- Medications: antibiotic drops such as quinolone, ofloxacin, and ciprofloxacin (see Table 10.1); analgesics and antipyretics such as acetaminophen and NSAIDs (see Table A.2) ▶

Treatment *(continued)*

- Small perforations of 25% or less: usually resolve within a month
- Larger injuries: may require tympanoplasty or myringoplasty

Nursing Interventions

- Do not irrigate the ears.
- Monitor for signs of a CSF leak, which is a clear/colorless drainage; may be suspected after a head injury or after brain or sinus surgery.
- Speak clearly to the patient on the unaffected side.

Patient Education

- Avoid blowing the nose.
- Do not clean the ears with cotton swabs.
- Do not submerge ears in water.
- If flying, try to equalize pressure in the ears by yawning or chewing gum to prevent a ruptured tympanic membrane.
- Keep the ears dry.
- Place petroleum jelly on the ear to repel water.
- Wear protective earplugs or earmuffs when working with loud machinery or when anticipating medium to very loud noises to prevent a ruptured tympanic membrane.

 POP QUIZ 10.3

A patient comes to the ED complaining of tinnitus aft a firecracker explosion. What condition does the nur suspect?

TEMPOROMANDIBULAR JOINT DISLOCATION

Overview

- *Temporomandibular joint (TMJ) dislocation*, or jaw dislocation, occurs when the condyle travels anteriorly along with articular eminence and becomes locked in the anterior-superior aspect of the eminence, preventing closure of the mouth.
- Risk factors for TMJ dislocation can include prolonged opening of the mouth (e.g., with dental procedures, when laughing or yawning), trauma, seizures, Ehlers-Danlos syndrome, Marfan syndrome, and dystonic reactions.

 COMPLICATIONS

Complications of TMJ dislocation can include dent problems, chronic pain, and limited jaw function.

Signs and Symptoms

- Difficulty chewing
- Drooling
- Inability to close the mouth
- Inability to talk
- Inability to swallow
- Muscle spasms
- Numbness
- Pain
- Swelling

Diagnosis

Labs

There are no lab tests specific to diagnosing TMJ dislocation.

Diagnostic Testing

- CT scan of the face to exclude mandibular fracture
- Panoramic jaw radiographs

Treatment

- Manual reduction under procedural sedation: extraoral techniques; supine position techniques; syringe method; traditional intraoral techniques; wrist pivot techniques
- Medications (see Table A.2): muscle relaxants such as diazepam; NSAIDs
- Oral and maxillofacial surgeon consult, if indicated

Nursing Interventions

- Assess and manage pain.
- Ensure safe swallowing practices; perform a swallow study.
- Gather supplies for procedural sedation.
- Monitor airway status during sedation.

Patient Education

- Avoid keeping the mouth in prolonged open or extreme positions.
- Eat a soft-food diet after the reduction.
- Follow up with an oral and maxillofacial surgeon 2 to 3 days after the reduction.

TRAUMA

Overview

- Soft-tissue trauma of the face can be from lacerations, animal or human bites, abrasions, ecchymosis from sports or motor vehicle crashes, intraoral trauma, and ear injuries. Animal bites and human bites carry large amounts of bacteria and debris. Ear trauma is classified as hematomas (e.g., cauliflower ear), lacerations, and avulsions. Facial nerve injuries can be present, but missed, due to the location of the wound and the dressings.

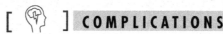 **COMPLICATIONS**

Complications of maxillofacial trauma can include airway obstruction, loss of teeth, infection, malocclusion, osteomyelitis, CSF leak, and TMJ disorders.

- Nasal fractures can cause airway obstruction and permanent disfiguration if not treated. Specifically, naso-orbital-ethmoid fractures can cause injury to the eye or the cribriform plate (resulting in a CSF leak).
- Maxillary fractures are classified as the following: Le Fort I involves the bottom third of the face and is a horizontal fracture of the maxilla. The upper teeth are moveable when the anterior teeth are grasped. Le Fort II involves the middle third of the face and is a fracture in which the pyramidal area is involved. The upper teeth are moveable, which causes movement of the nose and upper lip. Le Fort III is craniofacial disjunction in which there is total cranial facial separation. Airway obstruction is a life-threatening possibility as a result of this injury.
- Orbital blowout fractures and zygoma fractures are often found together.
- Mandibular fractures are categorized based on their location: body, condyle, angle, symphysis, coronoid, ramus, and alveolar ridge.
- Risk factors for maxillofacial trauma can include falls, motor vehicle crashes, assault, penetrating trauma, blunt trauma, and bicycle accidents.

Signs and Symptoms

- Bleeding
- Crossbite
- Diplopia
- Ecchymosis
- Edema
- Malocclusion
- Point tenderness
- Subcutaneous orbital emphysema
- Trismus

Diagnosis

Labs

- CBC
- CMP
- Lactate
- PT/PTT/INR
- Type and screen

Diagnostic Testing

- CT scan of head and face
- MRI
- Ocular ultrasound
- X-ray of the head and face

Treatment

- Assessment: broken teeth, bleeding, or bruising in the oral cavity
- Bleeding control: pressure and cold compress; head elevation 30 degrees if not contraindicated
- Closed nasal reduction
- Jaw reduction, fixation, and wiring
- Medications: antibiotics (see Table A.1); prophylactic tetanus vaccine; prophylactic rabies vaccine (see Table 10.1).
- Patent airway maintenance: possible intubation and mechanical ventilation. With airway edema: cricothyroidotomy or tracheostomy possible.
- Wound sutures, if indicated; no suture for puncture wounds

Nursing Interventions

- Apply ice to decrease swelling.
- Clean soft-tissue wounds with soap and water; be sure to flush with an adequate amount of saline.
- Ensure airway is patent; may need to use the jaw thrust maneuver if a cervical spine injury is also suspected. Do not place any nasal adjuncts, as there may be a cribriform plate fracture. This would increase the risk of penetrating the brain.
- If the patient is alert, oriented, and neurologically intact (no numbness/tingling to extremities), they may be in the upright position. Cervical collar should remain in place until cleared by imaging and the provider's order.
- Monitor for a CSF leak: halo test; beta-2-transferrin level.
- Monitor for intraocular injuries by assessing visual acuity.
- Monitor for signs of bleeding.
- Provide wound care dressing changes specific to injury; use antibiotic ointment if ordered.
- Suction excess secretions.

Patient Education

- Avoid blowing nose.
- Continue to keep wounds clean. Do not use harsh chemicals, such as hydrogen peroxide on wounds, as they are toxic to the tissues.
- Follow the prescribed medication regimen (e.g., antibiotic ointment).
- Follow up with rabies vaccinations if bit by an animal. Rabies immunoglobulin should be administered on day 0; unvaccinated immunocompetent patients should receive the rabies vaccine on days 0, 3, 7, and 14. Do not receive the vaccine and the immunoglobulin in the same anatomic location.

RESOURCES

Albrecht, M. A. (2019, October 21). Patient education: Shingles (beyond the basics). *UpToDate*. Retrieved August 1, 2021 from https://www.uptodate.com/contents/shingles-beyond-the-basics

Alotaibi, S., Haftel, A., & Wagner, N. (2021). Avulsed tooth. In *StatPearls*. StatPearls Publishing. https://www.uptodate.com/contents/shingles-beyond-the-basics

Cleveland Clinic. (n.d.). *Nosebleeds (epistaxis)*. Cleveland Clinic. https://my.clevelandclinic.org/health/diseases/13464-nosebleed-epistaxis

Dougherty, J. M., Carney, M., Hohman, M. H., & Emmady, P. D. (2022). Vestibular dysfunction. In *StatPearls*. StatPearls Publishing. https://www.ncbi.nlm.nih.gov/books/NBK558926

Furman, J. M. (2019, October 8). Patient education: Vertigo (beyond the basics). *UpToDate*. Retrieved August 1, 2021, from https://www.uptodate.com/contents/vertigo-beyond-the-basics

Galioto, N. J. (2017, April 15). Peritonsillar abscess. *American Family Physician*, 95(8), 501–506. https://www.aafp.org/afp/2017/0415/p501.html#afp20170415p501-t2

Gisness, C. M. (2020). Maxillofacial trauma. In V. Sweet & A. Foley (Eds.), *Sheehy's emergency nursing: Principles and practice*. (7th ed., pp. 424–430). Elsevier.

Mahoney, N. R. (n.d.). *Le Fort fractures*. American Academy of Ophthalmology. https://www.aao.org/oculoplastics-center/le-fort-fractures

Mayo Foundation for Medical Education and Research. (2021, October 12). *Ramsay Hunt syndrome*. Mayo Clinic. https://www.mayoclinic.org/diseases-conditions/ramsay-hunt-syndrome/symptoms-causes/syc-20351783

Mayo Foundation for Medical Education and Research. (2022, January 18). *Ruptured eardrum (perforated eardrum)*. Mayo Clinic. https://www.mayoclinic.org/diseases-conditions/ruptured-eardrum/symptoms-causes/syc-20351879

MedlinePlus. (n.d.-a). *Mastoiditis*. U.S. Department of Health and Human Services, National Institutes of Health, National Library of Medicine. https://medlineplus.gov/ency/article/001034.htm

MedlinePlus. (n.d.-b). *Broken or dislocated jaw*. U.S. Department of Health and Human Services, National Institutes of Health, National Library of Medicine. https://medlineplus.gov/ency/article/000019.htm

MedlinePlus. (n.d.-c). *Sinusitis*. U.S. Department of Health and Human Services, National Institutes of Health, National Library of Medicine. https://medlineplus.gov/ency/article/000647.htm

MedlinePlus. (n.d.-d). *Swimmer's ear*. U.S. Department of Health and Human Services, National Institutes of Health, National Library of Medicine. https://medlineplus.gov/ency/article/000622.htm

MedlinePlus. (n.d.-e). *Trigeminal neuralgia*. U.S. Department of Health and Human Services, National Institutes of Health, National Library of Medicine. https://medlineplus.gov/ency/article/000742.htm

National Institute of Neurological Disorders and Stroke. (n.d.-a). *Bell's palsy fact sheet*. U.S. Department of Health and Human Services, National Institutes of Health. https://www.ninds.nih.gov/Disorders/Patient-Caregiver-Education/Fact-Sheets/Bells-Palsy-Fact-Sheet

National Institute of Neurological Disorders and Stroke. (n.d.-b). *Herpes zoster oticus information page*. U.S. Department of Health and Human Services, National Institutes of Health. https://www.ninds.nih.gov/Disorders/All-Disorders/Herpes-Zoster-Oticus-Information-Page#disorders-r1

National Institute of Neurological Disorders and Stroke. (n.d.-c). *Trigeminal neuralgia fact sheet*. U.S. Department of Health and Human Services, National Institutes of Health. https://www.ninds.nih.gov/disorders/patient-caregiver-education/fact-sheets/trigeminal-neuralgia-fact-sheet#organization

National Institute on Deafness and Other Communication Disorders. (2017, February 13). *Ménière's disease*. U.S. Department of Health and Human Services, National Institutes of Health. https://www.nidcd.nih.gov/health/menieres-disease

Prescribers' Digital Reference. (n.d.-a). *Antivert* [Drug information]. https://www.pdr.net/drug-summary/Antivert-meclizine-hydrochloride-1822#14.

Prescribers' Digital Reference. (n.d.-b). *Boostrix (tetanus toxoid, reduced diphtheria toxoid and acellular pertussis vaccine, adsorbed)* [Drug information]. https://www.pdr.net/drug-summary/Boostrix-tetanus-toxoid--reduced-diphtheria-toxoid-and-acellular-pertussis-vaccine--adsorbed-179.5911.

Prescribers' Digital Reference. (n.d.-c). *Cefazolin sodium* [Drug information]. https://www.pdr.net/drug-summary/Cefazolin-Sodium-cefazolin-sodium-1193#10.

Prescribers' Digital Reference. (n.d.-d). *Children's Sudafed non-drowsy (pseudoephedrine hydrochloride)* [Drug information]. https://www.pdr.net/drug-summary/Children--39-s-Sudafed-Non-Drowsy-pseudoephedrine-hydrochloride-310

Prescribers' Digital Reference. (n.d.-e). *Diphenhydramine hydrochloride* [Drug information]. https://www.pdr.net/drug-summary/Diphenhydramine-Hydrochloride-diphenhydramine-hydrochloride-1140#14

Prescribers' Digital Reference. (n.d.-f). *HyperRAB S/D (rabies immune globulin (human))* [Drug information]. https://www.pdr.net/drug-summary/HyperRAB-S-D-rabies-immune-globulin--human--2985

Prescribers' Digital Reference. (n.d.-g). *Imovax (rabies vaccine)* [Drug information]. https://www.pdr.net/drug-summary/Imovax-rabies-vaccine-2914

Ronthal, M., & Greenstein, P. (2020, January 18). Patient education: Bell's palsy (beyond the basics). *UpToDate*. https://www.uptodate.com/contents/bells-palsy-beyond-the-basics

Sharma, N. K., Singh, A. K., Pandey, A., Verma, V., & Singh, S. (2015). Temporomandibular joint dislocation. *National Journal of Maxillofacial Surgery*, 6(1) 16–20. https://doi.org/10.4103/0975-5950.168212

Smith, T., Rider, J., Cen, S., & Borger, J. (2022). Vestibular neuronitis. In *StatPearls*. StatPearls Publishing. https://www.ncbi.nlm.nih.gov/books/NBK549866

Winter, J. L. (2020). Dental, ear, nose, throat, and facial emergencies. In V. Sweet & A. Foley (Eds.), *Sheehy's emergency nursing: Principles and practice* (7th ed., pp. 355–363). Elsevier.

11 OCULAR EMERGENCIES

ABRASIONS

Overview

- A *corneal abrasion* is a superficial scratch to the surface of the cornea, which is the protective layer of the eye.
- The damage exposes the nerves underneath the superficial layer of the cornea, which may cause discomfort.

Signs and Symptoms

- Blurry vision
- Pain
- Photophobia
- Redness of the eye(s)
- Sensation of something in the eye
- Tearing

Diagnosis

Labs

There are no lab tests specific to diagnosing corneal abrasions.

Diagnostic Testing

- Visual acuity examination
- Ocular examination
- Fluorescein sodium staining and cobalt light (slit lamp) examination

Treatment

- Anticholinergic eye drops such as cyclopentolate 1% (Table 11.1 for medications used for ocular emergencies)
- Topical anesthetics administered prior to fluorescein slit lamp (see Table 11.1); tetracaine 0.5%; proparacaine 0.5%.
- Topical antibiotics such as ointment or drops (see Table 11.1); sulfacetamide sodium; trimethoprim/ polymyxin B.
- Topical nonsteroidal anti-inflammatory drug (NSAID) drops (see Table 11.1); diclofenac; ketorolac
- Oral opioids or NSAIDs (see Table A.2)
- Gentle eye irrigation with a small amount of saline solution
- Consultation with ophthalmology if the abrasion is related to contact lens use or for significant symptoms
- Removal of the abrasive material

 COMPLICATIONS

Complications of corneal abrasion include infection and corneal erosion.

 ALERTS!

Corneal erosion is the loosening of the epithelium of the cornea. Treatment is similar to that for a corneal abrasion. However, surgery may be required if a corneal erosion occurs two or more times.

TABLE 11.1 Medications for Ocular Emergencies

INDICATIONS	MECHANISM OF ACTION	CONTRAINDICATIONS, PRECAUTIONS, AND ADVERSE EFFECTS
Alpha-adrenergic agonist ophthalmic drops (brimonidine ophthalmic drops)		
• Glaucoma • Intraocular hypertension	• Reduce aqueous humor production and stimulate humor outflow	• Use caution with antidepressant or Parkinson medications. • Adverse effects include change in eyesight, pain, and irritation.
Anesthetic ophthalmic drops (tetracaine ophthalmic, proparacaine ophthalmic)		
• Topical anesthetic	• Block intracellular sodium channels	• Do not use before driving or any other task that requires clear eyesight. • Adverse effects include sensitivity to light, tearing, blurred vision, throbbing pain, and bleeding.
Antibiotic ophthalmic drops and ointments (sulfacetamide, erythromycin, ciprofloxacin)		
• Treat or prevent bacterial eye infections	• Destroy bacterial cell wall	• Contraindicated in known allergy. • Discontinue and follow up with provider if symptoms are getting worse.
Anticholinergic ophthalmic drops (cyclopentolate HCL 1%, homatropine, scopolamine)		
• Dilate pupil • Control pain from ciliary spasms • Treat inflammation of the uveal tract	• Mydriatic effects by inhibiting parasympathetic pathways, causing pupil dilation • Cycloplegic effects by blocking acetylcholine and paralyzing sphincter muscles of the eye, causing pupil dilation	• Do not drive or participate in activities that require clear eyesight. • Discontinue for swelling, redness, or puffy eyelids. • Contraindicated for untreated closed-angle glaucoma. • Use caution in patients who are predisposed to IOP, such as those with Down syndrome.
Antiviral ophthalmic drops/ointment (acyclovir, trifluridine)		
• HSV of the eye • HZO	• Disrupt cellular DNA of viral infected cells and prevent its replication	• Contact provider if symptoms do not improve in 7 days. • Store in a refrigerator. • May cause blurred vision; use caution in situations where clear eyesight is needed.
Beta-blocker ophthalmic drops (timolol)		
• Open-angle glaucoma • IOP	• Decrease intraocular fluid production	• Allow 10 minutes between application of different eye drop medications • Use caution in patients with diabetes, narrow-angle glaucoma, or myasthenia gravis. • Do not use in patients with a history of asthma, COPD, or severe heart failure.
Carbonic anhydrase inhibitor ophthalmic drops (acetazolamide, methazolamide)		
• Glaucoma • Decrease IOP	• Decrease production of aqueous humor	• Side effects are burning sensation and inflammation of the conjunctivae. • Avoid with known hypersensitivity to sulfonamides.

(continued)

TABLE 11.1 Medications for Ocular Emergencies *(continued)*

INDICATIONS	MECHANISM OF ACTION	CONTRAINDICATIONS, PRECAUTIONS, AND ADVERSE EFFECTS
Nonsteroidal anti-inflammatory ophthalmic drops (diclofenac, ketorolac)		
• Reduce inflammation • Itchy eyes from allergies	• Inhibit activity of cyclooxygenase enzymes	• Monitor for development of keratitis and corneal erosion. • Use with caution in patients with diabetes. • Using beyond 14 days increases the risk of complications.
Prostaglandin analogs ophthalmic (bimatoprost)		
• Decrease IOP • Glaucoma	• Increases the uveoscleral outflow	• Contraindicated in patients with crystalloid macular edema and inflammatory glaucoma • Use at night to decrease the risk of hyperemia.
Rho kinase inhibitors ophthalmic (netarsudil)		
• Open-angle glaucoma • Ocular hypertension	• Increase fluid outflow and decrease production of aqueous humor	• Adverse effects are bloody eye, blurred vision, decreased vision, and pain. • Store bottle in refrigerator. • Wait at least 5 minutes before administering a different medication.
Corticosteroids ophthalmic (prednisolone acetate 1%, fluorometholone acetate 1%)		
• Relieve redness, itching, and swelling of the eyes	• Inhibit inflammatory signals • Decrease vasodilation and permeability of capillaries and decrease leukocyte activation	• May make existing infections worse, such as HSV or TB of the eye. • Alert prescriber to the presence of other medical conditions, such as cataracts and type 2 diabetes, as the drug can lead to or cause cataracts.

COPD, chronic obstructive pulmonary disease; HSV, herpes simplex virus; HZO, herpes zoster ophthalmicus; IOP, intraocular pressure; TB tuberculosis.

Nursing Interventions

- Administer medications as ordered to control pain and prevent infection.
- Gather equipment for slit lamp testing, including fluorescein strips and topical anesthetic.
- Irrigate the eyes if requested by the provider.
- Monitor for signs and symptoms of infection: redness, pus-like drainage, changes in vision, and photosensitivity.
- Perform visual acuity examination on arrival.

Patient Education

- Wear safety goggles when participating in activities during which abrasive material may come in contact with the eye.
- Do not aggressively rub the eyes.
- Keep fingernails short to prevent accidental injury to the cornea.
- Ensure proper hand hygiene prior to touching the eyes, such as when inserting or removing contact lenses.

BURNS

Overview

- Ocular or periorbital burns can threaten the vision. Timely treatment is critical.
- Ocular burns may be a result of exposure to chemical agents, radiation, or close contact with heat/flames (thermal burns).
- Chemical burns to the eye are a true ophthalmic emergency; timely treatment is important to prevent long-term damage. Any chemical can cause ocular damage, but strong alkaline or acidic injuries have the potential for permanent long-term complications. Injury from acids disrupts the pH, causing protein coagulation that creates a barrier to protect deeper layers, which makes the eye appear white and opaque. Strong alkaline substances may penetrate deeper into the cornea and anterior segment, raising intraocular pressures, which often causes permanent damage. The normal pH of ocular fluid is 7.0 to 7.3, with a goal of 7.5 after chemical exposure.
- Thermal burns often injure only the skin around the eye and usually avoid the globe. Eyelid contracture can occur, which can distort vision and prevent complete closure of the eye.
- Ultraviolet radiation burns (e.g., "arc flash") are extremely painful and can decrease visual acuity.
- Infrared burns can be the result of a laser pointed directly at the eye, causing a hole in the macula.

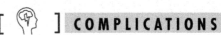

COMPLICATIONS

Complications of ocular burns include severe pain, eyelid contractures, infection, and vision loss.

POP QUIZ 11.1

A patient presents to the ED after having drain cleaner splashed into the eyes. Airway, breathing, circulation, and vital signs are intact and within normal limits. What interventions will the nurse anticipate?

Signs and Symptoms

- Impaired vision
- Pain
- Redness of the eye(s)
- Tearing

Diagnosis

Labs

There are no lab tests specific to diagnosing ocular burns.

Diagnostic Testing

- Visual acuity test
- Slit lamp examination
- pH test

Treatment

- Administer prophylactic broad-spectrum ophthalmic antibiotic drops or ointment (see Table 11.1): erythromycin, ciprofloxacin.
- Decrease intraocular pressure (IOP; see Table 11.1): methazolamide, diamox.
- Control pain and ciliary spasm with anticholinergic drops (see Table 11.1): homatropine drops, scopolamine ophthalmic drops.
- Administer corticosteroid drops (see Table 11.1): prednisone acetate 1%, fluorometholone acetate 1%.
- Administer oral opiates and NSAIDs for pain (see Table A.2).
- Administer tetanus vaccine.
- Flush chemicals, testing pH before and after.

Nursing Interventions

- Remove any powder chemicals that may be present.
- Test eye pH.
- Assess and manage pain as ordered prior to flushing.
- Assist with ocular irrigation. To flush, use a large syringe with normal saline at room temperature. Open the eyelids; use a retractor if needed; slowly syringe the fluid onto the eye from no more than 5 cm away on the front surface under the lower and upper eyelids. Have the patient move their eye in all directions while flushing.
- Use one of the following alternative methods to irrigate the eyes in the case of chemical burns: If eye wash station is available, use it for flushing. Spike a large bag of normal saline and connect the end of the intravenous tubing to a nasal cannula line; then place the nasal cannula on the bridge of the nose, turn the head toward the injured side, and run fluids wide open while draining into an emesis basin.
- Perform visual acuity examination with the Snellen chart.

Patient Education

- Wear protective lenses or a helmet when performing activities that can produce a bright light (e.g., welding).
- Wear sunglasses or protective lenses when participating in activities that may have a glare (e.g., boating, skiing).
- Limit exposure to UV lights to prevent periorbital burns. Use protective eyewear if using a tanning bed.
- Avoid looking directly at lasers.

FOREIGN BODIES

Overview

- Metallic objects can leave a rust ring if left in the conjunctiva or cornea longer than 12 hours.
- Intraocular foreign bodies are typically small and require a thorough examination to locate. They are often associated with a globe rupture.

[🧠] **COMPLICATIONS**

Complications of ocular foreign bodies include infection, corneal abrasion, and vision loss.

Signs and Symptoms

- Eye itching
- Eye pain
- Redness of the eye(s)
- Decreased visual acuity

Diagnosis

Labs

There are no lab tests specific to diagnosing foreign bodies.

Diagnostic Testing

- Visual acuity examination
- Ocular examination
- Ocular ultrasound
- Ocular CT
- Fluorescein sodium staining and cobalt light (slit lamp) examination

Treatment

- Pain control
- Topical proparacaine 0.5% (see Table 11.1)
- Opioids and NSAIDs (see Table A.2)
- Tetanus vaccine
- Antibiotics such as erythromycin ointment or drops to prevent infection (see Table 11.1)
- Removal of the foreign body if on the cornea
- Irrigation of the eye to flush out the foreign body, if indicated
- Use of a moistened cotton swab to remove the foreign body, if visualized by the provider
- Consult with an ophthalmologist to treat intraocular foreign bodies or globe penetration.

Nursing Interventions

- Apply analgesic eye drops prior to removal of foreign body if it is adhered to the cornea.
- Assist with ocular irrigation. To flush, use a large syringe with normal saline at room temperature. Open the eyelids; use a retractor if needed. Use an emesis basin to collect flushed fluids. Have the patient turn their head toward the eye being flushed; slowly syringe the fluid onto the eye from no more than 5 cm away on the front surface under the lower and upper eyelids. Have the patient move their eye in all directions while flushing.
- Perform visual acuity examination with the Snellen chart after irrigation.

Patient Education

- Do not rub the eyes if a foreign body is suspected.
- Use protective lenses when participating in activities or work that can cause a possible ocular foreign body (e.g., grinding metal, biking).
- Ensure proper hand hygiene prior to placement and removal of contact lenses.
- Do not try to remove a foreign body yourself; go to the ED to avoid further complications.

GLAUCOMA

Overview

- *Glaucoma* is an umbrella term for diseases that damage the optic nerve, usually because of increased IOP.
- Open-angle glaucoma is the result of an occluded or dysfunctional trabecular meshwork, which causes the buildup of fluid, increasing IOP on the optic nerve and leading to damage over time.
- Acute-angle closure glaucoma is an ocular emergency that results from a rapid increase in IOP due to outflow obstruction of aqueous humor. Often, the major factor is the structural anatomy of the anterior chamber, leading to a shallower angle between the iris and the cornea.

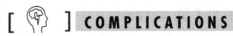 **COMPLICATIONS**

Complications of glaucoma include permanent vision loss and blindness.

Signs and Symptoms

- Blind spots (open-angle glaucoma)
- Vision loss and light halos (acute-angle closure glaucoma)
- Headache
- Eye pain
- Redness of the eyes
- Nausea and vomiting

Diagnosis

Labs

There are no lab tests specific to diagnosing glaucoma.

Diagnostic Testing

- Confocal scanning laser ophthalmoscopy
- Dilated-eye examination
- Gonioscopy
- Funduscopic examination
- Optical coherence tomography
- Visual acuity examination

Treatment

- Medications to decrease ocular pressure
- Prostaglandin analogs such as bimatoprost to increase fluid drainage (see Table 11.1)
- Beta-blocker eye drops such as timolol to decrease fluid production (see Table 11.1)
- Alpha agonists such as brimonidine to decrease fluid production and increase drainage (see Table 11.1)
- Carbonic anhydrase inhibitor such as dorzolamide to decrease production of intraocular fluid (see Table 11.1)
- Rho kinase inhibitors such as netarsudil to increase drainage (see Table 11.1)
- Systemic medications to decrease IOP with mannitol
- Pain medication such as acetaminophen and NSAIDs (see Table A.2)
- Antiemetics such as ondansetron to prevent vomiting, which increases IOP
- Urgent ophthalmic consultation for acute blockage, which is an ophthalmic emergency because vision loss and blindness may occur quickly
- Drainage tubes
- Filtering surgery
- Laser peripheral iridotomy for acute-angle closure glaucoma

Nursing Interventions

- Administer medications to decrease IOP.
- Instill eye drops.
- Reduce IOP by elevating the head of bed (HOB) or use a wedge pillow to raise the patient's head 20 degrees.
- Consult for surgery.

Patient Education

- Participate in routine eye examinations.
- Use eye drops as prescribed to reduce IOP.
- Be aware that vision loss from glaucoma is permanent and will require lifelong treatment and monitoring.
- Know that laser surgery may be an option to reduce pressure.
- Limit activities that increase IOP, such as ingesting caffeine, drinking large quantities of fluid at one time, and sleeping excessively.
- Avoid inverted exercises and those that increase pressure in the head, such as sit-ups.
- Remove tripping hazards and use large-screen electronic devices.

INFECTIONS

Overview

- Eye infections can affect any part of the eye, with the potential for serious complications such as permanent vision loss.
- Structures around the eye may become infected. Periorbital and orbital cellulitis cause impaired extraocular movement. Hordeolum, or a stye, involves an infection of the Zeis or Moll gland of the eyelashes. *Chalazion* is a lump inside the eyelid caused by an infected oil gland.
- Various tissues of the eye itself may become infected. *Endophthalmitis* is an infection of the tissues of the globe. *Conjunctivitis*, or pink eye, is the most common eye infection and is usually easy to treat. *Keratitis* is inflammation of the cornea caused by infection, injury, or wearing contact lenses for too long. *Keratoconjunctivitis* is inflammation of the cornea and conjunctiva. *Uveitis* is inflammation inside the eye, pertaining to the iris, ciliary body, and choroid. *Iritis*, also known as anterior uveitis, is inflammation of the iris.
- Herpes simplex virus (HSV) infection typically presents unilaterally and may include the eyelids, conjunctiva, and cornea.
- Herpes zoster ophthalmicus (HZO) is defined as viral involvement of the ophthalmic division (cranial nerve [CN] VI) of the trigeminal nerve (CN V). It occurs due to the reactivation of the latent varicella-zoster virus, a variation of herpes zoster that can cause ocular complications and requires urgent treatment.

Signs and Symptoms

- Redness
- Pain
- Burning
- Swelling
- Photophobia
- Purulent exudate
- Decreased vision
- Foreign body sensation
- Floaters in the vision (uveitis)

Diagnosis

Labs

- Blood cultures
- Complete blood count (CBC; if concern for systemic infection)
- Wound cultures

Diagnostic Testing

- Visual acuity test
- Fluorescein staining test
- Funduscopic examination

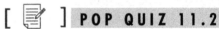

COMPLICATIONS

Complications of ocular infections include sepsis, vision loss, and blindness.

POP QUIZ 11.2

The nurse is assessing a patient who is complaining of a new-onset rash on the face. The patient reports being under a lot of stress lately and complains that the rash is itchy and draining to the left side of the face, nose, and eyelid. The patient has significant pain and photosensitivity to the left eye. Which infectious disease does the emergency nurse suspect?

NURSING PEARL

Cutaneous lesions on the tip of the nose (Hutchinson's sign) predict a high likelihood of ocular involvement during an HZO flare-up.

Treatment

- Medication management is specific to the condition.
- Orbital and periorbital cellulitis are treated with antibiotics (see Table A.1): Amoxicillin by mouth or cefotaxime IV. A significant infection may require surgery to drain abscess.
- Endophthalmitis is initially treated with broad-spectrum antibiotics, such as vancomycin and ceftazidime, that are injected directly into the vitreous (see Table 11.1).
- Bacterial conjunctivitis may be treated with antibiotic drops or ointments, such as erythromycin and moxifloxacin (see Table 11.1).
- Bacterial keratitis is treated with tobramycin, cefazolin, or vancomycin eye drops (see Table 11.1).
- Keratoconjunctivitis is treated by avoiding triggers and using artificial tears or topical corticosteroids (see Table 11.1).
- Uveitis is often treated with the following (see Table 11.1): corticosteroid eye drops; local anesthetic eye drops, such as proparacaine; mydriatic eye drops such as tropicamide; antibiotic eye drops.
- Iritis medications are used to control pain and infection: corticosteroid eye drops, such as prednisolone (see Table 11.1); antibiotic ointment or eye drops (see Table 11.1); anticholinergics (to block pain and light sensitivity; see Table 11.1); acetaminophen and NSAIDs (see Table A.2).
- HSV is treated with the following antiviral mediations (see Table 11.1): acyclovir oral or eye ointment; trifluorothymidine eye drops.
- HZO is treated with the following (see Table 11.1): antivirals such as acyclovir within 72 hours of onset; topical broad-spectrum antibiotics; cycloplegics if iritis is present; opiates for pain control (see Table A.2).
- Hordeolum should be treated with warm compresses and possible incision and drainage (I&D).
- Chalazions are treated with steroids or surgical incision and curettage.
- Ophthalmology consult and possible surgical intervention may be indicated based on condition.

Nursing Interventions

- Monitor for signs of a systemic infection.
- Administer warm compresses as indicated.
- Administer condition-specific medications and wait the appropriate time between applications of eye drops.
- Perform visual acuity examination with Snellen chart.

Patient Education

- Do not squeeze or pop abscesses; this can worsen the infection and spread the disease.
- Ensure proper and regular hand hygiene to avoid conjunctivitis.
- Obtain the shingles vaccine, if applicable, to prevent herpes zoster ophthalmicus.
- Pink eye is contagious, so avoid sharing pillowcases, towels, and other personal items.
- Take medications as prescribed, and follow up with a provider for worsening symptoms.
- Use proper technique for administering eye drops or ointment. Wash hands; for ointment, pull the lower lid away from the eye and lay a half-inch ribbon of ointment in the pocket of the lower lid. For eye drops, place the prescribed number of drops on the lower eyeball; blink eye a few times; wipe off excess ointment or tearing.

RETINAL ARTERY OCCLUSION

Overview

- There are two types of retinal artery occlusion: Central retinal artery occlusion (CRAO) is the sudden blockage of the central retinal artery, causing retinal ischemia and hypoperfusion, rapidly progressive cellular damage, and vision loss. Branch retinal artery occlusion (BRAO) is the blockage of small arteries that branch off the central artery, leading to partial vision loss.
- Timely diagnosis and treatment are essential to dislodge or lyse the offending embolus or thrombus in order to avoid irreversible retinal damage and blindness.

Signs and Symptoms

- Sudden, painless vision loss
- Loss of peripheral vision
- Vision changes
- Blind spots

Diagnosis

Labs

- Laboratory tests are necessary to assist in the exclusion of a cerebrovascular accident or transient ischemic attack: CBC, comprehensive metabolic profile (CMP), prothrombin time/international normalized ratio (PT/INR), partial thromboplastin time (PTT), point-of-care glucose, C-reactive protein, and erythrocyte sedimentation rate.

Diagnostic Testing

- Dilated-eye examination: A "cherry red" spot will be present in the macula with the surrounding retina appearing white, related to ischemia.
- Fluorescein angiography
- IOP examination
- Visual acuity examination
- Carotid ultrasound
- Echocardiogram
- Head CT without contrast (to rule out stroke)

Treatment

- No consensus about optimal treatment; goal is to restore retinal perfusion/oxygenation as soon as possible
- Immediate digital ocular massage to induce oscillations of IOP and dislodge the offending thrombus
- IOP reduction with acetazolamide (see Table 11.1), mannitol, topical timolol (see Table 11.1), or anterior chamber paracentesis (often recommended in conjunction with digital ocular massage)
- Hyperventilation into a paper bag or inhaled 10% carbon dioxide to induce respiratory acidosis and vasodilation
- Supplemental oxygen
- Thrombolytics to break up a clot
- Consultation with neurology and completion of a stroke workup

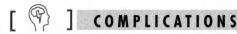 **COMPLICATIONS**

Complications of CRAO include temporary or permanent vision loss. It is a medical emergency. Patients with a CRAO have an increased risk of stroke in the first 4 weeks after the CRAO event.

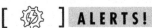 **POP QUIZ 11.3**

A patient arrives at the ED complaining of sudden blindness to the left eye and denies pain. What does the nurse suspect is happening to the patient, and what test will be ordered to rule out a stroke?

ALERTS!

Retinal circulation must be reestablished within 90 minutes to prevent permanent vision loss.

Nursing Interventions

- Anticipate and prepare for a rapid head CT.
- Obtain a thorough history, with time of onset and description of symptoms.
- Perform a neurologic examination and National Institutes of Health stroke scale.
- Assist patient with hyperventilating into a bag if indicated.
- Provide supplemental oxygen if ordered.
- Administer thrombolytics and closely monitor for signs of bleeding.

Patient Education

- Know the signs and symptoms of a stroke and when to call for help.
- Quit smoking, if applicable.
- Maintain routine follow up for diabetes mellitus, hypertension, and coronary artery disease.
- Know that vision loss may be permanent.

RETINAL DETACHMENT

Overview

- *Retinal detachment* is displacement of the retina from the back of the eye. It is considered a medical emergency.
- Retinal detachment is caused by the separation of two layers of the retina.

Signs and Symptoms

- Floaters in the eye
- Visualization of a "curtain falling" across the field of vision
- Flashes of light in one or both eyes

Diagnosis

Labs

There are no lab tests specific to diagnosing retinal detachment.

Diagnostic Testing

- Dilated-eye examination
- Ocular ultrasound

Treatment

- Cryopexy: freeze treatment to prevent the growth of abnormal retinal tissue
- Laser surgery

Nursing Interventions

- If a patient is suspected of having a retinal detachment in triage, expedite treatment.
- Assess for other ocular trauma.

Patient Education

- Recognize the signs and symptoms of retinal detachment.
- Seek medical attention immediately if retinal detachment is suspected.

[ ] **COMPLICATIONS**

Complications of retinal detachment include vision loss; it is a time-sensitive emergency and requires immediate medical attention.

TRAUMA

Overview

- The eye may receive blunt trauma, such as from a direct hit by a baseball or a fist, which may fracture the orbital and damage the eye.
- The orbit holds the eye in place. Significant force may cause the following types of fracture: A blowout fracture includes the floor or inner wall of the socket and can pinch muscles of the eyes, making them unable to rotate. An orbital rim fracture affects the outer-edge rim. Often with these injuries, there is damage to the optic nerve. An orbital floor fracture occurs when the rim is pushed back, forcing the bones of the eye socket to push down. It may affect the muscles and nerves, reducing eye movement.
- A tear in the iris or pupil may cause hyphema. It is often the result of a direct blow and may be mistaken for a subconjunctival hemorrhage, which is a painless broken blood vessel.
- An impaled object, such as an ice pick, may rupture the globe, causing significant bleeding that may lead to shock.
- Corneal abrasions are painful and involve epithelial damage to the cornea, creating a foreign body sensation. They are commonly seen with prolonged contact lens use or as a result of small particles like sand in the eye.

Signs and Symptoms

Table 11.2 shows signs and symptoms of eye trauma.

[🧠] **COMPLICATIONS**

Complications of ocular trauma include rebleeding, vision loss, loss of the eye, orbital compartment syndrome, and infection.

[🌐] **NURSING PEARL**

Do not mistake "raccoon eyes" for a sign of direct trauma to the eyes. They are a result of a basal skull fracture, which may accompany major head trauma.

[⚡] **ALERTS!**

Periorbital fat and extraocular muscles may become entrapped in a blowout fracture, which can lead to lateral gaze dysfunction and may require surgery.

TABLE 11.2 Signs and Symptoms of Eye Trauma

CONDITION	SIGNS AND SYMPTOMS
Corneal abrasion	Photophobia
	Redness
	Significant pain
Globe rupture	Decreased vision
	Irregular contour of globe
	Teardrop pupil
	Hyphema
Orbital floor fracture	Blurred vision
Orbital rim fracture	Bulging or sunken eyeballs
Blowout fracture	Difficulty moving eye
	Diplopia
	Facial numbness
	Periorbital ecchymosis and swelling
Subconjunctival hemorrhage	No pain
	No vision changes
	Red patch to the sclera

Diagnosis

Labs

There are no lab tests specific to diagnosing ocular trauma.

Diagnostic Testing

- CT scan (head, orbital, maxillofacial)
- Fluorescein staining (check for positive Seidel sign for globe rupture)
- MRI
- Visual acuity examination

Treatment

- Stabilize airway, breathing, and circulation.
- Control hemorrhage.
- Stabilize impaled objects and cover both eyes.
- Blunt trauma, if benign, resolves within 2 to 3 weeks. Apply cold packs to reduce swelling.
- Orbital fractures that affect the movement, function, or placement of the eye may require surgical intervention.
- Hyphemas may require medication to control swelling and IOP (see Table 11.1).
- Subconjunctival hemorrhages resolve within 2 to 3 weeks without intervention.
- Pain control, such as analgesic eye drops and oral medications, should be administered (see Table A.2).
- Small foreign bodies like sand particles may require saline irrigation.
- Oculoplastic surgery such as eyelid and tear duct repair may be used for periorbital wounds.

Nursing Interventions

- Monitor airway and apply cervical spine precautions for any major facial trauma. Control bleeding, stabilize any impaled objects in place, and cover both eyes with bulky dressing to decrease consensual movement.
- Keep the HOB elevated at 30 to 45 degrees.
- Apply cold pack for subconjunctival hemorrhages.
- Keep patient without oral intake (NPO) if surgery is expected.
- Do not irrigate the eye if globe rupture is suspected.
- Perform wound care for periorbital wounds.
- Give a prophylactic tetanus shot.

Patient Education

- Do not perform vigorous activity if a hyphema is present to prevent rebleeding.
- Do not strain to have a bowel movement or aggressively blow the nose to prevent increasing IOP.
- Follow up with an ophthalmologist.

RESOURCES

American Society of Retina Specialists. (n.d). *Retinal artery occlusion*. https://www.asrs.org/patients/retinal-diseases/32/retinal-artery-occlusion

Boyd, K. (2022). *Corneal abrasion and erosion*. American Academy of Ophthalmology. https://www.aao.org/eye-health/diseases/what-is-corneal-abrasion

Gappy, C., & Archer, S. M. (n.d.). Orbital cellulitis. *UpToDate*. https://www.uptodate.com/contents/orbital-cellulitis

Gudgel, D. T. (n.d.). *Eye pressure*. American Academy of Ophthalmology. https://www.aao.org/eye-health/anato my/eye-pressure

Harvard Medical School. (2019, March 22). *Foreign body in eye*. Harvard Health Publishing. https://www.health.harvard.edu/a_to_z/foreign-body-in-eye-a-to-z

Knoop, K. J., & Palma, J. K. (2021). Corneal abrasion. In K. J. Knoop, L. B. Stack, A. B. Storrow A.B, & R. Thurman (Eds.), *The atlas of emergency medicine* (5th ed.). McGraw Hill. https://accessemergencymedicine.mhmedical.com/content.aspx?bookid=2969&sectionid=250455847

Lazarus, R. (2021). *Retinal artery occlusion*. Optometrists network. https://www.optometrists.org/general -practice-optometry/guide-to-eye-conditions/guide-to-retinal-diseases/retinal-artery-occlusion

Mayo Foundation for Medical Education and Research. (2019, November 13). *Iritis*. Mayo Clinic. https://www.mayoclinic.org/diseases-conditions/iritis/symptoms-causes/syc-20354961

Mayo Foundation for Medical Education and Research. (2022a). *Glaucoma: Diagnosis & treatment*. Mayo Clinic. https://www.mayoclinic.org/diseases-conditions/glaucoma/diagnosis-treatment/drc-20372846

Mayo Foundation for Medical Education and Research. (2022b). *Glaucoma : Symptoms & causes*. Mayo Clinic. https://www.mayoclinic.org/diseases-conditions/glaucoma/symptoms-causes/syc-20372839

National Eye Institute. (n.d.-a). *Corneal conditions*. U.S. Department of Health and Human Services, National Institutes of Health. https://www.nei.nih.gov/learn-about-eye-health/eye-conditions-and-diseases/corneal-conditions

National Eye Institute. (n.d.-b). *Glaucoma*. U.S. Department of Health and Human Services, National Institutes of Health. https://www.nei.nih.gov/learn-about-eye-health/eye-conditions-and-diseases/glaucoma

National Eye Institute. (n.d.-c). *Uveitis*. U.S. Department of Health and Human Services, National Institutes of Health. https://www.nei.nih.gov/learn-about-eye-health/eye-conditions-and-diseases/uveitis#section-id-1096

National Eye Institute. (2020, December 18). *Retinal detachment*. U.S. Department of Health and Human Services, National Institutes of Health. https://www.nei.nih.gov/learn-about-eye-health/eye-conditions-and-diseases/retinal-detachment

Prescribers' Drug Reference. (n.d.-a). *Bion tears (dextran 70/hypromellose)* [Drug information]. https://www.pdr.net/drug-summary/Bion-Tears-dextran-70-hypromellose-1712#5

Prescribers' Drug Reference. (n.d.-b). *Ciloxan olution (ciprofloxacin hydrochloride)* [Drug information]. https://www.pdr.net/drug-summary/Ciloxan-Solution-ciprofloxacin-hydrochloride-1995

Prescribers' Drug Reference. (n.d.-c). *Cyclogyl (cyclopentolate hydrochloride)* [Drug information]. https://www.pdr.net/drug-summary/Cyclogyl-cyclopentolate-hydrochloride-1090#5

Prescribers' Drug Reference. (n.d.-d). *Isopto carpine (pilocarpine hydrochloride)* [Drug information]. https://www.pdr.net/drug-summary/Isopto-Carpine-pilocarpine-hydrochloride-2609#14

Singh, M., & Whitfield, D. (2021). Herpes zoster ophthalmicus. In K. J. Knoop, L. B. Stack, A. B. Storrow, & R. Thurman (Eds.), *The atlas of emergency medicine* (5th ed.). McGraw-Hill. https://accessmedicine.mhmedical.com/content.aspx?bookid=2969&sectionid=250454355

Turbert, D. (n.d.). *What is a corneal ulcer (keratitis)?* American Academy of Ophthalmology. https://www.aao.org/eye-health/diseases/corneal-ulcer

Ventocilla, M. (2022). Ophthalmologic approach to chemical burns. *Medscape*. https://emedicine.medscape.com/article/1215950-overview

12 MUSCULOSKELETAL EMERGENCIES

AMPUTATION

Overview

- Traumatic amputation occurs when bone and soft tissue are severed from the body. It requires immediate treatment to avoid further harm. These injuries are often related to machine operating, power tools, and motorcycle or car crashes.
- The most common amputated appendages are fingers, toes, arms, and legs. Reimplantation of the amputated appendage is possible depending on the following factors: availability of specialized treatment/reimplantation services; condition of the amputated part; location of amputation (upper extremity reimplantation is more successful); patient characteristics (age, occupation, and health status); time elapsed since the injury; type of cut involved (crush and avulsion injuries are harder to treat).

Signs and Symptoms

- Avulsion
- Bleeding
- Body part wholly or partially separated from the body
- Crush injury
- Laceration
- Pain

Diagnosis

Labs

Based on patient presentation, the following lab tests may be indicated:

- Arterial blood gases (ABGs)
- Complete blood count (CBC)
- Creatine kinase (CK; for crush injuries)
- Comprehensive metabolic panel (CMP)
- Prothrombin time (PT), activated partial thromboplastin time (aPTT)
- Type and screen

Diagnostic Testing

- CT scan
- X-ray

[🧠] **COMPLICATIONS**

Patients with a traumatic amputation are at high risk for uncontrolled hemorrhage. A pressure dressing should be applied, and the patient should be monitored closely for continued bleeding. Application of a tourniquet (or tourniquets) may be necessary to stop or slow bleeding from an extremity.

Treatment

- Ensure adequate airway, breathing, and circulation.
- Manage hemodynamic status, including immediate control of blood loss.
- Administer fluid resuscitation or consider massive transfusion protocol (MTP).
- Preserve severed body part.
- If partially attached, splint the limb in a position of anatomic function until operative fixation.
- Provide pain management such as acetaminophen, nonsteroidal anti-inflammatory drugs (NSAIDs), and opioids (see Table A.2).
- Administer antibiotics such as cefazolin or ceftriaxone (see Table A.1).
- Administer tetanus prophylaxis.
- Transfer to specialized trauma service for emergent surgery.

Nursing Interventions

- Perform trauma assessment. Perform a primary assessment and provide lifesaving interventions while assessing the patient's airway, breathing, circulation, and mentation (making sure to provide cervical spine precautions if indicated). Perform a secondary assessment by exposing and removing clothes to evaluate for all injuries head to toe, anterior and posterior.
- Administer high-flow oxygen, control bleeding (may require tourniquets), and stabilize hemodynamic status.
- Initiate two large-bore intravenous (IV) lines for crystalloid fluid and blood product administration.
- Clean and protect the amputation site (gentle irrigation with normal saline and occlusive dressing).
- Preserve the amputated part.
- Continually monitor hemodynamic status by maintaining a mean arterial pressure greater than 65 mmHg. The injury may require the use of MTP with uncrossed or unmatched blood products.
- Assess or manage pain.
- Administer antibiotics.
- Administer tetanus prophylaxis.
- Prepare the patient for emergent surgery or transfer to a higher level of care.

 NURSING PEARL

To preserve the amputated part, wrap it in saline-moistened gauze and place it in a plastic bag or container. Place the bag or container in an ice-water bath. Do not place the body part directly in ice water, which can damage the tissue.

 POP QUIZ 12.1

What should the nurse first assess in the patient with a traumatic amputation of the lower leg?

COMPARTMENT SYNDROME

Overview

- Compartment syndrome occurs when increased pressure within a myofascial compartment compromises the circulation and function of the tissues within that space.
- Increased compartmental pressure can result from two sources: internal bleeding or swelling within the compartment; external restrictions (edema, a dressing, or a splint). ▶

 COMPLICATIONS

Timely recognition and treatment of compartment syndrome are essential to avoid serious complications. Sustained, elevated pressure can lead to neurologic deficits, tissue ischemia and necrosis, infection, and delays in fracture healing. Complications of compartment syndrome may require amputation of the affected body part.

Overview *(continued)*

- Compartment syndrome is most often seen following trauma, long bone fracture, crush injuries, extensive soft tissue damage, surgery, or prolonged pressure injuries.
- It can occur anywhere a muscle is contained in a closed fascial space, most commonly the lower leg, forearm, foot, hand, gluteal region, and thigh. It can also develop in the abdomen after penetrating abdominal trauma or surgery.

Signs and Symptoms

- Delayed capillary refill
- Diminished pulses
- Swelling
- Weakness to the affected area
- The six Ps: **P**aralysis; **P**ain out of proportion to apparent injury and/or pain with passive stretch of muscles in the affected compartment; **P**aresthesia; **P**allor; **P**oikilothermia; **P**ulselessness.

Diagnosis

Labs

- Blood or urine testing to assess the degree of muscle damage, which may include the following: CBC; CMP; creatine phosphokinase urinalysis

Diagnostic Testing

- Doppler ultrasound
- Measurement of intercompartmental pressure
- X-ray, CT scan, and/or MRI as indicated for injuries

Treatment

- Prompt removal of any external dressing or splint (casts, bandages, dressings)
- Monitoring of intercompartmental pressure through needle manometry
- Emergency fasciotomy: The standard of treatment for acute compartment syndrome in most cases is to fully decompress all involved compartments. Fasciotomy is contraindicated when the muscle is already dead, at which point an amputation is indicated.
- Blood pressure support as needed in hypotensive patients; fluids (e.g., crystalloid, colloid); blood products
- Pain management with opioid analgesics (see Table A.2)

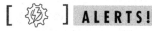 **ALERTS!**

With acute compartment syndrome, an intracompartment pressure of 30 mmHg or above is considered critical, and treatment with emergent surgical decompression should be initiated.

Nursing Interventions

- Assess for decreasing urine output, as this may indicate acute kidney injury or renal failure.
- Perform serial musculoskeletal and neurovascular assessments to extremity: edema, pain, peripheral vasculature.
- Carefully monitor vital signs of infection or shock: hypotension, increasing temperature, tachycardia.
- Elevate extremity no higher than heart level to facilitate venous drainage, reduce edema, and maximize tissue perfusion.
- Prevent compartment syndrome to other high-risk extremities by removing or loosening bandages, casting, and clothing/patient gown. ▶

Nursing Interventions *(continued)*

- Assess or manage pain.
- Prepare patient for surgery.

Patient Education

- Elevate the affected extremity to heart level (but not above).
- Seek treatment for worsening symptoms, including the following: increasing pain unrelieved by opioids; temperature changes in the affected limb; worsening paresthesia; worsening mobility or new-onset paralysis.
- Refrain from placing constricting items on affected limbs or extremities.

CONTUSIONS

Overview

- A *contusion* is a type of closed soft tissue injury that involves bleeding under the skin, resulting in discoloration (initially dark blue and purple, but the color changes over time).
- It is usually caused by a blunt force such as a fall or sports injury.
- Blunt trauma to the chest can cause underlying injuries to internal structures of the chest: Pulmonary contusions may lead to acute respiratory distress syndrome and pneumothoraxes. Cardiac contusions may lead to life-threatening arrhythmias, tachycardia, and hypotension.
- Renal and kidney contusion may lead to shock and organ failure.
- Continued bleeding under the skin can cause a hematoma. Small hematomas usually do not need additional treatment, but larger hematomas, such as those in certain areas as the head, or hematomas that continue to expand, need surgical treatment.

Signs and Symptoms

- Ecchymosis
- Swelling

Diagnosis

Labs

- CBC
- PT, aPTT

Diagnostic Testing

- CT scan
- EKG
- X-ray

Treatment

- Assess mental status and be alert for brain contusion (high risk if patient is on blood thinners).
- Provide oxygen and ventilatory support in case of pulmonary contusion.

[📝] POP QUIZ 12.2

A patient with a recently applied cast for a lower leg fracture complains of worsening pain and toe swelling. The patient has mottled toes and screams in pain with any leg movement. What is the priority intervention in this situation?

[🧠] COMPLICATIONS

Recurrent muscle contusions in athletic patients can caus[e] myositis ossificans, which causes tissue to calcify an[d] harden. Treatment is rest and gentle rehabilitation.

[🌐] NURSING PEARL

The RICE mnemonic describes appropriate care of [a] contusion as well as other orthopedic injuries:

- Rest the involved area.
- Ice the involved area.
- Compression in the form of a bandage or splint will hel[p] decrease swelling.
- Elevation will decrease swelling.

Treatment *(continued)*

- Perform the following as required for myocardial contusion: blood pressure support; monitoring for arrhythmia; oxygen; pacemaker; surgical repair.
- Rest, ice, and elevate the injured area.
- Assess underlying structures.
- Consider the mechanism of injury and evaluate for multiple and underlying injuries.
- Provide pain management with acetaminophen and opioids (see Table A.2).
- Assess for maltreatment or abuse of patient.
- Consult appropriate services (e.g., neurology, cardiology, orthopedics).

Nursing Interventions

- Perform trauma assessment. Perform a primary assessment and provide lifesaving interventions while assessing the patient's airway, breathing, circulation, and mentation (being sure to provide cervical spine precautions if indicated). Perform a secondary assessment by exposing and removing clothes to evaluate for all injuries head to toe, anterior and posterior.
- Establish IV access and draw blood if ordered.
- Perform EKG and cardiac monitoring.
- Provide fluid resuscitation if indicated.
- Assess mechanism of injury; consider abuse.
- Monitor for renal and kidney contusion that may lead to shock and organ failure.
- Assess medical history and consider prescribed medications, such as blood thinners.
- Perform a focused assessment of the injury area, including neurovascular status.
- Assess and manage pain.
- Apply ice or cold compresses and elevate the injury.

Patient Education

- Follow RICE protocol. Do not put ice directly on the skin. Ice packs should be covered with a cloth and used for 15 to 20 minutes several times a day for the first 2 to 48 hours.
- Expect the contusion to be painful, swollen, and dark purple or red for a few days. As the blood is absorbed, the color will change to yellowish and should resolve in 2 weeks.
- Report worsening swelling, numbness, or tingling to the involved extremity.
- Wear a seatbelt and use protective equipment during sports.
- Remove tripping hazards in the home.

COSTOCHONDRITIS

Overview

- *Costochondritis* is an inflammation of the cartilage in the rib cage that causes chest wall pain.
- It is caused by repeated coughing, chest injury, or respiratory infection.
- Pain can be mild or severe but is usually self-limiting.

Signs and Symptoms

- Chest pain: usually sharp and associated with coughing or deep breathing
- Chest wall tenderness to palpation

[🧠] **COMPLICATIONS**

Costochondritis causes chest pain that can mimic cardiac conditions. Patients who report chest pain should always be evaluated for cardiac problems first, even if the symptoms appear mild.

Signs and Symptoms *(continued)*

- Cough
- Fever
- Shortness of breath

Diagnosis

Labs

- Cardiac enzymes: troponin
- CBC
- CMP
- PT, aPTT (if indicated)

Diagnostic Testing

- Chest x-ray
- EKG

Treatment

- Pain management: acetaminophen and NSAIDs (see Table A.2); pain-relieving creams or patches such as lidocaine (Table 12.1).
- EKG and cardiac enzymes to rule out cardiac etiology
- Chest x-ray to rule out underlying respiratory etiology

TABLE 12.1 Orthopedic Medications		
INDICATIONS	MECHANISM OF ACTION	CONTRAINDICATIONS, PRECAUTIONS, AND ADVERSE EFFECTS
Xanthine oxidase inhibitors (e.g., allopurinol sodium)		
• Gout	• Interfere with purine catabolism and reduce uric acid production in the body	• Gout symptoms temporarily worsen after initiating allopurinol therapy; do not discontinue therapy but instead manage acute symptoms concurrently with colchicine.
Disease-modifying anti-rheumatic drugs (etanercept, methotrexate)		
• Rheumatoid arthritis • Psoriatic arthritis • Autoimmune diseases	• Tumor necrosis factor inhibitor • Block inflammation by targeting specific immune proteins	• Live vaccines need to be avoided. • May cause pregnancy complications; possible side effects are fever, chills, flu-like symptoms, and easy bruising. • Adverse effects include shortness of breath, swelling to legs, and chest pain.
Skeletal muscle relaxants (e.g., cyclobenzaprine hydrochloride)		
• Muscle strains, spasms • Reduce pain	• Centrally acting muscle relaxant that works on the brainstem to reduce spasms (exact mechanism unknown)	• Can cause drowsiness, dry mouth, dizziness • Short-term use only • Contraindicated with MAOIs because it may cause serotonin syndrome

MAOIs, monoamine oxidase inhibitors.

Nursing Interventions

- Perform focused cardiac and respiratory assessments.
- Assess or manage pain.
- Administer antibiotics and cough medication as indicated.
- Provide patient education on incentive spirometer use: Sit upright; take a deep breath in and out; inhale slowly through the mouthpiece until hitting the target mark; hold the breath for 3 seconds, then exhale; repeat this 10 times per hour.

Patient Education

- Avoid activity or movement that makes the pain worse.
- Take medications as prescribed.
- Report any signs of infection.
- Take deep breaths periodically or use incentive spirometry if prescribed to decrease the risk of a respiratory infection.
- Participate in stretching exercises or place a heating pad on the painful area.

 POP QUIZ 12.3

While the nurse is assessing a patient with chest pain, the patient reports that the pain worsens with palpation and movement. What diagnostic testing should be performed?

FOREIGN BODIES

Overview

- Foreign bodies, such as splinters, bullets, or pieces of metal, glass, or plastic, may be found in bone and overlying tissue because of an accidental or intentional injury.
- The path the projectile travels can cause secondary cavitation injuries, such as fractures, damaged tissues, or ruptured organs or vessels.
- Foreign bodies may be superficial and able to be removed under local anesthesia, or they may be deep and require surgical intervention to remove. Artificial hips and orthopedic hardware are considered foreign bodies; occasionally, the body rejects them, and the equipment needs to be removed.
- If untreated, foreign bodies may cause inflammation and infection.

COMPLICATIONS

Controlling bleeding should be a priority because the risk of hemorrhage is high with penetrating and high-velocity injuries. In some cases, embedded foreign bodies may compress vasculature and lead to significant bleeding once removed. A deceptively small wound may mask significant internal damage.

Signs and Symptoms

- Bleeding
- Evidence of the object (either palpable or visible)
- Pain and tenderness at the site
- Varying symptoms, from minor localized symptoms to significant trauma, depending on the mechanism of injury

Diagnosis

Labs

- Trauma workup for significant penetrating trauma: CBC, CMP, PT, aPTT, type and screen, ABGs
- Wound cultures

Diagnostic Testing
- CT scan
- X-ray

Treatment
- Perform a trauma assessment and provide lifesaving interventions.
- Monitor for neurologic complications (as with bullet or knife wound to the head).
- Assess for underlying injury before removing an object. Removal of large and deep objects, such as a knife, may need to be done in the operating room.
- Provide pain management such as acetaminophen, NSAIDs, and opioids (see Table A.2).
- Provide local anesthesia such as lidocaine or bupivacaine (see Table 12.1) prior to foreign body retrieval.
- Stabilize the involved body part.
- Give tetanus prophylaxis if indicated.
- Treat infection with antibiotics such as cephalexin (see Table A.1).
- With gun shot wounds (GSWs) or stabbings, refer the patient to treatment for trauma.

Nursing Interventions
- Perform a trauma assessment, if indicated, or a focused examination including neurologic assessment of an extremity.
- Assess and manage pain.
- Assess and monitor hemodynamic stability.
- Assess and monitor neurovascular status.
- Administer tetanus immunization.
- Stabilize the involved body part for an impaled object.
- Clean and disinfect the wound.
- Facilitate evidence collection in crime situations, including collection of clothing and belongings in paper bags, descriptive documentation of wounds, and maintenance of the chain of custody.
- Prepare patient for surgical removal of object, if indicated.

Patient Education
- Seek treatment for any signs and symptoms of infection from a retained foreign body, such as pain, tenderness, or development of papules or abscesses.
- Follow up for any uncontrolled bleeding; minimal bleeding may be normal.
- Alert security staff of retained bullets when going through a metal detector.

FRACTURES AND DISLOCATIONS
Overview
- Dislocations occur when joint surfaces are no longer intact. Joint dislocations reduced in the ED frequently require analgesia and sedation.
  A common dislocation in the pediatric population involves the subluxation of the radial bone from the elbow joint.
- Fractures involve a break in bone continuity. Fractures can be open (with an associated break in the skin) or closed. Because of the surrounding ▶

 COMPLICATIONS

Rapid identification of fracture/dislocation followed by immobilization and/or surgical repair is indicated to prevent severe complications and lifelong disability. Unstable injuries can continue to bleed, as well as cause additional damage to surrounding tissues. Long bones, particularly the femur, are at high risk for significant hemorrhage. Additionally, prompt identification of an open fracture is important to permit early administration of antibiotics.

Overview *(continued)*

tissue, musculature, and organs, femoral and pelvic fractures are associated with significant bleeding, concomitant internal injuries, and high mortality rate.

- Special considerations vary depending on the location of the fracture. Common locations for fractures are as follows: skull fracture; spinal fracture; clavicular fracture; scapular fracture; upper extremity fractures; pelvic fractures; hip fractures; lower extremity fractures. Additional fracture types are described in Table 12.2.

Signs and Symptoms

- Abnormal movement or range of motion (ROM)
- Bruising
- Crepitus
- Deformity
- Immobility
- Inability to bear weight on affected extremity
- Pain
- Swelling
- Tenderness

Diagnosis

Labs

- Trauma workup may be indicated: CBC, CMP, PT, aPTT, and type and screen

Diagnostic Testing

- CT scan of the affected area
- X-rays: include the joints above and below the injury site to rule out related dislocations or additional fractures

TABLE 12.2 Types of Fractures

TYPE	MECHANISM OF INJURY	DESCRIPTION
Avulsion	Forceful contraction of a muscle (third-degree strain)	Bone fragment is displaced at muscle insertion point
Comminuted	Severe direct force	Two or more bone fragments are present
Compression	Severe force to head, sacrum, or heels (e.g. from a jump); secondary to osteoporosis-related bone loss	Vertebral bones collapse; may cause displaced fragments
Depressed	Blunt trauma to a flat bone	Bone fragment is displaced below the rest of the bone surface
Greenstick	Compression force to an extremity, causing it to bend and break	Usually occurs in children; the break is present on one side of a long bone but does not extend through the bone
Impacted	Severe force that causes bone ends to come together	Ends are jammed together and may or may not be comminuted
Oblique	Twisting force	Complete fracture usually oblique to the long axis of a bone
Spiral	Twisting force with the extremity planted	Fracture can resemble a corkscrew
Transverse	Sharp, direct blow	Complete fracture perpendicular to the bone's axis

Treatment

- Stabilize the injured extremity above and below the joint or apply traction for a femur fracture. Check neurologic function after every intervention. Minor closed long bone fractures that are not displaced may require casting followed by physical therapy/occupational therapy. Major long bone and open fractures require surgery for debridement and possible placement of implanted hardware followed by physical therapy/occupational therapy. Open fracture of a joint or long bone requires antibiotics to prevent osteomyelitis (see Table A.1).
- Administer fluid resuscitation as indicated for hemodynamic instability.
- Administer pain medication such as acetaminophen, NSAIDs, and opioids (see Table A.2).
- Prepare patient for conscious sedation if indicated to reduce dislocations.
- Realign the extremity to maintain neurovascular function.
- Give tetanus prophylaxis for open fractures.
- Consult with the appropriate surgical specialty, such as orthopedic or hand specialists.

Nursing Interventions

- Perform a focused assessment, and check for neurologic function before and after every intervention.
- Assist with stabilizing injury to proper alignment, including cast splinting.
- Assess and treat pain.
- Ensure that signed or implied consent is documented.
- Perform monitoring during sedation, which includes: end-tidal monitoring, SpO_2, frequent blood pressure monitoring, and continuous cardiac monitoring; patent IV access; having reversal medications available; having emergent airway interventions available.

Patient Education

- Follow prescribed activity restrictions, including crutch use and weight-bearing restrictions.
- Follow up with physical therapy/occupational therapy.
- Follow up with the provider to ensure adequate healing and repeat imaging in a few weeks.
- Follow RICE instructions.
- Keep the cast clean and dry, if applicable; do not insert items into the cast.
- Report increased pain, numbness, or tingling in the affected area.

[🔩] ALERTS!

Frequently, patients with lower extremity fractures are discharged with crutches. Instruct the patient on safe crutch-walking techniques to avoid additional injuries. Adjust the crutches to the patient's height and have them demonstrate safe use before discharge.

[📝] POP QUIZ 12.4

A splint is to be applied to a patient with a tibia/fibula fracture. What should the nurse assess before and after splint application?

INFLAMMATORY CONDITIONS

Overview

- Common inflammatory conditions include rheumatoid arthritis, osteoarthritis, gout, and tendonitis.
- *Rheumatoid arthritis* is a chronic, systemic, autoimmune, inflammatory condition that primarily involves synovial joints. The arthritis is of unknown etiology and is typically symmetrical, leading to the destruction of joints and causing joint deformities if left untreated.
- *Osteoarthritis* is the degenerative breakdown of cartilage that occurs gradually. It can happen in any joint but occurs more frequently in the fingers, spine, hips, and knees.
- *Gout*, another form of arthritis, develops when urate crystals accumulate in a joint. It most often occurs in the big toe and comes on suddenly. Common foods that trigger gout are seafood, red meat, alcohol, and sugar.

Overview *(continued)*

- *Tendonitis* is the painful inflammation of a tendon, which is the tissue connecting the bone to muscle. It may occur around any joint in the body, but common sites are the elbow, shoulder, and wrist.
- Patients with inflammatory conditions may seek treatment for worsening or uncontrolled pain.
- Underlying infection should be ruled out as a cause for the inflammation.

[🧠] **COMPLICATIONS**

Septic arthritis is a joint infection that can develop from a penetrating wound to the joint or from bacteria that travel from another part of the body. The signs and symptoms initially resemble a typical arthritis exacerbation. However, worsening pain and fever will develop. Prompt treatment is required to avoid joint damage.

Signs and Symptoms

Table 12.3 shows signs and symptoms of inflammatory conditions.

Diagnosis

Labs

- Antibody factors (rheumatoid arthritis)
- CBC
- C-reactive protein (CRP)
- Cultures (blood, aspirate to rule out septic arthritis)
- Erythrocyte sedimentation rate (ESR)
- Uric acid level (gout)

Diagnostic Testing

- X-rays

Treatment

- Pain management with NSAIDs (see Table A.2)
- Steroids such as prednisone (see Table A.4)
- Allopurinol for gout (see Table 12.1)
- Disease-modifying antirheumatic drugs (DMARDs) such as etanercept and infliximab and nonbiologic drugs, such as methotrexate (see Table 12.1)
- Ruling out of underlying injuries and infection
- Use of splints, braces, and elastic bands if appropriate
- Surgery for arthroplasty or joint replacement
- Referral to a specialist, such as a rheumatologist, orthopedist, or pain doctor

TABLE 12.3 Signs and Symptoms of Inflammatory Conditions			
RHEUMATOID ARTHRITIS	**OSTEOARTHRITIS**	**GOUT**	**TENDONITIS**
• Decreased appetite • Fever • Fatigue • Painful joints • Stiffness in joints that is generally worse in the morning	• Painful joints (may be mild with little impact on activities of daily living or debilitating) • Pain increases with higher-impact activities • Sensation of crunching or grinding in joints	• Severe localized pain • Redness and swelling • Often affects the great toe	• Dull ache to affected joint or extremity that is worse with movement • Swelling • Tenderness

Nursing Interventions

- Assess and manage pain; consider comfort measures such as heat or cold, apply supportive splints, and facilitate position changes.
- Perform a focused musculoskeletal assessment.

Patient Education

- Avoid activities that make the pain worse, such as running.
- Attend physical therapy/occupational therapy therapy to promote joint movement and muscle strength and to learn appropriate stretching exercises.
- Use braces, splints, and canes, if indicated.
- Apply cold compresses to decrease pain and swelling.
- Perform ROM exercises as prescribed to promote mobility.
- Report uncontrolled pain or signs and symptoms of infection to the provider.

JOINT EFFUSIONS

Overview

- A *joint effusion* is a collection of fluid in a joint commonly caused by infection, trauma, and inflammation.
- The knee is most frequently affected.
- A joint effusion is associated with osteoarthritis, rheumatoid arthritis, gout, and bursitis.

Signs and Symptoms

- Decreased ROM/compromised ambulation
- Fever
- Pain/stiffness
- Redness
- Swelling
- Warmth at joint

Diagnosis

Labs

- Antinuclear antibody titers (rheumatoid arthritis)
- CBC
- Cultures (of aspirate)
- ESR
- Uric acid (for gout)

Diagnostic Testing

- CT scan
- X-rays

Treatment

- Application of cold compress, elevation of joint, and encouragement of rest of the extremity
- Arthrocentesis or aspiration of joint fluid to relieve pressure and for diagnosis to guide treatment
- Pain management with NSAIDs (see Table A.2)

[ ]   **COMPLICATIONS**

Untreated effusions can limit ROM and mobility and affect surrounding tissues. Joint aspirations may be necessary if conservative treatment is unsuccessful or to determine the etiology if unknown (e.g., to rule out a septic joint or abscess).

Treatment *(continued)*

- Steroid injection, such as hydrocortisone, given directly into the joint to block inflammation (see Table A.4)
- Antibiotics (see Table A.1)
- Allopurinol for gouty joint effusion (see Table 12.1)

Nursing Interventions

- Perform focused musculoskeletal assessment.
- Monitor neurovascular assessment of the affected limb.
- Immobilize the affected area.
- Elevate and apply ice to the affected area.
- Assess and manage pain.
- Draw blood for lab tests, as ordered.
- Assist with joint aspiration procedure. Gather supplies and medications; witness consent; provide sample of aspirated fluid to the laboratory.
- Administer ordered medications specific to the condition.

Patient Education

- Follow activity restrictions, including weight-bearing limitations, as instructed.
- Report increased pain, numbness, or tingling.
- Report signs and symptoms of infection.

LOW BACK PAIN

Overview

- Low back pain is a common complaint in the ED. It may be benign or an emergent critical condition.
- Chronic low back pain is aggravated by inappropriate body mechanics, lifting, straining, twisting, contusions, or torsion.
- Emergent conditions, such as infection, malignancy, fracture, and cauda equina may cause compression on the spinal cord, which should be treated emergently as it can lead to permanent damage. Signs of spinal cord compression include numbness, tingling, and weakness in the extremities. Cauda equina affects the root nerves and presents with bilateral leg weakness and loss of control of the bowel and/or bladder.
- *Sciatica*, which may cause debilitating pain, is the impingement of the sciatic nerve in the low back and is usually caused by a herniated disk or bone spur in the spine. Pain is generally unilateral.

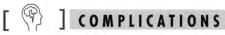

COMPLICATIONS

Low back pain may indicate an abdominal aortic aneurysm. This condition should be considered in older patients who present with low back pain. If undetected, a ruptured aneurysm can cause a life-threatening hemorrhage.

Signs and Symptoms

- Difficulty ambulating
- Numbness or tingling of the lower extremities
- Pain in the lower back, possibly radiating to one or both legs
- Positive Babinski sign (cord compression)
- Spasticity

Diagnosis

Labs

- Urinalysis to check for nephrolithiasis or pyelonephritis
- Urine pregnancy test as appropriate to rule out ectopic pregnancy and guide future imaging

Diagnostic Testing
- CT scan
- MRI
- X-rays

Treatment
- Muscle relaxants (see Table 12.1)
- Pain management with acetaminophen or NSAIDs (see Table A.2)
- Pain management with opioids and tramadol for more severe pain (see Table A.2)
- Topical pain medication, such as lidocaine
- Ruling out of neurologic conditions or other medical causes
- Antibiotics to prevent or treat vertebral osteomyelitis (see Table A.1)
- Neurosurgical consult for epidural abscess
- Emergent neurologic consult for decompression surgery with cauda equina
- Pain services for unresolved or long-term pain control
- Physical therapy/occupational therapy for proper body mechanics teaching

Nursing Interventions
- Assess and manage pain. Try alternative measures like repositioning.
- Use ice or heat on the sore area.
- Perform a head-to-toe examination with a thorough neurologic assessment.
- Administer prescribed medications.
- Prepare for surgery if indicated.

Patient Education
- Apply heat or ice to the area to relieve pain.
- Take prescribed medications; do not operate a car or heavy machinery while on opioids or muscle relaxers.
- Follow up with physical therapy/occupational therapy if indicated.
- Follow prescribed activity limitations and use optimal body mechanics.
- Return to the ED for new or worsening pain, numbness, tingling, or loss of control of bowel or bladder.

OSTEOMYELITIS
Overview
- *Osteomyelitis* is an infection involving bone. It may be classified based on the mechanism of infection (hematogenous vs. nonhematogenous) and the duration of illness (acute vs. chronic).
- It can result from an open fracture, orthopedic surgery, or an infection that travels from another part of the body.
- Patients with diabetes or end-stage renal disease, those who have a history of IV drug use, and those who have compromised circulation are at an increased risk of developing osteomyelitis.
- Most frequently, this bone infection is caused by *Staphylococcus aureus*.
- Early identification and prompt initiation of IV antibiotic therapy are needed to prevent deteriorating condition and complications.

 COMPLICATIONS

Untreated osteomyelitis can lead to tetanus, necrotizing fasciitis, and sepsis, resulting in permanent disability, bone damage, and death. It is a common cause of amputation in patients with diabetes, who may not identify wounds until advanced infection develops due to neuropathy.

Signs and Symptoms

- Fever
- Pain
- Decreased movement of affected extremity
- Erythema, warmth, and edema at infected site
- Wound drainage

Diagnosis

Labs

- Blood cultures
- CBC
- CMP
- Lactic acid (sepsis)
- Procalcitonin (sepsis)
- CRP and ESR
- Wound cultures

Diagnostic Testing

- Imaging of the infected area: CT scan, MRI, x-ray
- Bone biopsy

Treatment

- Administration of antibiotics such as penicillin, ceftriaxone, or clindamycin (see Table A.1)
- Assessment and treatment of sepsis if present
- Surgical intervention: irrigation and drainage; debridement for removal of necrotic material and culture of involved tissue and bone; removal of orthopedic hardware, if applicable; amputation if infection cannot be managed
- Pain management, such as with NSAIDs and opioids (see Table A.2)
- Hyperbaric therapy: adjunctive therapy in patients with refractory osteomyelitis

Nursing Interventions

- Perform musculoskeletal assessment.
- Assess for sepsis.
- Monitor neurovascular status.
- Administer tetanus prophylaxis, if indicated.
- Assess and treat pain as ordered.
- Assess wound and dressing status. Change wound dressing as needed/ordered. Inform provider of any wound drainage changes, including new foul smell and color or consistency changes.
- Administer antibiotics. Monitor side effects. Monitor dosages and trough levels.
- If patient is taking oral nutrition, encourage dietary choices with high protein and vitamin content.
- Offload pressure with repositioning, padding, and turning every 2 hours.
- Promote mobility of unaffected joints/extremities as tolerated.

Patient Education

- Complete all antibiotics as prescribed.
- Report worsening pain or signs and symptoms of infection.
- If diabetes is present, maintain tight glycemic control, inspect skin and feet daily, bathe feet in warm (not hot) water, dry feet completely, and apply lotion.
- If using IV drugs, follow up with prescribed resources to treat addiction. If continuing to use, do not share or reuse needles.

STRAINS AND SPRAINS

Overview

- Both strains and sprains are minor musculoskeletal injuries that result from traumatic movement.
- A *strain* involves an overstretched muscle that stretches or tears a tendon.
- A *sprain* involves an overextended joint that stretches or tears a ligament.
- Damage and treatment vary depending on the extent of injury (first, second, or third degree).
- Muscle or tendon ruptures are usually sports-related injuries. For example, an Achilles tendon rupture can occur when a patient steps abruptly with the knee forced in extension.

[ ] **COMPLICATIONS**

A severe strain (third degree) causes complete disruption of the muscle of tendon, which can result in an avulsion fracture. In addition to splinting and non–weight-bearing status, surgery may be necessary to reconnect the tendon.

Signs and Symptoms

- Decreased ROM (second or third degree)
- Ecchymosis
- Erythema
- Muscle spasm (strain)
- Pain
- Swelling
- Tenderness

Diagnosis

Labs

Laboratory tests are not indicated unless the patient has sustained other trauma.

Diagnostic Testing

- X-rays to exclude fracture

Treatment

- Stabilization of the injury (splint or cast)
- Pain management (see Table A.2)
- RICE protocol

Nursing Interventions

- Perform focused musculoskeletal assessment.
- Assess neurovascular status (especially before and after splint application).
- Elevate affected extremity.
- Apply ice.
- Assess and manage pain.
- Wrap or splint the injury.

Patient Education

- Follow RICE protocol.
- Report increased pain or numbness and tingling.
- Use crutches with light to no weight bearing, if prescribed.
- Follow safe crutch-walking techniques to prevent additional injuries (i.e., look forward, not down, when walking; let hands support body weight, and move crutches together close to the body).
- Follow up with provider for reevaluation if needed.
- Follow up with physical therapy/occupational therapy.

[🧠] **COMPLICATIONS**

Massive trauma can cause significant hemorrhage with hypovolemic shock related to internal and external bleeding. The patient will present with altered mental status, hypotension, tachycardia, and diaphoresis. Emergent treatment with fluid resuscitation and MTP is anticipated.

TRAUMA

Overview

- The priority in trauma is to provide lifesaving interventions and prevent the loss of limbs. The provider should not be distracted by musculoskeletal injuries that do not involve circulatory compromise.
- The mechanism of injury is very important when anticipating the type of orthopedic injuries that may be present.
- The ED nurse should gather a detailed description of the traumatic event: motor vehicle crash (MVC)—damage to the vehicle, rate of speed, presence of broken windshield, patient ejection, use of seatbelt, death of another person in the same vehicle; motorcycle crash—use of helmet and other protective clothing, rate of speed, impact with an object, patient ejection; burns—involvement of a fall (e.g., from window of burning building), length of exposure to fire, depth of burns; falls—height of fall, surface of landing, position of patient's body on impact; GSW—caliber of bullet, distance from the shooter, type of gun, predicted trajectory of the bullet after entering the body, potential exit wound.
- Blast injury may cause musculoskeletal injuries and traumatic amputation, among other injuries, not only from the initial wave but from projectiles.

Signs and Symptoms

- Altered mental status
- Amputation
- Burns
- Diaphoresis
- Ecchymosis
- Hypotension
- Lacerations
- Obvious deformities
- Punctures
- Significant pain
- Swelling
- Tachycardia
- Uncontrolled hemorrhage

Diagnosis

Labs

- ABG
- CBC
- CMP
- Lactate
- Point-of-care testing glucose test
- PT, aPTT
- Type and crossmatch

Diagnostic Testing

- CT scan
- Focused assessment with sonography in trauma (FAST) to check for pericardial effusion and hemoperitoneum
- X-rays

Treatment

- Stabilize airway, breathing, and circulation while using cervical spine precautions until cleared.
- Control external hemorrhage.
- Ensure adequate IV access, intraosseous access, or central line (cordis) if needed.
- Assess for additional injuries.
- Stabilize broken bones with traction/splints.
- Provide fluid resuscitation with crystalloids (cautiously) or colloids; activate MTP if needed.
- Provide pain management (see Table A.2).
- Give tetanus prophylaxis if indicated.
- Administer antibiotics if indicated (see Table A.1).
- Consult with appropriate services; patient may require emergent surgery.

Nursing Interventions

- Perform trauma assessment with interventions as follows: Take cervical spine precautions; apply cervical collar if not already in place. Perform an across-the-room assessment of mental status. Assess and manage airway, breathing, and circulation, including assisting with intubation, applying oxygen, and gathering supplies for needle decompression. Control hemorrhage with direct pressure or tourniquet. Establish two large-bore IV lines, intraosseous access, or assist with central line placement. Administer fluid resuscitation if indicated; use crystalloids cautiously. Administer MTP in a ratio of 1 packed red blood cells to 1 platelets to 1 fresh frozen plasma to avoid dilution coagulopathy; use rapid infuser if indicated. Remove all clothing and perform a head-to-toe assessment, both anterior and posterior. Identify and document deformity, contusions, abrasions, penetration, ecchymosis, tenderness, lacerations, and swelling, which may indicate underlying orthopedic injuries. Assess pulses and neurologic function of extremities. Apply splints and traction to properly realign extremity and restore blood flow. Draw blood for lab tests including ABG; may need to assist with femoral blood draw. Administer pain medications. Give tetanus vaccine if indicated. Administer antibiotics urgently for open fractures or GSW/penetration to the abdomen.
- Provide an update to the family if the patient agrees.
- Establish medical history; include medications currently taken and allergies.
- Evaluate mechanism of injury.
- Continuously reevaluate patient for change in condition.
- Prepare patient for surgery if indicated.

Patient Education

- Report any signs or symptoms of infection and perform regular dressing changes and wound care as ordered.
- Report worsening pain or any numbness or tingling that develops.
- Wear a seatbelt when driving or riding in a car.
- Wear a helmet and protective clothing when on a motorcycle.
- Remove tripping hazards in the home.
- Take medications as prescribed and follow up as ordered.

[📝] 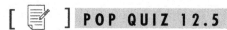 **POP QUIZ 12.5**

A patient involved in a high-velocity MVC is unresponsive and hemodynamically unstable secondary to apparent internal injuries. Why is it important to complete a secondary head-to-toe assessment on this patient?

RESOURCES

American College of Surgeons. (2018). *ATLS advanced trauma life support*. Author.

Blank-Reid, C. (2020). Epidemiology and mechanisms of injury. In V. Sweet & A. Foley (Eds.), *Sheehy's emergency nursing: Principles and practice* (7th ed., pp. 378–400). Elsevier.

Casey, P. E. (2014). Low back pain. In S. C. Sherman, J. M. Weber, M. A. Schindlbeck, & R. G. Patwari (Eds.), *Clinical emergency medicine*. McGraw-Hill. https://accessemergencymedicine.mhmedical.com/content.aspx?bookid=991&sectionid=55139213

Centers for Disease Control and Prevention. (2003, March 18). *Explosions and blast injuries*. https://www.cdc.gov/masstrauma/preparedness/primer.pdf

Cerepani, M. (2020). Orthopedic and neurovascular trauma. In V. Sweet & A. Foley (Eds.), *Sheehy's emergency nursing: Principles and practice* (7th ed., pp. 477–502). Elsevier.

Choudharym, S., Pasrija, D., & Mendez, M. (2021). Pulmonary contusion. In *StatPearls*. StatPearls Publishing. https://www.ncbi.nlm.nih.gov/books/NBK558914

Cleveland Clinic. (2019, September 26). *Osteoarthritis*. https://my.clevelandclinic.org/health/diseases/5599-osteoarthritis

Halpern, J. (2013). Musculoskeletal trauma. In B. Hammond & P. Zimmerman (Eds.), *Sheehy's manual of emergency care* (7th ed., pp. 427–437). Elsevier Mosby.

Khan, I., & Kahwaji, C. (2021). Cyclobenzaprine. In *StatPearls* Publishing. https://www.ncbi.nlm.nih.gov/books/NBK513362

MedlinePlus. (n.d.) *Traumatic amputation*. U.S. Department of Health and Human Services, National Institutes of Health, National Library of Medicine. https://medlineplus.gov/ency/article/000006.htm

Morelli, J. (2021). *Rheumatoid arthritis (RA) medications*. RxList. https://www.rxlist.com/rheumatoid_arthritis_ra_medications/drugs-condition.htm#what_are_effective_over-the-counter_medications_for_rheumatoid_arthritis

Prescribers' Digital Reference. (n.d.-a). *Allopurinol sodium*[Drug information]. https://www.pdr.net/drug-summary/Aloprim-allopurinal-sodium-847.897

Prescribers' Digital Reference. (n.d.-b). *Colchicine*[Drug information]. https://www.pdr.net/drug-summary/Colcrys-colchicine-592

Prescribers' Digital Reference. (n.d.-c). *Cyclobenzaprine hydrochloride*[Drug information]. https://www.pdr.net/drug-summary/Cyclobenzaprine-Hydrochloride-cyclobenzaprine-hydrochloride-3089.1153

Prescribers' Digital Reference. (n.d.-d). *Diphtheria and tetanus toxoids adsorbed*[Drug information]. https://www.pdr.net/drug-summary/Diphtheria-and-Tetanus-Toxoids-Adsorbed--For-children-6-weeks-through-6-years-of-age--diphtheria-and-tetanus-toxoids-adsorbed-3293

Roberts, N. W. (2022). Joint aspiration or injection in adults: Technique and indications. *UpToDate*. https://www.uptodate.com/contents/joint-aspiration-or-injection-in-adults-technique-and-indications/print

Weiser, T. G. (2020, May). *Blunt cardiac injury: Cardiac contusion*. Merck Manual. https://www.merckmanuals.com/professional/injuries-poisoning/thoracic-trauma/blunt-cardiacinjury

13 WOUND EMERGENCIES

ABRASIONS
Overview
- *Abrasions* are friction wounds that develop when skin rubs against a hard surface. They may be classified as follows: *linear*—simple abrasions, such as a scratch, that are typically able to heal by primary intention; *graze*—superficial abrasions from the body rubbing against a rough surface (e.g., "road rash"); *patterned*—abrasions that leave a characteristic impression of the object that caused the injury, such as ligature abrasions.
- Superficial abrasions involve the epidermis, while partial-thickness abrasions extend into the dermis.

Signs and Symptoms
- Bleeding
- Exposed underlying layers of skin
- Tenderness

Diagnosis
Labs

There are no lab tests specific to diagnosing abrasions. However, tests may be indicated if the patient has additional trauma.

Diagnostic Testing

There are no diagnostic tests specific to abrasions. However, imaging such as x-rays may be indicated to rule out a foreign body in the wound and to assess for underlying injury.

Treatment
- Antibiotics if indicated (see Table A.1)
- Cleaning and debridement of the wound
- Pain management, including local anesthesia if indicated
- Tetanus prophylaxis (see Table 13.1)

Nursing Interventions
- Perform a focused injury assessment.
- Thoroughly clean the wound as ordered.
- Apply antibacterial ointment and dressing (see Table 13.1).

[ ] **COMPLICATIONS**

Thorough cleansing of an abrasion is vital to remove all dirt, debris, and bacteria. An abrasion that is poorly cleaned is at high risk of becoming infected. "Tattooing" occurs when debris is left in a wound, causing staining and permanent scarring of the skin.

[ ] **ALERT!**

Nonadherent dressings are often used directly on the abrasion to prevent the dressing material from sticking to the wound, which may cause secondary trauma on removal.

TABLE 13.1 Wound Medications

INDICATIONS	MECHANISM OF ACTION	CONTRAINDICATIONS, PRECAUTIONS, AND ADVERSE EFFECTS
Antibiotics, topical ("triple antibiotic ointment": bacitracin/neomycin/polymyxin B sulfate)		
• Infection prophylaxis for minor burns and abrasions	• Provide bactericidal and bacteriostatic activity to inhibit bacterial growth and prevent infection	• There are limited interactions and contraindications, as systemic absorption is minimal when applied topically. • Use with caution in patients with renal impairment. • Long-term use increases risk for neomycin hypersensitivity.
Antifibrinolytic therapy (TXA)		
• Hemorrhage (trauma, obstetric bleeding)	• Hemostatic agent to bind the lysine binding site for fibrin on the plasmin molecule	• Antifibrinolytic therapy is contraindicated in intracranial bleeding and thrombolytic disease. • Use caution in renal impairment, seizure disorders, and surgery. • Adverse effects include thrombosis, thromboembolism, pulmonary embolism, renal thrombosis, visual impairments, and seizures.
Tetanus prophylaxis (Td vaccine)		
• Diphtheria and tetanus prophylaxis	• Promotes development of antibodies and antitoxins in response to diphtheria and tetanus toxoids	• Td preparation is indicated only for patients age 7 years and older; children should receive combination vaccine, which includes pertussis immunization (TdaP), unless otherwise contraindicated. • Td vaccine is indicated for both primary immunization and infection prophylaxis for potentially contaminated wounds.
Topical anesthetics (lidocaine)		
• Local anesthetic for wound cleansing and repair	• Provide a reversible nerve conduction blockade	• Medication is administered subcutaneously or topically. • Medication can be combined with epinephrine to enhance absorption and decrease bleeding. • Preparations with epinephrine may compromise blood flow to areas such as the fingertips, toes, and nose.

Note: All agents are contraindicated in the presence of hypersensitivity to the medication or one of its components.
Td, tetanus/diphtheria; TdaP, tetanus, diphtheria, pertussis; TXA, tranexamic acid.

Nursing Interventions *(continued)*

- Assess neurovascular status if circumferential dressing is applied.
- Administer tetanus prophylaxis (see Table 13.1).

Patient Education

- Perform wound care as directed.
- Report signs and symptoms of infection, such as increased redness, swelling, or drainage. ▶

[📝] **POP QUIZ 13.1**

How does irrigating a deep abrasion promote wound healing?

Patient Education *(continued)*

- Seek emergent care for worsening symptoms such as uncontrolled bleeding or fever.
- Use sunscreen on the area once the wound has healed to minimize scarring.

AVULSIONS

Overview

- Avulsion injuries cause full-thickness injury, in which most of the skin is torn away but remains attached to the body in one area.
- Proximal-based avulsions have better circulation than distal-based avulsions, which increases the chance that the avulsed tissue will survive.
- The wound edges are unable to be approximated for closure; severe injuries may require grafting.
- Degloving injuries are severe avulsion injuries in which the skin is pulled away from the underlying muscle and fascia, usually circumferentially.
- Degloving injuries frequently involve the fingers but can also affect other parts of the body.
- Less frequently, degloving injures can be a closed injury when shearing causes creation of a cavity between tissues, which fills with blood and fat (Morel-Lavalée injury).

[🧠] **COMPLICATIONS**

Finger degloving injuries can occur when a patient's ring gets caught on an object (ring avulsion). Complications include open fractures and amputation of the finger.

Signs and Symptoms

- Bleeding
- Pain
- Wound that cannot be approximated because of missing tissue

Diagnosis

Labs

- As indicated per severity; trauma workup may be needed.

Diagnostic Testing

- CT (for closed degloving injury)
- X-ray to rule out foreign body or underlying fracture

Treatment

- Antibiotics if indicated (see Table A.1)
- Pain management (see Table A.2)
- Surgical grafting if indicated
- Tetanus prophylaxis (see Table 13.1)
- Thorough wound cleaning, irrigation, and debridement

Nursing Interventions

- Perform a focused wound assessment, including neurovascular assessment of affected area.
- Clean and irrigate the wound.
- Assess/manage pain.
- Apply antibiotic ointment and dressing if indicated (see Table 13.1).
- Administer tetanus prophylaxis (see Table 13.1).

Patient Education

- Perform wound care as directed.
- Report any signs or symptoms of infection, such as redness, swelling, and drainage.

FOREIGN BODIES

Overview

- Foreign bodies include metallic objects, fiberglass particles, glass shards, plastic fragments, and wood or other organic material.
- These can cause soft tissue damage and infection if not removed.
- Many, but not all, are radiopaque.

Signs and Symptoms

- Bleeding
- Bruising
- Open wound
- Palpable or visible object
- Redness
- Swelling
- Tenderness

Diagnosis

Labs

There are no lab tests specific to diagnosing foreign bodies. However, tests are indicated if infection is suspected or other trauma is present.

Diagnostic Testing

- CT
- Ultrasound
- X-ray

Treatment

- Cleaning and disinfection of wound
- Object removal
- Pain management, if indicated (for local anesthetics, see Table 13.1; for additional pain medications, see Table A.2)
- Antibiotics, if indicated (see Table A.1)
- Tetanus prophylaxis (see Table 13.1)

Nursing Interventions

- Administer medications as ordered.
- Administer tetanus prophylaxis (see Table 13.1).
- Perform focused wound assessment, including neurovascular assessment of the affected limb.
- Perform wound care.

[📝] **POP QUIZ 13.2**

What is the priority assessment in a degloving injury?

[🧠] **COMPLICATIONS**

A thorough assessment for foreign bodies is important. Retained foreign bodies are an infection risk and can initially cause localized pain, swelling, and redness. If untreated, this can lead to chronic or recurrent infections, as well as permanent scarring. Wounds from foreign bodies may not be sutured because of the risk of infection.

 [🌐] **NURSING PEARL**

Indications for imaging vary depending on composition of the suspected foreign body because materials have different levels of radiolucency. Radiopaque materials, such as metal, glass, stone, and most bones, are visible on x-ray, while intermediate to radiolucent materials, such as plastics and wood, may not be visible. Ultrasound may be used to find foreign bodies that are not visible on x-ray or CT.

Patient Education

- Perform wound care as instructed.
- Report signs and symptoms of infection, such as redness, swelling, and drainage.

INFECTIONS

Overview

- Skin is an important barrier against infection.
- Skin infections result from a break in skin integrity from some type of wound or injury.
- Wounds in the mouth, on the perineum, and on the soles of the feet are at higher risk for wound infections because of bacterial flora normally present on those parts of the body.

[ ] **COMPLICATIONS**

Complications of cellulitis include permanent tissue damage and gangrene at the infection site, necessitating amputation. The infection can also spread to the blood and to other body parts, resulting in septic shock or death.

- Wounds that are contaminated at the time of the injury are at a higher risk for infection, including injuries from farming-related accidents, wounds exposed to contaminated water, and animal and human bites.
- Thorough wound cleaning is the best prophylaxis for infection. Other than topical antibiotic ointment (see Table 13.1), routine antibiotics are not recommended unless the wound is high-risk.
- Antibiotics are recommended for puncture wounds, open fractures, heavily contaminated wounds, major soft tissue injuries, and bites. Antibiotics are also indicated for most wounds for which the patient delayed seeking care (typically for greater than 12–24 hours).
- Individuals who are immunocompromised or have chronic health problems may require prophylactic antibiotics for other injury types.
- An *abscess* is a collection of pus beneath tissue.
- Abscesses develop when the body's immune system mobilizes to surround the collection of leukocytes and necrotic tissue, creating a wall to seal off the area and limit the spread of infection.
- *Cellulitis* is non-necrotizing inflammation of the skin and subcutaneous tissue usually caused by streptococcus or staphylococcus. Risk factors for cellulitis include a history of cellulitis or skin problems, peripheral vascular disease, diabetes, a history of skin trauma or open wounds, or being immunocompromised.

Signs and Symptoms

- Blisters
- Drainage
- Fever
- Pain and tenderness
- Redness
- Swelling
- Warmth

Diagnosis

Labs

- Blood cultures
- Complete blood count (CBC)
- Comprehensive metabolic panel (CMP) ▶

Labs (continued)

- Lactic acid (sepsis)
- Wound cultures

Diagnostic Testing

- CT
- X-rays

Treatment

- Antibiotics (see Table A.1)
- Assessment and treatment of sepsis, if present
- Incision, drainage, and debridement of the wound if indicated
- Pain management (see Table A.2)
- Severe infections: may require hospital admission
- Tetanus prophylaxis (see Table 13.1)

Nursing Interventions

- Administer antibiotics as ordered
- Administer tetanus prophylaxis (see Table 13.1).
- Assess and manage pain.
- Perform focused wound assessment.
- Perform sepsis assessment.
- Perform wound care.

Patient Education

- Perform wound care as directed.
- Report worsening signs and symptoms of infection, including fever and increased pain, redness, swelling, or drainage.
- Take all antibiotics as prescribed.

INJECTION INJURIES

Overview

- Injection injuries are caused by paint or grease guns and usually involve the hand.
- Only a small area of damage may be visible on the skin, but these injuries can cause significant internal tissue damage.
- In addition to the tissue damage caused by the physical force of the injury, there can be toxic effects from the chemical injected.

Signs and Symptoms

- Bleeding
- Drainage of the injected substance
- Pain
- Puncture wound

[ ]   COMPLICATIONS

Injection injuries are likely to become infected, cause chronic pain, and decrease mobility and function of the injured area. These wounds require urgent surgical exploration and treatment to reduce the risk of complications. Oil-based paint injection and solvent injection are the most damaging to tissues and frequently result in amputation.

Diagnosis

Labs

- CBC
- CMP
- Type and screen

Diagnostic Testing

- CT
- X-rays

Treatment

- Broad-spectrum antibiotics
- Pain management
- Tetanus prophylaxis (see Table 13.1)
- Surgical debridement

Nursing Interventions

- Administer antibiotics.
- Administer tetanus prophylaxis (see Table 13.1).
- Assess and monitor neurovascular status for potential compartment syndrome.
- Assess and manage pain.
- Perform focused injury assessment.
- Prepare patient for surgery.

Patient Education

- Change or remove dressing as directed.
- Take all antibiotics as prescribed.
- Report increasing pain, numbness and tingling, and loss of function to the affected body part.
- Report signs and symptoms of infection.

LACERATIONS

Overview

- A *laceration* is a tissue tear as a result of blunt trauma, caused by crushing or shearing forces. Superficial lacerations involve the epidermis and dermis.
- Sutures or staples may be necessary to close deep lacerations or lacerations over joints. Local anesthetics are used to decrease pain during the procedure.
- Superficial lacerations may be closed with closure strips or tissue adhesives.

[ ] **POP QUIZ 13.3**

A patient presents to the ED after shooting themselves in the hand with a grease gun. How should the nurse proceed?

[🧠] **COMPLICATIONS**

Thorough cleaning, debridement, and appropriate wound closure are the best way to prevent an infection. The recommended maximum timeline for wound closure varies depending on wound location and mechanism of injury; generally, primary wound closure is recommended for up to 18 hours for most lacerations and up to 24 hours for head wounds. Topical antibiotic ointment is usually sufficient for simple lacerations. The routine use of prophylactic antibiotics is not recommended for healthy patients with uncomplicated wounds.

Signs and Symptoms

- Bleeding
- Open area in the skin: edges can be uneven or smooth but usually can be approximated.
- Pain

Diagnosis

Labs

- Dependent on severity; may require trauma workup

Diagnostic Testing

- X-rays as indicated to detect a foreign body

Treatment

- Antibiotics as indicated
- Cleaning, irrigation, and debridement
- Nonadherent dressing
- Pain management
- Tetanus prophylaxis as indicated (see Table 13.1)
- Wound closure using closure strips, staples, or sutures

Nursing Interventions

- Administer antibiotics as indicated (see Table A.1).
- Administer tetanus prophylaxis (see Table 13.1).
- Apply nonadherent dressing.
- Assess/manage pain (see Table A.2).
- Assess neurovascular status after wound closure and if circumferential dressing is applied.
- Clean and irrigate the wound.

Patient Education

- Perform wound care as directed
- Report any signs or symptoms of infection, such as fever, redness, drainage, and swelling.
- Return for suture or staple removal as directed.
- If tissue adhesive was used, do not apply ointments or get the wound wet. The adhesive will fall off in 5 to 10 days.
- If adhesive strips were used, do not apply ointments or get the wound wet. The strips will fall off on their own.

MISSILE INJURIES

Overview

- *Missile injuries* are injuries from projectiles such as bullets.
- Injuries from gunshots may be accidental or intentional and may occur as a result of suicidal ideation, crime, or interpersonal violence. ▶

 NURSING PEARL

The time frame for suture removal varies depending on the location of the sutures. Sutures on the face are removed after 3 to 5 days. Sutures on the scalp, torso, hands, and feet are removed in 7 to 10 days. Sutures in the arms and legs and over any joints must stay in place for 10 to 14 days. Staple removal follows similar recommendations, with removal recommended as follows: scalp at 7 to 10 days, trunk/upper extremities at 7 days, and lower extremities at 8 to 10 days.

 POP QUIZ 13.4

The patient has a laceration repair that requires tissue adhesive care for the wound at home. How can the patient keep it from getting infected?

 COMPLICATIONS

Injuries sustained from gunshot wounds vary from minor to life threatening. Critical injuries require aggressive fluid resuscitation and emergent surgical intervention to control hemorrhaging and reduce mortality risk.

Overview *(continued)*

- Follow local laws for reporting these injuries.
- Note that patients may delay seeking treatment or provide an inconsistent history of events due to concerns about gunshot wounds being reported to police.
- The location, size, and appearance of any visible wounds should be documented; however, when assessing for injuries, the size and location of external wounds will not necessarily correlate with the location and extent of internal trauma.
- The amount of injury is related to the speed and path of the missile and its shape and composition.
- Bullet wounds can be high or low velocity and can involve tumbling (twisting/turning of the projectile), yawing (traveling at an angular path), and fragmentation (breaking apart), which increase the amount of tissue damage.
- Nail gun injuries are usually accidental and occupation related.
- Additional trauma and complications may be caused by the patient attempting to remove the object themselves.

Signs and Symptoms

- Abrasions
- Bleeding
- Burn marks
- Bruising
- Pain
- Puncture wound
- Signs of hemodynamic instability and shock
- Visible/palpable foreign body

Diagnosis

Labs

- CBC
- CMP
- Prothrombin time (PT), activated partial thromboplastin time (aPTT)
- Type and crossmatch

Diagnostic Testing

- CT
- Ultrasound
- X-rays

Treatment

- Driven by the extent of the injury: localized interventions to full trauma resuscitation
- Antibiotics as indicated
- Control of hemorrhage
- Fluid resuscitation as indicated
- Pain management
- Surgical removal of foreign body
- Tetanus prophylaxis (see Table 13.1)

Nursing Interventions

- Perform trauma assessment. Preservation of forensic evidence should be considered when providing lifesaving interventions, although evidence collection should not delay care. Handle patient clothing carefully with clean gloves, and place individual items in a separate paper bag. Place a paper bag over the patient's hands to preserve gunshot residue. If a bullet is found and removed, place it in a sterile specimen cup. Carefully document patient assessment, noting all evidence collected, and maintain chain of custody until evidence is transferred to police.
- Control bleeding. Apply pressure to wounds to control bleeding. Application of a tourniquet is indicated for uncontrolled bleeding from an extremity. Patients are likely to experience hemodynamic compromise and shock due to acute blood loss. See Chapter 2 for further information regarding management of hypovolemic shock.
- Initiate two large-bore intravenous (IV) lines for crystalloid fluid and blood product administration.
- Monitor neurovascular function and hemodynamic status.
- Administer medications (see Table 13.1).
- Prepare patient for emergent surgery or transfer to trauma unit.

Patient Education

- Report signs and symptoms of infection.
- Perform wound care as instructed.
- Follow up as instructed for continued treatment after discharge (with mental health resources if applicable for suicidal ideations, with victim support, or with outpatient physical therapy as indicated).

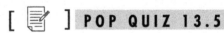

POP QUIZ 13.5

Why is it necessary to perform a head-to-toe assessment on patients with gunshot wounds?

PRESSURE ULCERS

Overview

- Pressure ulcers result from excess pressure on the skin.
- Severity ranges from nonblanching erythema (stage 1) to open wounds with major tissue loss and even bone exposure (stage 4).
- Pressure ulcers are more common over bony prominences.
- Patients with limited mobility and comorbid conditions are at the highest risk.
- Other risk factors frequently seen in patients that the nurse can address include incontinence, poor nutritional status, dehydration, and use of medical devices (e.g., cervical collar, nasal cannula, and bilevel positive airway pressure [BIPAP] machine).

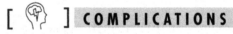

COMPLICATIONS

Advanced stage pressure ulcers can be very painful and difficult to treat. Usually, they require surgical debridement and extensive wound care measures.

Signs and Symptoms

- Drainage
- Erythema (stage 1)
- Open wound: stage 2—shallow, basin-like wound or blister; stage 3—deep, crater-like wound with exposed fat tissue; stage 4—major deep tissue loss; unstageable—covered by necrotic tissue/eschar
- Pain

Diagnosis

Labs

- CBC
- CMP
- Serum albumin levels
- Wound cultures as indicated

Diagnostic Testing

CT scan may be indicated for severe wounds.

Treatment

- Antibiotic administration (see Table A.1)
- Cleansing and debridement of the wound
- Nutritional consult
- Pain management (see Table A.2)
- Relief of pressure on the area
- Wound specialist consult

Nursing Interventions

- Assess and treat pain.
- Assess other at-risk areas.
- Measure and document wound size and characteristics.
- Pad bony prominences or other areas with pressure from medical devices.
- Perform focused wound assessment.
- Perform wound care.
- Turn and reposition patient frequently.

Patient Education

- Maintain good nutritional intake.
- Perform wound care as directed.
- Turn and reposition frequently.

PUNCTURE WOUNDS

Overview

- *Puncture wounds* are caused by an object that penetrates the skin and underlying tissues, resulting in a wound that is deeper than it is wide.
- These wounds range in severity from minor (e.g., wood splinter in finger), which requires only localized treatment, to severe (e.g., large impaled object), which requires a trauma workup and emergent surgery.
- Bites (from humans or animals) are also considered puncture wounds and are associated with a very high risk for infection.

 ALERT!

Frequently, ED patients have comorbidities that increase their risk for pressure injuries. Additionally, ED stretchers typically have thin mattresses, and some patients are placed on long backboards. Remember to perform a skin assessment on all patients who are at risk for developing pressure injuries. Turn and reposition these patients frequently and apply padding to reduce their risk.

 COMPLICATIONS

Patients may develop severe complications related to puncture wounds. Punctures overlying a joint may lead to the development of septic arthritis, a serious condition in which the joint space becomes infected. Punctures that penetrate bone may lead to the development of osteomyelitis. Certain puncture injuries, such as needlesticks, may lead to the development of diseases such as HIV infection and hepatitis.

Signs and Symptoms

Presentation varies depending on the mechanism of injury and may include the following:

- Bleeding or discharge
- Foreign body (may or may not be present in wound)
- Pain

Diagnosis

Labs

- CBC
- Cultures if indicated

Diagnostic Testing

- X-ray (to assess for foreign body in wound)

Treatment

- Antibiotics (see Table A.1)
- Pain management (see Table A.2)
- Removal of object: may require surgical intervention
- Tetanus prophylaxis (see Table 13.1)

Nursing Interventions

- Administer antibiotics as ordered (see Table A.1).
- Administer tetanus prophylaxis (see Table 13.1).
- Assess and treat pain.
- Perform focused wound assessment, including neurovascular assessment of the affected area.
- Perform wound care as indicated, including wound irrigation, application of antibiotic ointment (if indicated), and dressing as ordered.
- If a foreign body is present in the wound, removal may be performed by the emergency provider. Patients with large foreign bodies may require stabilizing treatment and surgical intervention to remove the object. Penetrating injuries to the chest are covered in greater depth in Chapter 2 and penetrating abdominal trauma is covered in Chapters 5 and 6.
- Document and report animal bites per local regulations.

[🌐] **NURSING PEARL**

Typically, puncture wounds are not closed by primary intention due to significant risk for infection. Ensure that the wound has been irrigated and dressed properly to prevent infection. When providing discharge teaching, emphasize the importance of proper wound care and monitoring for signs of infection to prevent complications.

Patient Education

- Perform wound care as instructed.
- Return for evaluation if signs of infection occur, such as redness, swelling, drainage, or tenderness.

TRAUMA

Overview

- Understanding the mechanism of injury helps identify potential injuries.
- The immediate concern for traumatic wounds is blood loss.

[🧠] **COMPLICATIONS**

Infection is a frequent complication of traumatic wounds. The mechanism of injury may involve a source of contamination. Additionally, thorough cleaning of wounds may be delayed by resuscitation efforts.

Overview *(continued)*

- Uncontrolled hemorrhage should be treated during the primary survey.
- Methods of controlling arterial bleeding include application of direct pressure, application of pressure to a proximal artery, elevation of the extremity, and application of tourniquets (for extremity bleeding).

Signs and Symptoms

- Bleeding/hemorrhage
- Pain
- Signs of hemodynamic instability
- Wounds: lacerations, avulsions, puncture wounds, bites, abrasions, injection injuries, gunshot or other missile/projectile injuries

Diagnosis

Labs

- CBC
- CMP
- PT, aPTT
- Type and crossmatch

Diagnostic Testing

- CT
- Ultrasound
- X-rays

Treatment

- Priority treatment: controlling external hemorrhage
- Cleaning and disinfection of wounds
- Possible administration of a hemostatic agent, such as tranexamic acid (see Table 13.1)
- Fluid resuscitation (crystalloid fluids or blood products)
- Pain management
- Stabilization of airway, breathing, and circulation
- Surgical intervention (possibly emergent)
- Trauma assessment
- Tetanus prophylaxis (see Table 13.1)

Nursing Interventions

- Administer tetanus prophylaxis (see Table 13.1).
- Assess and treat pain.
- Clean and disinfect wounds.
- Initiate two large-bore IV lines for fluid resuscitation.
- Monitor hemodynamic status.
- Perform trauma assessment.
- Prepare patient for surgical intervention.

Patient Education

- Follow prescribed activity limitations.
- Perform wound care as directed.
- Report any signs or symptoms of infection.

RESOURCES

American College of Surgeons. (2018). *ATLS advanced trauma life support*. Author.

Blank-Reid, C. (2020). Epidemiology and mechanisms of injury. In V. Sweet & A. Foley (Eds.), *Sheehy's emergency nursing: Principles and practice* (7th ed., pp. 378–400). Elsevier.

Boyse, T. D., Fessell, D. P., Jacobson, J. A., Lin, J., van Holsbeeck, M. T., & Hayes, C. W. (2001). US of soft-tissue foreign bodies and associated complications with surgical correlation. *RadioGraphics*, *21*(5), 1251–1256. https://doi.org/10.1148/radiographics.21.5.g01se271251

Cerepani, M. (2020). Orthopedic and neurovascular trauma. In V. Sweet & A. Foley (Eds.), *Sheehy's emergency nursing: Principles and practice* (7th ed., pp. 477–502). Elsevier.

Denke, N. (2020). Wound management. In V. Sweet & A. Foley (Eds.), *Sheehy's emergency nursing: Principles and practice* (7th ed., pp. 93–111). Elsevier.

Halpern, J. (2013). Musculoskeletal trauma. In B. Hammond & P. Zimmerman (Eds.), *Sheehy's manual of emergency care* (7th ed., pp. 427–437). Elsevier Mosby.

Herr, R. (2013). Wound management. In B. Hammond & P. Zimmerman (Eds.), *Sheehy's manual of emergency care*. (7th ed., pp. 147–166). Elsevier Mosby.

Prescribers' Digital Reference. (n.d.-a). *Bacitracin/neomycin/polymyxin B sulfate* [Drug nformation]. https://www.pdr.net/drug-summary/Neosporin-Original-Ointment-bacitracin-neomycin-polymyxin-B-sulfate-2743

Prescribers' Digital Reference. (n.d.-b). *Lidocaine hydrochloride* [Drug information]. https://www.pdr.net/drug-summary/Xylocaine-injection-lidocaine-hydrochloride-2454

Prescribers' Digital Reference. (n.d.-c). *Tetanus and diphtheria toxoids adsorbed* [Drug information]. https://www.pdr.net/drug-summary/Tetanus-and-Diphtheria-Toxoids-Adsorbed--For-age-7-years-and-older--tetanus-and-diphtheria-toxoids-adsorbed-884

Prescribers' Digital Reference. (n.d.-d). *Tranexamic acid* [Drug information]. https://www.pdr.net/drug-summary/Cyklokapron-tranexamic-acid-1885

14 ENVIRONMENTAL EMERGENCIES

BURNS

Overview

- Burns are caused by fire, chemicals, hot liquids or gases, electricity, lightning, radiation, or frostbite.
- Location, extent, and duration of exposure are key factors influencing patient outcomes.
- Thermal burns are the most common and are caused by exposure to hot liquid (scald burn), fire (flame burn), explosions (flash burn), or a hot object (contact burn).
- Electrical burns take the path of least resistance and may cause significant internal injuries involving the heart, muscle, and nerve tissue.
- Local reaction includes vascular changes and aggressive inflammatory response.
- The systemic response to severe burns is the release of inflammatory mediators causing systemic capillary leaking, large intervascular fluid shifts, and intervascular fluid loss.
- Complications from the systemic inflammatory response are coagulation, fibrinolysis, cardiovascular changes, and a hypermetabolic state.
- Burn shock is the result of fluid shifts, decreased cardiac output, and increased vascular resistance that is treated with early, aggressive intravenous (IV) therapy.
- Burns are classified according to depth (degree; may change over time) and extent (% total body surface area [TBSA]).
- Indications for transfer to a burn center: partial-thickness/full-thickness burns greater than 10% TBSA; burns involving the face, hands, feet, genitalia, perineum, or major joints; full-thickness burns; electrical or chemical burns; inhalation injury; existing comorbidities; concomitant trauma (fractures); pediatric patients or patients with special needs; patients who require special social or emotional care, often associated with traumatic burns; patients who will need significant physical rehabilitation due to loss of function.

[ ] **COMPLICATIONS**

Inhalation injury is the most common cause of death from fire. It involves three different problems: CO intoxication, upper airway obstruction, and chemical injury to the lower airways and lungs. Signs of inhalation injury should be treated aggressively. Patients with these injuries usually require early intubation and ventilation with 100% oxygen to prevent serious respiratory complications (acute respiratory distress syndrome) and death.

Signs and Symptoms

See Table 14.1.

Diagnosis

Labs

- Arterial blood gases (ABGs) with carboxyhemoglobin measurement
- Complete blood count (CBC): elevated white blood cells, low hemoglobin and hematocrit
- Creatine kinase (CK) elevated in rhabdomyolysis ▶

TABLE 14.1 Signs and Symptoms of Burns

SUPERFICIAL (FIRST-DEGREE) EPIDERMIS	PARTIAL-THICKNESS (SECOND-DEGREE) DERMIS: PAPILLARY REGION	FULL-THICKNESS (THIRD-DEGREE) DERMIS/HYPODERMIS OR SUBCUTANEOUS TISSUE
• Possible blistering • Mild to moderate pain • Redness • Sunburn appearance	• Blistering • Blanchable • Mottled appearance • Swelling • Painful	• Deep-partial thickness: white and leathery with slight pain • Full thickness: charred, loss of sensation and eschar • Painless

Labs (continued)

- Comprehensive metabolic panel (CMP) to determine hyperkalemia/hypocalcemia resulting from damaged muscle cells, blood urea nitrogen/creatine to assess for acute renal insufficiency
- Lactic acid: elevated
- Type and crossmatch
- Urinalysis (UA)
- Urine myoglobin

Diagnostic Testing

- Bronchoscopy (inhalation injury)
- Chest x-ray (inhalation injury)
- Compartment pressure monitoring
- EKG
- X-rays as indicated for other trauma

Treatment

- Airway/respiratory management: assessment for carbonaceous debris or sputum or singed nasal hairs and changes in voice, which may indicate inhalation injury; assessment for circumferential burns to head, neck, and chest; determination of inhalation injury likelihood; emergent intubation before edema worsens and obstructs airway; head of bed (HOB) elevated to 30 degrees; high-flow O_2 via non-rebreather mask if patient not intubated (humidified preferred)
- Circulatory management: assessment of circumferential burns and risk of compartment syndrome; monitoring for dysrhythmias, hypotension, and burn shock; assessment/management for hypovolemic, distributive, and cardiogenic shock; fluid guidelines for burns greater than 20% TBSA; monitoring urine output; burn patients treated as trauma patients first
- Chemical burns on skin flushed with copious amounts of water unless contraindicated
- Emergent transfer to a burn unit if indicated

 ALERT!

Immediately stop the burning process by removing the patient's clothing. Be aware that chemical burns may require a hazardous materials response before initiating treatment except in lifesaving interventions. This response may include staff wearing chemical-resistant suits and a breathing apparatus.

NURSING PEARL

Do not apply ice to any burns, as this may cause further damage to the skin. Leave all blisters intact.

Treatment *(continued)*

- Hyperbaric oxygenation
- Infection prevention using sterile nonadherent dressings and sterile sheets or towels
- Monitoring for compartment syndrome with pressures over 30 mmHg; may require emergent escharotomy or fasciotomy
- Pain management such as with acetaminophen, nonsteroidal anti-inflammatory drugs (NSAIDs), and opiates (see Table A.2)
- Partial-thickness burns: cleaned with soap; blisters left intact; antibiotic ointment and dressing; *no* delay of transfer for diagnostic or wound care
- Regulation of body temperature to prevent hypothermia with large partial- and full-thickness burns (keep patient dry)
- Specialty dressing
- Tetanus prophylaxis
- Topical antibiotics such as silver sulfadiazine (see Table 14.2)
- Treatment of other injuries as indicated

TABLE 14.2 Environmental Medications

INDICATIONS	MECHANISM OF ACTION	CONTRAINDICATIONS, PRECAUTIONS, AND ADVERSE EFFECTS
Antibiotics (silver sulfadiazine, sulfadiazine)		
• Minor burns	• Stop growth of bacteria	• Medication belongs to the sulfa drug class; use caution in patients with sulfa allergy.
Anticholinergics (atropine sulfate)		
• Cholinergic crisis induced by organophosphate exposure	• Inhibit autonomic postganglionic cholinergic receptors • Decrease secretions to help maintain airway; increase HR	• Administer IV or IM and repeat every 20–30 minutes until symptoms dissipate. • Maintain HR of 100 bpm. • Medication is considered the first-line antidote.
Antifungals, topical (clotrimazole, miconazole)		
• Ringworm	• Fungistatic agents that alter the fungal cell membrane	• Wash hands before and after use. • Clean area before applying.
Antihistamines (cyproheptadine hydrochloride)		
• Scabies	• H1-receptor blockers	• Do not administer to infants. • Medication can be sedating.
Antiprotozoals (metronidazole, tinidazole, nitazoxanide)		
• Giardiasis and other protozoal infections	• Amebicidal, bactericidal and trichomonacidal	• Medication can be given PO or IV. • Use IV administration by intermittent or slow infusion only in dedicated line. • Medication can cause headache and metallic taste in mouth.

(continued)

TABLE 14.2 Environmental Medications *(continued)*

INDICATIONS	MECHANISM OF ACTION	CONTRAINDICATIONS, PRECAUTIONS, AND ADVERSE EFFECTS
Antivenin, snake (crotalidae polyvalent immune fab ovine)		
• North American crotalid envenomation (rattlesnakes, copperheads, water moccasins)	• Binds and neutralize venom toxins	• The best response occurs if initiated within 6 hours of bite. • Initiate first dose at a slow rate for the first 10 minutes. If no signs of allergic reaction occur, increase the infusion rate up to 250 mL/hr. • Observe patient for 1 hour after first dose. If symptoms persist, administer 4–6 additional doses.
Antivenin, spider (black widow spider antivenin equine)		
• Envenomation (black widow spider)	• Neutralizes symptomatic toxic effects of bite	• Administer IV or IM. • Perform sensitivity testing prior to administration. • Monitor for signs of allergic reaction.
Pralidoxime chloride		
• Organophosphate poisoning	• Reverses muscle paralysis	• Medication must be administered concomitantly with atropine. • Medication can be given IV or IM.
Rabies immune globulin		
• PEP for rabies	• Provides immediate passive immunity to rabies	• Medication is not indicated if patient has adequate rabies antibodies. • Medication is administered by infiltration around the wound and IM. • Wounds should be thoroughly cleaned before administration. • Side effects include malaise and headache. • Medication is administered in conjunction with the rabies vaccine.
Rabies vaccine		
• PEP for rabies	• Induces production of specific neutralizing antibodies against the rabies virus	• Use IM administration only. • Side effects include malaise and headache. • Medication can cause localized reaction at injection site. • Administer in conjunction with rabies immune globulin.

Note: All agents are contraindicated in the presence of hypersensitivity to the medication or one of its components.
bpm, beats per minute; HR, heart rate; IM, intramuscular; IV, intravenous; PEP, postexposure prophylaxis; PO, orally.

Nursing Interventions

- Administer antibiotics if ordered (see Table A.1).
- Administer pain medications as ordered. Burn patients have a higher metabolism, so dosing will need to be more frequent.
- Administer tetanus prophylaxis as indicated.
- Assess/manage airway, breathing, and circulation.
- Assess type, location, extent, and depth of burns.
- Implement infection prevention measures to minimize wound contamination.

 ALERT!

The rule of nines, which breaks down sections of the body into multiples of 9%, can be used to quickly estimate burn size (Table 14.3).

TABLE 14.3 Rule of Nines	
Anterior head	4.5%
Posterior head	4.5%
Anterior arm	4.5%
Posterior arm	4.5%
Anterior torso	18%
Posterior torso	18%
Anterior leg	9%
Posterior leg	9%
Perineum	1%

Nursing Interventions (continued)

- Initiate two large-bore IV lines for fluid resuscitation (preferably in nonburned tissue) and draw blood for lab tests.
- Monitor for compartment syndrome and assist in gathering equipment for intervention.
- Monitor hemodynamic status.
- Monitor input/output (I/O) as minimum output: should be 0.5 to 1 mL/kg/hr. Significant burns may require a Foley catheter for accurate recording.
- Monitor/maintain temperature and minimize heat loss: Ideal temperature is between 98.6°F (37°C) and 101.3°F (38.5°C).
- Monitor neurovascular status.
- Perform wound care as indicated.
- Prepare for transfer to a burn unit as indicated.
- Remove all patient clothing and assess need for hazardous materials intervention.

Patient Education

- Do not break blisters if developed.
- Do not scratch skin during the healing process, as this may lead to increased scarring and infection; an antihistamine may be suggested by the provider.
- First- and second-degree burns generally heal in 1 to 2 weeks with little chance of scarring, but skin may appear darker for up to 6 to 9 months.
- Follow prescribed activity guidelines to promote safe movement and prevent contractures; attend physical/occupational therapy if ordered.
- Follow up with the burn center if recommended.
- Learn burn prevention: Use water no hotter than 120°F (48.8°C), keep candles and matches away from children, ensure smoke detectors are working, and prevent sunburn by using sunscreen liberally and frequently.
- Maintain adequate nutritional intake to promote wound healing. Focus on a high-protein and low-sugar diet.
- Prevent infection by washing hands before touching wound, do not apply home topicals unless approved by doctor, and perform dressing changes as ordered. ▶

[ ] **POP QUIZ 14.1**

An adult patient fell into a fire pit and sustained a circumferential third-degree burn to the right leg from the knee to the toes, as well as second-degree burns to the entire right anterior arm. How would the nurse assess and treat this patient?

Patient Education *(continued)*

- Report signs or symptoms of infection such as increasing redness, pain, pus-like drainage, and temperature over 100.4°F (38°C).
- Take antibiotics appropriately if ordered.
- Take prescribed pain medication as ordered.
- Use incentive spirometry if prescribed.

CHEMICAL EXPOSURES

Overview

- Chemical exposures may be a result of terrorism or accidental exposure to industrial or domestic chemicals; identification of the substance is critical for appropriate treatment.
- They occur through inhalation, contact, ingestion, or injection.
- Traditional weapons of mass destruction: blood agents (cyanide); incapacitating agents (anticholinergic agents); nerve agents (tabun, sarin, soman); pulmonary agents (chlorine, phosgene); vesicants (blister agents such as sulfur mustard).
- Crowd control weapons: pepper spray; tear gas.
- Toxic industrial chemicals (may be found residentially and/or mixed): ammonia; formaldehyde; hydrogen fluoride; hydrogen sulfide; phosphene; sulfuric acid.
- Organophosphates such as insecticides, herbicides, and nerve gases (sarin) are cholinesterase inhibitors that cause accumulation of acetylcholine, leading to immediate, life-threatening symptoms.
- Chemicals may produce burns, dermatitis, allergic reaction, thermal injury, and/or systemic toxicity.

[🧠] COMPLICATIONS

Damage from chemical burns continues to progress after the initial injury. Chemical burns should be treated aggressively to reduce the risk of scarring and infection. For severe burns, skin grafting may be required.

Signs and Symptoms

- Skin: itching, redness, blistering, open wound, and necrosis
- Respiratory: cough, bloody sputum, shortness of breath, and adventitious lung sounds
- Nausea/vomiting/diarrhea
- Tearing of the eyes
- Runny nose
- Mild/moderate exposure to nerve agent: behavioral changes, constricted pupils, diaphoresis, dyspnea, fasciculations, increased secretions, nausea/vomiting, polyuria, weakness
- Severe exposure to nerve agents: apnea, convulsions, flaccid paralysis, seizures, unconsciousness

[🌐] NURSING PEARL

The SLUDGEM mnemonic describes the signs and symptoms caused by exposure to a nerve agent:

S: Salivation and increased secretions
L: Lacrimation
U: Urinary incontinence
D: Defecation, incontinence
G: Gastrointestinal distress
E: Emesis
M: Miosis

Diagnosis

Labs

- ABG
- Calcium, magnesium, and potassium for hydrofluoric exposure
- CBC ▶

Labs (continued)
- CMP
- Creatine phosphokinase (CPK)
- pH/litmus test
- Prothrombin time (PT)/coagulation panel
- UA: pseudocholinesterase; PT/coagulation panel

Diagnostic Testing
- Chest and/or abdomen x-ray if signs of peritonitis
- EKG
- Further imaging as indicated for exposure

Treatment

- Priority: airway maintenance; first intervention or done simultaneously with decontamination
- Identification of causative agent and decontamination/hazardous materials procedures to safely remove contaminant and protect ED staff from exposure. Staff should be protected from off-gassing (when a patient breathes out inhaled chemicals). Dry substances should be carefully removed and appropriately discarded. Unidentified chemicals most likely require flushing copiously with water. Cover with mineral oil if exposure to metallic lithium, sodium, potassium, or magnesium is suspected or confirmed. Use eyewash station when available and appropriate.
- Basic life support care only until decontamination is complete; remove dressings, tubes, or catheters placed before decontamination, as they are now contaminated.
- Airway, breathing, and circulation management (intubation and sedation likely indicated).
- Antibiotics as indicated (see Table A.1).
- Assessment for signs of shock and initiation of fluid resuscitation.
- Bronchoscopy if burns to the airway need to be assessed.
- Consultation with appropriate services such as GI, ear-nose-throat, or ophthalmology.
- Consultation with hazmat resources or poison control to find antidote (epinephrine, activated charcoal, neutralizing agents).
- Pain management (see Table A.2).
- Chemical burns: Brush off dry substances before irrigating skin. Remove clothing carefully, as skin may be adhered to clothes. Irrigate wet chemical burn (acidic irrigation for 30 minutes; alkali continuous irrigation until neutral pH achieved). Follow treatment strategies for burns.
- Nerve agents: Control seizure activity. Administer antidotes (atropine and pralidoxime chloride).

Nursing Interventions

- Don appropriate personal protective equipment (PPE), which may include a powered air purifier, a chemical suit with foot coverings, and double gloves.
- Airway maintenance and lifesaving interventions are a priority and should be the first intervention.
- Identify agent and decontaminate patient after lifesaving interventions are complete.
- Administer fluid resuscitation if ordered.
- Administer medications as ordered for sedation and seizures (see Table A.2).
- Administer tetanus vaccine if indicated.
- Assess and manage pain (see Table A.2).
- Assess and document burn, and perform burn care if indicated.
- Assess for systemic toxicity.
- Assess/maintain airway, breathing, and circulation (frequent suctioning may be needed for organophosphate exposure). ▶

Nursing Interventions *(continued)*

- Establish IV access and draw blood for lab tests.
- Frequently monitor vital signs and neurologic status.
- If cause is known, give antidote as soon as it is available.
- Initiate suicide precautions if the exposure was self-induced/intentional.

Patient Education

- Follow burn and wound care instructions and learn how to change dressings.
- Follow up as directed for continued management of side effects.
- Learn proper use of pain medications and antibiotics.
- Monitor for signs and symptoms of infection.

ELECTRICAL INJURIES

Overview

- Electrical injuries may range from mild to severe, and internal damage may be significantly worse than anticipated based on the path of conduction between two points.
- High-voltage and arching sources of electricity are a prevalent occupational hazard for electricians and power-line workers.
- Common sources of electrical injuries are downed power lines, often encountered at the scene of a car crash; lightning; tasers/stun guns; and electrical appliances.
- Electrical injuries may involve any tissue of the body, including the central nervous system (CNS).
- Complications are related to amount, duration, and type of current (alternating [AC] or direct [DC]).

Signs and Symptoms

- Altered mental status or unconsciousness
- Altered vision and hearing
- Burns/necrosis
- Cardiac arrest
- Dark urine
- Dysrhythmias/tachycardia
- Fractures
- Muscle spasms, tetany
- Pain
- Paralysis
- Seizures
- Shortness of breath

Diagnosis

Labs

- ABG
- Cardiac enzymes ▶

[📝] **POP QUIZ 14.2**

A patient has sustained a splash of an unknown cleaning chemical to the face and is experiencing blurry vision. What is the initial assessment and treatment upon arrival to the ED?

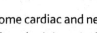

[🧠] **COMPLICATIONS**

Some cardiac and neuromuscular complications appear soon after the injury, including cardiac dysrhythmias, and others may be delayed, such as rhabdomyolysis.

[🤲] **NURSING PEARL**

Flash burns are a result of heat being released from arcing wires that causes thermal burns to the body without electricity actually entering the body. Skin burns and eye injuries result.

Labs (continued)

- CBC
- CMP to monitor for acute kidney injury, electrolyte abnormalities
- CPK
- Myoglobin (for rhabdomyolysis)
- UA

Diagnostic Testing

- CT
- EKG
- Ultrasound (focused assessment with sonography in trauma, cardiac)
- X-rays

Treatment

- Airway, breathing, and circulation maintenance
- Antibiotics for burns (see Table A.1)
- Anticipation of internal burns in high-voltage electrical events
- External burn wounds treated with dry sterile dressing
- Fasciotomy to improve tissue perfusion and prevent further necrosis/compartment syndrome
- Fluid resuscitation if indicated: crystalloid fluid infused at 75 to 100 mL/hr with goal of urine output 1 to 1.5 mL/kg/hr or clear urine; colloids for internal hemorrhage
- Monitoring/treatment of dysrhythmias; continuous monitoring required for any abnormalities on EKG
- Pain management (see Table A.2.)
- Seizure medications
- Treatment of electrolyte abnormalities

Nursing Interventions

- Administer antibiotics and/or seizure medications.
- Administer fluid resuscitation.
- Assess and treat pain.
- Assess and manage airway, breathing, and circulation.
- Establish IV access and draw blood for lab testing.
- Monitor I/O.
- Perform a thorough neurologic assessment.
- Perform wound/burn care.
- Place patient on cardiac monitor, perform EKG, and treat any abnormal rhythms.
- Remove clothing and perform a head-to-toe assessment (including visual acuity).

Patient Education

- Chronic pain syndrome may be a result of electrical injury. Take prescribed pain medications and follow up with the provider if pain persists.
- Make sure appliances are in good working order, replace frayed wires, keep electrical sources away from water, do not approach downed power lines, and stay indoors away from windows during lightning storms. ▶

[ ] **POP QUIZ 14.3**

A bystander at the scene of a car and utility pole crash rushed to assist the victim but received a shock and was thrown a few feet back when they opened the car door. Upon arrival at the ED, the patient has severe chest and abdomen pain. What does the nurse suspect is the cause, and what are the anticipated injuries?

Patient Education *(continued)*

- Seek treatment for any neurologic changes, including confusion, weakness, or muscle twitching.
- Seek treatment for chest pain, palpitations, or syncope.
- Treat burns as directed, including dressing changes and antibiotics if prescribed.

ENVENOMATION EMERGENCIES

Overview

- Death from envenomation is rare. The most potentially toxic or lethal causes are the result of bites by reptiles, arthropods, and insects: snakes such as pit vipers, rattlesnakes, and copperheads; arthropods such as widow spiders, recluse spiders, and scorpions; insects such as bees, wasps, and fire ants.
- The extent of injuries from envenomation is based on location and depth of bite, amount of venom injected, and number of sites.
- Stingrays (which have a venom-coated barb at the end of the tail) and jellyfish (which have stinging capsules on tentacles) also cause venom-induced injuries.

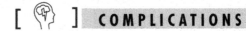 **COMPLICATIONS**

Most black widow spider bites produce only localized symptoms, including pain and skin lesions. But children and immunocompromised patients are at a higher risk for systemic effects and complications, including muscle pain, spasms, and hypertension. Antivenin use should be reserved for severe or high-risk cases.

Signs and Symptoms

See Tables 14.4, 14.5, and 14.6.

Diagnosis

Labs

- CBC
- CK
- CMP
- PT, activated partial thromboplastin time (aPTT)
- UA
- Wound culture

Diagnostic Testing

- EKG
- X-rays (rule out foreign body—stingray; chest x-ray for respiratory symptoms)

TABLE 14.4 Signs and Symptoms of Venomous Snake Bites

LOCAL	SYSTEMIC
Fang marks	Abdominal pain
Pain	Altered mental status
Bruising	Coagulopathies
Blistering	Hypotension
Swelling	Nausea/vomiting
	Parethesias

TABLE 14.5 Signs and Symptoms of Venomous Spider Bites	
LOCAL	**SYSTEMIC (BLACK WIDOW)**
Pain	Pain: abdomen, back, chest
Redness	Headache
Swelling	Hypertension
Itching	Nausea/vomiting
Blue-gray macule (brown recluse)	Respiratory distress
	Seizures

TABLE 14.6 Signs and Symptoms of Stingray and Jellyfish Injuries	
LOCAL	**SYSTEMIC**
Pain	Headache
Redness	Nausea/vomiting
Swelling	Neurologic symptoms (stingray)

Treatment

- Management of life-threatening symptoms; respiratory distress common
- Identification of species
- Poison control contact
- Immobilization/elevation of bite site to heart level
- Tourniquet removal if in place once IV access is secured
- Antidote if available
- Monitoring of site for changes in condition or infection
- Exploration for retained foreign bodies/fangs
- Pain management (no NSAIDs for snake bites)
- Tetanus prophylaxis if indicated
- Monitoring, as envenomation injury can worsen over time
- Snakebite treatment: antivenin (pit viper; see Table 14.2); immobilization of involved extremity near heart level; monitoring of swelling; no ice, tourniquets, or venom removal kits; patient exertion minimized; removal of constrictive jewelry/clothing
- Spider bite treatment: antivenin (black widow; see Table 14.2); benzodiazepines for muscle spasms (black widow; see Table A.2); ice to bite area
- Stingray treatment: antibiotics if indicated (see Table A.1); barb removal if indicated; immersion of wound in hot water for 30 to 90 minutes
- Jellyfish treatment: hot water soak; pain control; tentacle removal, if present; white vinegar rinse

[ ] **NURSING PEARL**

Tourniquets should be avoided, as they are considered ineffective and dangerous; it is better to immobilize the affected limb and keep it at heart level.

Nursing Interventions

- Administer antidote (see Table 14.2).
- Administer fluid resuscitation if indicated. ▶

Nursing Interventions (*continued*)

- Administer pain medications as prescribed (see Table A.2).
- Administer tetanus prophylaxis.
- Assess and assist with maintenance of airway, breathing, and circulation.
- Establish IV access with lab draw if ordered.
- Monitor frequently for 12 hours, as symptoms may progress slowly.
- Outline redness and swelling around site and monitor for changes.
- Perform frequent neurovascular reassessments.
- Perform thorough cleaning of site and provide wound care.
- Remove clothing and jewelry.
- Repeat lab studies every 4 to 6 hours if ordered.

Patient Education

- Perform wound care as directed.
- Seek treatment if urine becomes dark or if decreased urine output occurs.

[📝] **POP QUIZ 14.4**

What is the treatment for a stingray envenomation?

FOOD POISONING

Overview

- Food poisoning results from eating food contaminated with bacteria, viruses, or parasites.
- Contamination can occur at any point in the food preparation process.
- Norovirus, *Salmonella*, *Clostridium perfringens*, *Campylobacter*, and *Staphylococcus aureus* are the most common causes of food-borne illness.
- *Clostridium botulinum*, *Listeria*, *Escherichia coli*, and *Vibrio* are not as commonly diagnosed but are more likely to lead to hospitalization.

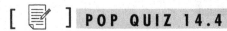

[🧠] **COMPLICATIONS**

Most food-borne illnesses are self-limiting and require minimal treatment. However, very young and older adult patients, as well as immunocompromised patients, are at high risk for complications, including dehydration and severe electrolyte disturbance.

Signs and Symptoms

- Abdominal pain/cramping
- Bloody stools
- Diarrhea
- Fever/chills
- Nausea/vomiting

Diagnosis

Labs

- CBC
- CMP
- Stool culture
- Stool for ova and parasites
- UA

Diagnostic Testing

- CT if indicated to rule out other GI issues

Treatment

- Antibiotics if indicated (see Table A.1)
- IV hydration
- Symptomatic treatment

Nursing Interventions

- Administer IV hydration.
- Administer prescribed medications.
- Perform focused GI assessment, including history of exposure.

Patient Education

- Advance diet as tolerated, starting with bland foods.
- Practice good hand hygiene.
- Practice safe food-handling techniques to prevent recurrence.
- Return for further evaluation if unable to tolerate oral intake.

PARASITE AND FUNGAL INFECTIONS

Overview

- Giardiasis is caused by the parasite *Giardia,* which is found on surfaces or in food and water contaminated with feces from infected people or animals. It is transmitted via food, contaminated drinking water, or person-to-person contact.
- *Ringworm,* or tinea, is a fungal skin infection.
- *Scabies* is a contagious condition caused by *Sarcoptes scabiei*, a mite that burrows into skin. It is transmitted via direct contact.

Signs and Symptoms

- Giardiasis: abdominal pain and cramps; bloating and foul-smelling gas; diarrhea; nausea; vomiting; weight loss
- Ringworm: hair loss; itchiness; peeling skin; redness; ring-shaped rash
- Scabies: blisters; burrow tracks; itching (usually worse at night); wheals

Diagnosis

Labs

- Blood smear
- CBC
- CMP
- Stool culture (giardiasis)
- Stool for ova and parasites (giardiasis)

Diagnostic Testing

- CT
- Endoscopy/colonoscopy (parasites)

[⚡] **ALERT!**

When treating patients with food poisoning, verify local reporting requirements, as many food-borne illnesses must be reported to local health departments. Obtain as many details as possible regarding the exposure to assist the health department in identifying potential outbreaks.

[🧠] **COMPLICATIONS**

Giardiasis can cause long-term complications, including weight loss, malnutrition from chronic diarrhea, and lactose intolerance.

Treatment

- Giardiasis: supportive (including fluid and electrolyte replacement); antibiotics for severe cases
- Ringworm: antifungal medications
- Scabies: permethrin cream; oral antihistamines
- Decontamination of patient environment/isolation precautions

Nursing Interventions

- Perform GI assessment (giardiasis).
- Perform skin assessment (ringworm, scabies).
- Administer crystalloid fluids (giardiasis).
- Administer medication as indicated (see Table 14.2).

Patient Education

- Avoid close contact with others until symptoms have resolved.
- Practice good hand hygiene.

RADIATION EXPOSURE

Overview

- Radiation injury occurs when a person inhales, ingests, or comes into physical contact with a radioactive source.
- Harmful exposure can result from an accident or an act of war.
- Side effects can result from use as cancer therapy.
- *Acute radiation syndrome* is the acute illness that develops from a significant exposure. It initially affects hematopoiesis and then, at higher doses, affects digestion and finally the CNS. Symptoms are progressive, and death is likely to occur up to weeks later depending on level of exposure.

Signs and Symptoms

- Hematopoietic: bleeding, bruising, infection
- GI: abdominal pain, diarrhea, fever; GI bleeding, nausea/vomiting
- CNS: altered LOC, confusion, convulsions

Diagnosis

Labs

- Amylase
- CBC (repeat to monitor lymphocytes)
- CMP
- Human leukocyte antigen
- Type and screen
- UA

Diagnostic Testing

Dosimetry

[📝] **POP QUIZ 14.5**

When triaging a pediatric patient who has had diarrhea for the past 2 weeks, the nurse learns that the child has been swimming in the neighbor's pond. What condition should the nurse suspect?

[ ] **COMPLICATIONS**

Significant radiation exposure affects the CNS, causing nervousness, altered level of consciousness (LOC), and convulsions. These are ominous signs indicating that the patient has experienced a fatal level of exposure.

Treatment

- Decontamination
- Consultation with specialists (hospital radiation safety officer or community experts)
- Notification of public health and law enforcement
- Stem cell or platelet transfusions as indicated
- Supportive treatment

Nursing Interventions

- Decontaminate the patient.
- Follow interventions for chemical burns.
- Use PPE to prevent contaminating staff.

Patient Education

- Avoid sunlight and extremes in temperature.
- Return for continued treatment if chest pain, respiratory distress, or uncontrolled nausea/vomiting develop.

SUBMERSION INJURY

Overview

- Patients with submersion injury may be asymptomatic initially but subsequently experience more serious complications.
- Hypoxia is the cause of death in drowning victims, regardless of water type.
- Identify the cause of the drowning event (e.g., neurologic event, abuse/trauma, suicide attempt) and treat related injuries or complications as indicated.

[🧠] **COMPLICATIONS**

In a drowning patient, water contaminants, including chlorine, microorganisms, and other substances, can worsen the pulmonary injury. Contaminants can exacerbate hypoxia and increase the risk of pneumonia and respiratory failure.

Signs and Symptoms

- Bronchospasm
- Dysrhythmias
- Hypotension
- Hypothermia
- Altered LOC
- Respiratory distress

Diagnosis

Labs

There are no labs specific to diagnosing submersion injuries. However, labs may be indicated to differentiate etiology of the event or to manage the resulting injuries.

Diagnostic Testing

- Chest x-ray
- EKG
- Other testing as indicated for injuries

Treatment

- Airway, breathing, and circulation management
- Associated injury treatment as indicated
- Close monitoring of respiratory status, as symptoms can be progressive
- Hypothermia monitoring if appropriate
- Mandatory reporting of suspected abuse/neglect as appropriate

Nursing Interventions

- Administer IV crystalloid fluids and medications as ordered.
- Manage other injuries or underlying causes as indicated.
- Monitor core temperature and implement warming measures as needed.
- Monitor respiratory status.
- Perform trauma assessment.

Patient Education

- Monitor for new or worsening symptoms, as these can manifest days after the initial injury.
- Seek urgent treatment for fevers, chest pain, and shortness of breath.

TEMPERATURE-RELATED INJURIES

Overview

- Temperature-related injuries involve situations in which the body is too hot or too cold and is unable to maintain normothermia.
- *Hyperthermia* usually develops from environmental exposure or strenuous exercise in a warm or hot environment. Hyperthermia ranges from heat exhaustion to heatstroke. Heatstroke is life threatening and usually occurs from passive exposure. Exertional heatstroke occurs among individuals with a barrier to heat dissipation (e.g., wearing thick clothing). Consider other causes of hyperthermia (e.g., infection, thyroid storm, drug-induced hyperthermia).
- *Hypothermia* usually occurs in cold or wet weather or in cold-water immersion but can occur in warmer conditions if heat loss exceeds body production. It usually occurs as a result of outdoor activities, disasters, homelessness, or substance use. It can occur secondary to trauma, sepsis, hypoglycemia, and other medical conditions.
- Iatrogenic hypothermia can occur within the ED. It is intentional with temperature management for certain medical conditions. It is unintentional when patients are not adequately protected from heat loss.
- *Frostbite* is a freezing injury of the skin and underlying tissues. Frostbite occurs from cold weather exposure, contact with cold objects, evaporative cooling, or convective cooling from wind chill. Risk factors include inadequate insulation from cold or wind, constrictive clothing or footwear, circulatory disease, fatigue, alcohol or drug misuse, smoking, injuries, dehydration, and hypothermia.

[ ] **COMPLICATIONS**

Patients who are mildly hypothermic will have stressed but intact thermoregulatory systems. As the patient's condition worsens, these systems will decompensate. The patient's respiratory and heart rates will decrease, and neurologic changes will develop.

Signs and Symptoms

- Hyperthermia: heat exhaustion, heat stroke
- Hypothermia: mild hypothermia, moderate hypothermia, severe hypothermia
- Frostbite: blisters with milky fluid (with thawing); cold and firm to palpation; numbness; pale, waxy appearance; eventually becoming necrotic and requiring amputation

Diagnosis

Labs

- CBC
- CMP
- Ethyl alcohol/drug screen if indicated
- PT, aPTT
- UA

Diagnostic Testing

- EKG
- Ultrasound (frostbite)

Treatment

- Airway, breathing, and circulation management
- Associated injury treatment
- Core temperature management
- Gentle handling of patient with hypothermia or frostbite
- Hypothermia-related arrhythmias treatment; ventricular fibrillation most common
- Hyperthermia: heat exhaustion, heat stroke
- Hypothermia: mild, moderate, severe
- Frostbite: hypothermia treatment; rapid thawing by immersion of tissue in warm-water bath at 99°F (37°C) to 102°F (39°C); rewarming until area becomes erythematous and pliable (20–45 minutes); NSAIDs to reduce tissue damage; pain management (opioids, nerve blocks, epidurals); protection of damaged tissue from further injury with padding

Nursing Interventions

- Address psychosocial issues contributing to environmental exposure (e.g., homelessness).
- Assess airway, breathing, and circulation.
- Assess and manage pain (see Table A.2).
- Monitor core temperature and implement cooling or rewarming measures.
- Monitor for cardiac dysrhythmias.
- Perform wound care as indicated for frostbitten areas.

[⚡] **ALERT!**

Minimize patient movement whenever possible when treating hypothermia. In severe hypothermia, the patient is at increased risk for developing ventricular fibrillation, which can be triggered by movement.

[🌐] **NURSING PEARL**

When rewarming a hypothermic patient, monitor core temperature to prevent rewarming the patient too rapidly, which can alter intracranial pressure and cause adverse neurologic effects. Afterdrop can occur when the cooler peripheral blood returns to the core, causing further vasodilation and drop in temperatures during rewarming. The recommended rewarming rate is 0.5°C to 2°C/hr.

Patient Education

- Avoid alcohol and substance use in warm or cold environments.
- Avoid temperature extremes.
- Drink plenty of fluids (monitor urine color: should remain diluted and light colored).
- Follow up if frostbitten area turns black or if sensation is lost.

VECTOR-BORNE ILLNESSES

Overview

- Vector-borne diseases are transmitted by blood-feeding arthropods such as mosquitoes, ticks, and fleas.
- Common vector-borne diseases are Lyme disease (from tick bites), malaria, Rocky Mountain spotted fever *(Rickettsia rickettsii)*, West Nile virus, and Zika virus.
- *Rabies* is a deadly viral disease spread from wild animals and from domesticated animals not immunized against it.

Signs and Symptoms

- Fatigue
- Fever
- Headache
- Insect bite
- Paralysis
- Lyme disease specific: flu-like symptoms; joint pain, stiffness; red "bulls-eye" rash; symptoms starting 5 to 7 days after tick bite
- Rocky Mountain spotted fever: petechial skin lesions
- Rabies: agitation, confusion, dysphagia, excessive salivation, fever, hallucinations, headache, hyperactivity, nausea/vomiting, paralysis

Diagnosis

Labs

- CBC
- CMP
- CSF sampling
- Serologic testing or staining of skin biopsy
- Lyme titer
- Tick-borne disease antibodies

Diagnostic Testing

- CT (head)
- EKG

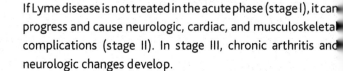

POP QUIZ 14.6

Which signs and symptoms would lead the nurse to suspect that a patient is suffering from heat stroke instead of heat exhaustion?

COMPLICATIONS

If Lyme disease is not treated in the acute phase (stage I), it can progress and cause neurologic, cardiac, and musculoskeletal complications (stage II). In stage III, chronic arthritis and neurologic changes develop.

Treatment

- Rabies: rabies postexposure prophylaxis (PEP; see Table 14.2)
- Tick-borne illnesses: tick removal, antibiotics

Nursing Interventions

- Administer PEP and other medications as indicated (see Table 14.2).
- Assess and manage airway, breathing, and circulation.
- Notify appropriate government agencies (animal control, health department).
- Perform focused neurologic, skin, and wound assessments.

Patient Education

- Report any new or worsening symptoms, including neurologic changes or signs and symptoms of infection.
- If rabies PEP is initiated, it is essential that the administration schedule is followed to ensure proper coverage.
- If awaiting animal testing, follow up as instructed to obtain the test results.

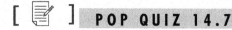

NURSING PEARL

The incubation period for rabies is 3 to 8 weeks. If the animal can be tested promptly, PEP can be deferred until the results are received. PEP should be administered if the animal cannot be found.

POP QUIZ 14.7

A patient is discharged after being bitten by an animal suspected of having rabies. What discharge instructions are essential for this patient?

RESOURCES

American Burn Association. (2018). *Advanced burn life support course: Provider manual 2018 update*. Author. http://ameriburn.org/wp-content/uploads/2019/08/2018-abls-providermanual.pdf

American College of Surgeons. (2018). *ATLS advanced trauma life support*. Author.

Blansfield, J. S. (2020). *Provider manual eighth edition TNCC trauma nursing core course: Provider manual*. Jones & Bartlett.

Centers for Disease Control and Prevention. (n.d.-a). *About the division of vector-borne diseases*. U.S. Department of Health and Human Services. https://www.cdc.gov/ncezid/dvbd/about.html

Centers for Disease Control and Prevention. (n.d.-b). *Food safety*. U.S. Department of Health and Human Services. https://www.cdc.gov/foodsafety/index.html

Centers for Disease Control and Prevention. (n.d.-c). *Parasites*—Giardia. U.S. Department of Health and Human Services. https://www.cdc.gov/parasites/giardia/index.html

Centers for Disease Control and Prevention. (n.d.-d). *Ringworm*. U.S. Department of Health and Human Services. https://www.cdc.gov/fungal/diseases/ringworm/index.html

Cooper, M. (2022). Lightning injuries clinical presentation. *Medscape*. https://www.medscape.com/article/770642

Danzl, D. F. (2022). Hypothermia and peripheral cold injuries. In J. Loscalzo, A. Fauci, D. Kasper, S. Hauser, D. Longo, & J. Jameson (Eds.), *Harrison's principles of internal medicine* (21st ed., pp. 3630–3634). McGraw-Hill. https://accessmedicine.mhmedical.com/content.aspx?bookid=3095&sectionid=264098884

De Laby, M. (2020). Chemical, biological, radiologic, nuclear (CBRN) threats. In V. Sweet & A. Foley (Eds.), *Sheehy's emergency nursing: Principles and practice* (7th ed., pp. 170–180). Elsevier.

Denke, N. (2020). Wound management. In V. Sweet & A. Foley (Eds.), *Sheehy's emergency nursing: Principles and practice* (7th ed., pp. 93–111). Elsevier.

Foley, A., & Sweet, V. (2020). Respiratory emergencies. In V. Sweet & A. Foley (Eds.), *Sheehy's emergency nursing: Principles and practice* (7th ed., pp. 216–226). Elsevier.

Katz, K. (2020). Organophosphate toxicity. *Medscape*. https://www.medscape.com/article/167726

Logee, K. (2020). Pediatric emergencies. In V. Sweet & A. Foley (Eds.), *Sheehy's emergency nursing: Principles and practice* (7th ed., pp. 556–575). Elsevier.

Oliver, R., Jr. (2021). Burn resuscitation and early management. *Medscape*. https://www.medscape.com/article/1277360

Prescribers' Digital Reference. (n.d.-a). *Atropine sulfate* [Drug information]. https://www.pdr.net/drug-summary/Atropine-sulfate-injection-atropine-sulfate-684.4376

Prescribers' Digital Reference. (n.d.-b). *Black widow spider antivenin equine* [Drug information]. https://www.pdr.net/drug-summary/Antivenin--latrodectus-Mactans--black-widow-spider-antivenin--equine--330

Prescribers' Digital Reference. (n.d.-c). *Crotalidae polyvalent immune fab ovine* [Drug information]. https://www.pdr.net/drug-summary/Crofab-crotalidae-polyvalent-immune-fab--ovine--2650

Prescribers' Digital Reference. (n.d.-d). *Cyproheptadine hydrochloride* [Drug information]. https://www.pdr.net/drug-summary/Cyproheptadine-hydrochloride-syrup-cyproheptadine-hydrochloride-2646

Prescribers' Digital Reference. (n.d.-e). *Fluconazole* [Drug information]. https://www.pdr.net/drug-summary/Fluconazole-injection-fluconazole-3458

Prescribers' Digital Reference. (n.d.-f). *Metronidazole* [Drug information]. https://www.pdr.net/drug-summary/Metronidazole-injection-metronidazole-1728.4200

Prescribers' Digital Reference. (n.d.-g). *Miconazole* [Drug information]. https://www.pdr.net/drug-summary/Oravig-miconazole-2287.2366

Prescribers' Digital Reference. (n.d.-h). *Pralidoxime chloride* [Drug information]. https://www.pdr.net/drug-summary/Protopam-Chloride-pralidoxime-chloride-1131

Prescribers' Digital Reference. (n.d.-i). *Rabies immune globulin human* [Drug information]. https://www.pdr.net/drug-summary/Imogam-rabies-immune-globulin--human--2915.3591

Prescribers' Digital Reference. (n.d.-j). *Rabies vaccine* [Drug information]. https://www.pdr.net/drug-summary/Imovax-rabies-vaccine-2914.1916

Prescribers' Digital Reference. (n.d.-k). *Silver sulfadiazine* [Drug information]. https://www.pdr.net/drug-summary/Silvadene-silver-sulfadiazine-2781

Schaefer, T. J., & Nunez Lopez, O. (2022). Burn resuscitation and management. In *StatPearls*. StatPearls Publishing. https://www.ncbi.nlm.gov/books/NBK430795

Sedlak, S. (2013a). Bite and sting emergencies. In B. Hammond & P. Zimmerman (Eds.), *Sheehy's manual of emergency care* (7th ed., pp. 345–352). Elsevier Mosby.

Sedlak, S. (2013b). Environmental emergencies. In B. Hammond & P. Zimmerman (Eds.), *Sheehy's manual of emergency care* (7th ed., pp. 333–343). Elsevier Mosby.

Wiktor, A., & Richards, D. (2022). Patient education: Skin burns (beyond the basics). *UpToDate*. https://www.uptodate.com/contents/skin-burns-beyond-thebasics

Worley, G. (2020). Environmental emergencies. In V. Sweet & A. Foley (Eds.), *Sheehy's emergency nursing: Principles and practice* (7th ed., pp. 321–339). Elsevier.

Wraa, C. (2020). Burns. In V. Sweet & A. Foley (Eds.), *Sheehy's emergency nursing: Principles and practice* (7th ed., pp. 503–516). Elsevier.

15 TOXICOLOGIC EMERGENCIES

ACIDS AND ALKALIS

Overview

- Acidic substances that are ingested can cause systemic toxicity, such as coagulation necrosis. Examples of acidic substances include hydrochloric acid, sulfuric acid, and nitric acid.
- Alkaline substances that are ingested can cause direct tissue necrosis. Examples of alkaline substances include discoid batteries, laundry detergent, disinfectant materials, and lye.
- Both acidic and alkaline substances may damage prominent airway structures, such as the bronchi, larynx, and trachea, when ingested.
- Suicidal or intentional actions should be considered when caring for the patient who was exposed.

Signs and Symptoms

- Abdominal pain
- Changes in voice
- Drooling
- Dysphagia
- Hematemesis
- Nausea

Diagnosis

Labs

- Arterial blood gases (ABGs), venous blood gases (VBGs)
- Complete blood count (CBC)
- Comprehensive metabolic panel (CMP)
- Coagulation panel
- Lactate level
- Toxicology levels (e.g., salicylate, acetaminophen, and ethanol)
- Type and screen
- Urine drug screen

Diagnostic Testing

- Chest x-ray
- CT scan of chest and abdomen
- EKG
- Endoscopic procedures

[🧠] **COMPLICATIONS**

Complications of ingesting acidic and alkaline substances often include perforation, peritonitis, stricture formation, and ulceration.

[⚡] **ALERT!**

After patient ingestion of an acidic or alkaline substance, death may result from acid-base disruption, hemolysis, coagulopathy, and renal failure.

Treatment

- Airway management with intubation or tracheostomy: may be required
- Endoscopy: may be indicated
- Fluid resuscitation
- Medications as indicated (see Table 15.1; see also Table A.1): activated charcoal; antibiotics; antiemetics such as ondansetron; proton pump inhibitors such as omeprazole.
- Nothing by mouth (NPO) with consideration of alternative nutrition sources
- Poison control center consult
- Psychiatric services consult and suicidal precautions if indicated
- Respiratory support
- Significant exposure: may require admission to hospital or ICU
- Surgical intervention: may be needed for exploration or repair of perforation to the esophagus or peritoneum

Nursing Interventions

- Administer fluid resuscitation if ordered.
- Assist with airway, breathing, and circulation interventions.
- Consider suicide precautions.
- Establish intravenous (IV) access and draw blood for lab tests.
- Follow poison control center directions.
- Give antidotes/medications (see Table 15.1): activated charcoal, antiemetics.
- Keep patient NPO.
- Monitor intake and output (I/O).
- Perform decontamination, and wear appropriate personal protective equipment (PPE).
- Prepare the patient for procedures or surgical intervention.

TABLE 15.1 Medications for Toxic Conditions

INDICATIONS	MECHANISM OF ACTION	CONTRAINDICATIONS, PRECAUTIONS, AND ADVERSE EFFECTS
Acetylcysteine		
• Acetaminophen overdose	• Increases synthesis of glutathione in the liver and has antioxidant effects	• Medication may cause nausea, vomiting, GERD, and anaphylactoid reactions.
Activated charcoal		
• Minimizes systemic absorption of toxins	• Absorbs and binds to toxins that are in the dissolved liquid phase	• Medication does not work for alcohol. • Monitor for pulmonary aspiration and emesis. • Complications may include bowel obstruction.
Alkalizing agents (sodium bicarbonate)		
• Correct acid-base disorders	• Increase plasma bicarbonate level and systemic alkalizer	• Medication may exacerbate CHF. • Side effects are cerebral hemorrhage, high blood sodium levels, and low potassium levels.

(continued)

TABLE 15.1	Medications for Toxic Conditions *(continued)*	
INDICATIONS	**MECHANISM OF ACTION**	**CONTRAINDICATIONS, PRECAUTIONS, AND ADVERSE EFFECTS**
Antidote (calcium chloride)		
• To treat calcium channel blocker overdose	• Supplement	• Side effects include low blood pressure, hypomagnesemia, nausea, and vasodilation.
Antidote for cyanide poisoning (amyl nitrate, sodium nitrate, sodium thiosulfate, hydroxocobalamin)		
• Cyanide poisoning	• Binds with cyanide and is excreted in urine	• Adverse effects are hypertension, reddish brown skin, and anaphylactoid reactions.
Antidote for digoxin overdose (digoxin immune fab)		
• Antidote for digoxin overdose	• Digoxin-specific antibody	• Use caution with heart or kidney disease and known allergy to antibiotics.
Antidote for warfarin overdose (vitamin K)		
• Warfarin overdose	• Promotes blood clotting	• Medication takes several hours to reverse anticoagulation.
Antidote for organophosphate poisoning (2-PAM, pralidoxime)		
• Organophosphate overdose • Antidote for chemical weapons like sarin, tabun, soman, and cyclosarin	• Binds to organophosphates and breaks alkyl phosphate-cholinesterase bond	• Side effects are slurred vision, dizziness, and headaches. • Loading dose is to be given slowly. • Patients with myasthenia gravis may have a myasthenic crisis.
Antiemetics		
• Prevent nausea and vomiting	• Inhibit stimulation of GI tract by blocking receptors that trigger vomiting.	• Side effects are headache, fatigue, dizziness, dry mouth, and changes in bowel movement.
Antihypertensives (clonidine)		
• Hypertension associated with alcohol or opiate withdrawal	• Alpha-antagonist effect in the posterior hypothalamus and medulla • Reduced sympathetic outflow from the CNS, decreasing arterial blood pressure	• Do not give barbiturates, phenothiazines, benzodiazepine, or opioids with clonidine. • Mixing with tricyclic antidepressants will increase blood pressure.
Benzodiazepine antagonist (flumazenil)		
• Benzodiazepine overdose	• Blocks GABA receptors and inhibits the activity of benzodiazepine	• Serious adverse effects are neurologic effects, seizures, and arrhythmias. • Medication is contraindicated when benzodiazepines are being used to control intracranial pressure or status epilepticus.
Cathartics		
• To accelerate defecation	• Stimulate intestinal motility by irritating the mucosal lining	• Monitor for dehydration and excessive electrolyte loss.

(continued)

TABLE 15.1 Medications for Toxic Conditions *(continued)*

INDICATIONS	MECHANISM OF ACTION	CONTRAINDICATIONS, PRECAUTIONS, AND ADVERSE EFFECTS
Heavy metal antagonist (deferoxamine)		
• Overdose on heavy metals	• Binds with free iron or aluminum in the bloodstream to assist with elimination	• Use caution with cataracts, seizures, renal disease, and tinnitus. • Do not give to patients who are breastfeeding. • Medication is contraindicated in renal disease and anuria.
Opioid antagonists (naloxone, methadone, buprenorphine, naltrexone)		
• Reversal of narcotic	• Block activation of opioid receptors	• Monitor for signs of pulmonary edema. • Repeat doses may be needed, as the effects of the opioid overdose last longer than the reversal agent.
Proton pump inhibitors (omeprazole, esomeprazole)		
• GERD	• Block gastric secretion	• Adverse effects are IBS, atrophic gastritis, and vitamin and mineral malabsorption.
Thiamin/vitamin B₁ supplements		
• Thiamine for alcohol withdrawal and intoxication	• Combine with ATP to form thiamine diphosphate	• Use caution in pregnant patients. • Avoid if history of hypersensitivity to thiamine

ATP, adenosine triphosphate; CHF, congestive heart failure; CNS, central nervous system; GABA, gamma-aminobutyric acid; GERD, gastroesophageal reflux disease; GI, gastrointestinal; IBS, irritable bowel syndrome; PAM, pralidoxime.

Patient Education

- Return for new or worsening of symptoms like vomiting, blood in the stool, or inability to tolerate food and drink.
- Keep chemicals and cleaning supplies out of reach of children.
- Treat wounds as instructed and return if there are signs and symptoms of infection.

[📝] POP QUIZ 15.1

An adult patient reportedly drank a cup of hand sanitizer 2 hours ago to "get a buzz." The patient now feels nauseated and has vomited one time. What interventions will the nurse anticipate?

CARBON MONOXIDE

Overview

- *Carbon monoxide* is a by-product of incomplete combustion. Common sources are faulty furnaces and exhaust from cars.
- Carbon monoxide is colorless, odorless, and tasteless, and prolonged exposure can be lethal.
- Carbon monoxide has a higher affinity to hemoglobin than to oxygen, so oxygen becomes displaced, allowing the red blood cells to be saturated with carbon monoxide.

 COMPLICATIONS

Patients who are rescued from a house fire and present unresponsive and hypotensive may have concurrent cyanide toxicity.

Signs and Symptoms

- Altered mental status
- Cherry-red skin
- Confusion
- Dizziness
- Headache
- Lack of coordination
- Nausea and vomiting
- Tachypnea

Diagnosis

Labs

- ABG/VBG
- Basic metabolic panel
- Carboxyhemoglobin level
- Serum lactate level
- Urine pregnancy test

Diagnostic Testing

- Chest x-ray
- CT scan of the head
- EKG

[🌐] **NURSING PEARL**

Do not rely on a pulse oximetry monitor for a true oxygen saturation reading; it will be inaccurate. The pulse oximetry monitor will read that the hemoglobin is saturated, but it will not indicate if it is saturated with oxygen or carbon monoxide, giving a false reading.

Treatment

- 100% oxygen via non-rebreather mask (NRB) or intubation, if severe, to reduce the half-life of carboxyhemoglobin
- Airway maintenance
- Carbon monoxide exposure with cyanide toxicity: evaluation and possible treatment for rhabdomyolysis
- Cardiac workup on any patients with preexisting cardiovascular history
- Patients with carboxyhemoglobin under 25% most likely discharged from the ED
- Poison control center consult for carboxyhemoglobin over 25%, which may require hyperbaric oxygenation

Nursing Interventions

- Apply high-flow oxygen via NRB.
- Assist the patient to a high Fowler's position to facilitate better airflow with respirations.
- Assist with airway maintenance.
- Monitor cardiac status and perform an EKG for patients with cardiac history.
- Draw blood sample for lab testing.
- Refer for psychiatric evaluation as required for intentional exposure to carbon monoxide.
- Prior to discharge, ensure that patient is returning to a safe location; if there was a carbon monoxide leak in the home, assist patient with finding an alternative place to go.

Patient Education

- Do not smoke cigarettes, as they give off carbon monoxide.
- Follow up in 4 to 6 weeks for a cognitive evaluation after significant exposure.
- Perform safety measures in the home to reduce the chance of exposure. Clean and inspect the chimney yearly. Do not block exhaust outlets. Do not burn charcoal indoors. Do not use generators inside the house. Do not use the stove to heat the house. Inspect the furnace yearly. Install carbon monoxide detectors in the home. Keep the garage door open when the car is running.

CYANIDE

Overview

- *Cyanide* is an extremely toxic chemical that affects the ability of the blood to transport oxygen, often leading to cellular hypoxia and death.
- Cyanide can be found as a gas, liquid, or solid and may be absorbed by direct contact, ingestion, or inhalation.
- Common sources: cigarette smoke; combustion of synthetic materials; house fires; parts of certain foods, such as lima beans, apricot pits, and apple seeds, which are metabolized into cyanide; laboratories; vermin extermination materials.
- Cyanide has been used in chemical warfare.

Signs and Symptoms

- Altered mental status
- Bradycardia/tachycardia
- Dizziness
- Headache
- Hypotension
- Nausea/vomiting
- Smell of bitter almonds
- Tachypnea

Diagnosis

Labs

- ABG/VBG
- EKG
- Lactate level
- Whole blood cyanide level

Diagnostic Testing

- Chest x-ray

[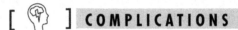] **POP QUIZ 15.2**

A patient arrives to the ED via emergency medical services after being rescued from a house fire. The patient pushes the NRB away, stating, "Look at my oxygen level! I am fine." The nurse looks at the monitor and notes that the pulse oximetry is 100%. Should the nurse still apply oxygen? Why or why not?

[ ] **COMPLICATIONS**

Severe cyanide poisoning may present with confusion, hyperventilation, hypotension, and bradycardia.

[ ] **NURSING PEARL**

Significant cyanide exposure causes impaired oxygenation and anerobic metabolism, which will be reflected by an anion gap and elevated lactate level.

Treatment

- Antidotes (see Table 15.1): amyl nitrate; sodium thiosulfate; hydroxocobalamin; activated charcoal if ingestion within 2 hours
- Carboxyhemoglobin level check if patient exposed to smoke
- Cyanide poisoning: report to law enforcement and public health personnel
- Delayed toxicity monitoring
- Hospital admittance for observation of delayed toxicity
- Lifesaving interventions for airway, breathing, and circulation
- Poison control center consult
- Possible fluid resuscitation
- Possible hazardous materials response and appropriate PPE
- Removal of all patient clothing and washing with soap and water in case of skin contamination
- Supplemental oxygen if indicated

Nursing Interventions

- Administer appropriate antidotes.
- Administer fluid resuscitation when indicated.
- Administer supplemental oxygen therapy.
- Decontaminate by: removing clothing; washing with soap and water; flushing eyes.
- Establish IV access and draw blood for lab tests.
- Monitor and support airway, breathing, and circulation interventions.
- Monitor for delayed toxicity.
- Provide continuous cardiac monitoring.

Patient Education

- Beware of side effects related to treatment of hydroxocobalamin, which include photosensitivity and red discoloration of urine.
- Follow up with provider for a neurologic evaluation if indicated because of a significant exposure.
- Implement safe work practices and follow all Occupational Safety and Health Administration (OSHA) guidelines.
- Report exposure to work site occupational safety department.

DRUG INTERACTIONS

Overview

- Coadministration of two or more drugs, as well as other substances like herbs and home remedies, can have devastating, if not fatal, consequences.
- Drug interactions may change the way a medication is metabolized and excreted, altering the desired effects.
- Home remedies and herbal substances, as well as nicotine, food or drinks, alcohol, and vitamins, can have an impact on drug interactions (Table 15.2).

 A L E R T !

The vasodilator nitroprusside sodium may be a source of toxic blood concentrations of cyanide when used in high doses over many days. Symptoms manifest as confusion and combativeness. Treatment is coadministration of hydroxocobalamin or sodium thiosulfate.

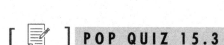 **P O P   Q U I Z   1 5 . 3**

An ambulance arrives to triage with a patient who is awake and alert and being transported for possible cyanide exposure. What is the priority intervention?

 A L E R T !

The term "skittling" refers to taking a handful of unknown medications with the intent to achieve pleasurable effects. This has become a more common activity among younger people and can have lethal and unpredictable complications.

TABLE 15.2   Common Drug, Herb, and Food Interactions

	DRUG	COMPLICATION
Ephedra	• MAOIs • Sympathomimetic drugs	• Additive effects • Increased toxicity
Ginkgo	• Aspirin • Warfarin	• Increased risk of bleeding
Grapefruit juice	• Amiodarone • Benzodiazepines • Calcium channel blockers • Carbamazepine • Clomipramine • Cyclosporine • Dextromethorphan • Ethinyl estradiol • Quinidine • Sertraline • Statins	• Vital intestinal enzyme not properly metabolized, causing more of the drug to enter the blood, taking longer to excrete
Levothyroxine	• Aluminum-containing antacids • Calcium • Chromium • Carbamazepine • Diazepam • Estrogen therapy • Furosemide • Heparin • Iron • Phenytoin • Phosphate binders • PPIs • Raloxifene • Sucralfate	• Decreased or unpredictable absorption of thyroid medication • Interferes with protein binding
MAOIs	• Meperidine • Dextromethorphan • Tramadol • Linezolid • Propoxyphene • SSRIs	• Life-threatening interactions • Tyramine reaction when mixed with sympathomimetics • Serotonin syndrome; may be fatal
NSAIDs	• Antihypertensives • Aspirin • Ibuprofen • Warfarin	• Inhibits the therapeutic effects of aspirin • Decreases the effectiveness of antihypertensive medications • Increases risk of bleeding with warfarin
Vitamin K	• Warfarin	• Altered metabolism of warfarin • Results in subtherapeutic levels
St. John's wort	• Cyclosporine • Digoxin • Indinavir	• Decreases serum level of the drugs • Increases risk of transplant rejection (cyclosporine)

MAOI, monoamine oxidase inhibitor; NSAID, nonsteroidal anti-inflammatory drug; PPI, proton pump inhibitor; SSRI, selective serotonin reuptake inhibitor.

Signs and Symptoms
- Decreased therapeutic effects of medication
- Increased effects of medication
- Unexpected or adverse symptoms

Diagnosis
Labs
- CBC
- CMP
- Coagulation panel
- Specific drug levels (e.g., seizure medications)
- Thyroid levels

Diagnostic Testing
There are no diagnostic tests specific to drug interactions.

Treatment
- Adequate airway, breathing, and circulation
- Cardiac monitoring, if indicated
- Corrective medications: vitamin K (see Table 15.1); seizure medication
- Fluid resuscitation
- Symptomatic treatment (see Table 15.1): antiemetics, antihypertensives, cardiac stabilizing medications, electrolyte replacement

Nursing Interventions
- Assist with any life-threatening airway, breathing, or circulatory issues.
- Consult with a pharmacist for safe use and evaluation of potential interactions between home medications and herbs and vitamins.
- Establish an IV line and draw blood for ordered lab tests.
- Give corrective doses of medications.
- Give fluid resuscitation if ordered.
- Perform EKG or place patient on cardiac monitoring for arrhythmias, if indicated.
- Treat complications and adverse effects as ordered.

Patient Education
- Have medications filled at the same pharmacy.
- Follow dietary and other drug restrictions found on the drug insert. Avoid alcohol and tobacco consumption. Avoid common over-the-counter (OTC) medications with high potential for complications, such as nonsteroidal anti-inflammatory drugs (NSAIDs). Do not drink grapefruit juice while on certain medications. Eat about the same amount of vitamin K daily. Vitamin K is found in many green, leafy vegetables and in fish, liver, meat, and eggs.

 COMPLICATIONS

Patients with decreased renal function who receive IV contrast and take metformin run a higher risk of developing contrast-induced neuropathy. Renal function should be checked 48 hours after contrast to determine when to restart medication.

 NURSING PEARL

Follow the Six Rights of medication administration:
- Right route
- Right patient
- Right documentation
- Right dose
- Right time
- Right medication
- Confirmation of IV compatibility

 POP QUIZ 15.4

What is a serious complication of taking St. John's wort and cyclosporine?

▶

Patient Education *(continued)*

- Inform providers and pharmacists of all herbal, prescribed, supplemental, and OTC medications that are being taken.
- Keep all medications in the original bottle.
- Read all medication labels and ingredients.

OVERDOSE AND INGESTION

Overview

- Overdose or ingestion of drugs or other substances may require immediate intervention to stop their absorption by the body.
- Determining time and amount of ingestion will help anticipate effects and length of observation until excreted from the body.
- Overdose and ingestion may have serious toxic effects on the liver and kidneys that may require hemodialysis.
- All patients who present to the ED should be screened for suicidal intentions.

[ ]   **NURSING PEARL**

Establish the following as soon as possible:

- Amount
- Combined use of alcohol or other drugs
- Comorbidities that will affect drug excretion
- Dose
- Home interventions
- Route
- Time of ingestion

Signs and Symptoms

Table 15.3 shows signs and symptoms of toxic overdose with antidotes.

TABLE 15.3 Signs and Symptoms of Toxic Overdose With Antidotes		
SUBSTANCE	**SIGNS AND SYMPTOMS**	**ANTIDOTE**

Acetaminophen	• Four stages to acetaminophen toxicity:
	  ◦ Stage I (0–24 hours): asymptomatic, or gastric upset and lethargy
	  ◦ Stage II (24–48 hours): asymptomatic, or abnormal LFTs, prolonged aPTT, and RUQ pain
	  ◦ Stage III (72–96 hours): encephalopathy, hypoglycemia, jaundice, liver failure; can progress to death
	  ◦ Stage IV (recovery phase; 4 days to 2 weeks): healing process of hepatic dysfunction
		• Acetylcysteine administered orally or IV (see Table 15.1)

Benzodiazepines (alprazolam, diazepam, clonazepam)	• Amnesia • Confusion • Drowsiness • Hallucinations • Hypotension • Hypotonia/hyporeflexia • Slurred speech • Respiratory depression	• Flumazenil, may cause seizures (see Table 15.1)

(continued)

TABLE 15.3 Signs and Symptoms of Toxic Overdose with Antidotes *(continued)*

SUBSTANCE	SIGNS AND SYMPTOMS	ANTIDOTE
Beta-blockers and calcium channel blockers	• Arrhythmias (e.g., heart blocks) • Bradycardia • Bronchospasms • Delirium • Hypotension • Vasodilation	• Glucagon (see Table 15.1) • Atropine, as needed • Transcutaneous pacing: may be required
CNS stimulants (e.g., cocaine, methamphetamines)	• AMI • Coagulopathies • Hypertension • Hyperthermia • Paranoia • Rhabdomyolysis • Tachycardia • Stroke	• Calcium chloride or calcium gluconate (see Table 15.1)
Digitalis glycosides	• Arrhythmias • Coma • Lethargy • Nausea and vomiting • Visual changes (e.g., yellow or green halos)	• Digoxin immune Fab (see Table 15.1)
Heavy metals (e.g., arsenic, lead, mercury, zinc)	Overdoses typically related to chronic inhalation or ingestion • Anemia • Neuropathies • Pulmonary edema • Renal failure • Seizures • Tremors	• Activated charcoal contraindicated • Chelation therapy for heavy metal toxicities
Hydrocarbons (glues, paints, solvents, gasoline, fluorocarbons); inhalation often called "huffing" or "bagging"	• Arrhythmias • Chemical pneumonitis • Coughing • Headache • Liver failure • Renal failure • Wheezing	• No antidote

Iron	• Doses less than 20 mg/kg: typically no symptoms
	• Doses between 20 and 40 mg/kg: symptoms of GI upset
	• Doses greater than 40 mg/kg: serious
	• Doses greater than 60 mg/kg: can be lethal
	• Symptoms of iron toxicity:
	  ◦ Acidosis
	  ◦ Gastric hemorrhage
	  ◦ GI upset
	  ◦ Liver failure
	  ◦ Seizures
		• Deferoxamine for iron poisoning 15 mg/kg/hr, in serious intoxication (see Table 15.1)
		• May turn urine red/orange; watch for adequate dilution when urine returns to normal color

(continued)

TABLE 15.3 Signs and Symptoms of Toxic Overdose with Antidotes *(continued)*

SUBSTANCE	SIGNS AND SYMPTOMS	ANTIDOTE

NSAIDs (e.g., ibuprofen)	• Abdominal pain
	• Ingestion of large quantities causes
	  · Bradycardia
	  · Coma
	  · Renal failure
		• Hemodialysis for resultant AKI
		• Patients who have ingested 10 or more tablets of NSAIDs: activated charcoal
		• Sodium bicarbonate for severe metabolic acidosis

Opiates (e.g., fentanyl, oxycodone, heroin)	• Apnea • Coma • Drowsiness • Hypothermia • Miosis • Respiratory depression	• Naloxone: intranasal or IV (see Table 15.1) • Repeat doses of naloxone or drip possibly indicated, related to half-life of 30 minutes to 2 hours
Organophosphates (e.g., insecticides, sarin, soman, tabun)	Signs of cholinergic toxicity: • Blurred vision and miosis • Bradycardia • Coma • Diarrhea • Emesis • Lacrimation • Mental confusion, slurred speech • Respiratory arrest	• Wash skin thoroughly • If insecticide ingested: activated charcoal • 2-PAM (see Table 15.1) • Atropine: drug of choice for organophosphate toxicity

Salicylates (e.g., aspirin, oil of wintergreen, bismuth subsalicylate)	Acute ingestion
	• Mild ingestion (dose more than 150 mg/kg):
	  · Nausea and vomiting
	  · Tinnitus
	• Moderate ingestion (dose more than 250 mg/kg):
	  · Ataxia
	  · Hyperpyrexia
	  · Sweating
	  · Tachypnea
	• Severe ingestion (dose more than 500 mg/kg):
	  · Coma
	  · Hypotension
	  · Metabolic acidosis
	• Chronic ingestion (100 mg/kg/day for 2 or more days):
	  · Hallucinations
	  · Lethargy
	  · Pulmonary edema
	  · Renal failure
		• Sodium bicarbonate IV to correct severe acidosis (see Table 15.1)

Sedative-hypnotics and barbiturates	• CNS depression • Coma • Hypothermia • Poor judgment • Slurred speech	• No antidote

(continued)

TABLE 15.3 Signs and Symptoms of Toxic Overdose with Antidotes *(continued)*

SUBSTANCE	SIGNS AND SYMPTOMS	ANTIDOTE
Toxic alcohols (ethylene glycol/antifreeze, methanol, isopropanol)	• Acetone breath (isopropanol ingestion) • Acidosis • Arrhythmias • CNS depression • Confusion, hallucinations, blurred vision • Hypotension, tachycardia, dysrhythmias • Hypothermia • Respiratory depression • Seizures • Urinary retention	• Antidote for ethylene glycol and methanol: fomepizole (see Table 15.1) • IV ethanol for toxic alcohol overdoses, except isopropanol, at 100 mg/kg/hr during dialysis • Hemodialysis
Toxic plants (lily of the valley, poinsettia)	• Potential for anticholinergic or cardiac complications	• Dependent on the type of plant; poison control center consult
Tricyclic antidepressants (amitriptyline and trazodone)	• Arrhythmias (e.g., heart block, torsades de pointes, VF, VT) • CNS depression • Coma • Mydriasis • Tachycardia • Vasodilation	• Sodium bicarbonate to counter dysrhythmias and maintain pH (see Table 15.1) • Benzodiazepines (e.g., diazepam) as needed to control seizures (see Table A.2) • Serotonin syndrome: treated with dantrolene sodium; clonazepam used to treat rigor; cooling blankets to control temperature

AKI, acute kidney injury; AMI, acute myocardial infarction; aPTT, activated partial thromboplastin time; CNS, central nervous system; GI, gastrointestinal; IV, intravenous; LFTs, liver function tests; NSAIDs, nonsteroidal anti-inflammatory drugs; PAM, pralidoxime; RUQ, right upper quadrant; VF, ventricular fibrillation; VT, ventricular tachycardia.

Diagnosis
Labs
- ABG/VBG
- CBC
- CMP
- Coagulation panel
- Drug levels as indicated: acetaminophen level: every 4 hours after ingestion; digoxin level; iron level; salicylate level
- Ethyl alcohol level
- Serum drug screen
- Troponin
- Urine drug screen

Diagnostic Testing
- Chest x-ray
- CT scan of head
- EKG
- X-ray of abdomen

 ALERT!

Gastric lavage will rarely be ordered because it has been shown to cause complications such as aspiration pneumonia and life-threatening electrolyte disturbances. It will be ordered only when the benefits outweigh the risks and when it can be performed within 1 hour of ingestion.

 NURSING PEARL

Consider administering naloxone to the patient suspected of opioid overdose before intubation to potentially avoid this airway intervention.

Treatment

- Adequate airway, breathing, and circulation
- Antidote (see Table 15.2)
- Blood pressure support
- Core body temperature monitoring
- Fluid resuscitation
- Gastrointestinal (GI) decontamination by one of the following methods: activated charcoal (see Table 15.1) for oral ingestion within 2 hours unless contraindicated; cathartics (see Table 15.1); whole-bowel irrigation
- Hemodialysis for overdoses causing acute kidney injury
- Oxygen if ordered
- Poison control center consult
- Psychiatric and social work consults for suicidal patients

Nursing Interventions

- Assist and monitor airway, breathing, and circulation interventions.
- Contact poison control center and administer prescribed antidote (see Table 15.3).
- Ensure proper decontamination procedures if indicated.
- Establish IV line and draw blood for lab tests and repeat as necessary.
- Monitor and treat for seizures: seizure medications such as lorazepam; padded side rails; suction available.
- Monitor for progressive signs and symptoms of acute liver and kidney failure that may require aggressive measures, such as liver failure: jaundice, ascites, confusion; kidney failure: decreased urine output, fluid retention, shortness of breath, confusion.
- Monitor urine output to ensure adequate hydration and to assess kidney function.
- Perform psychosocial assessment and suicide precautions if self-induced/intentional overdose.
- Place nasogastric tube if indicated to administer activated charcoal.
- Place on cardiac monitoring; perform EKG if ordered.
- Provide a quiet environment for patient with overdose of drug that affects CNS.
- Provide bowel decontamination as ordered; give activated charcoal within 2-hour time frame (see Table 15.1).
- Provide fluid resuscitation if indicated.
- Take patient weight in kg because dosage of many antidotes is weight based.

Patient Education

- Chronic opioid or heroin users may be discharged with naloxone or be referred to an outpatient provider to receive it. The patient's family should learn proper, lifesaving use of naloxone.
- Do not take other people's prescription medication.
- Family and significant others should learn about relapse and signs and symptoms to watch for.
- Follow up with outpatient psychiatric service if referrals are made. ▶

[ ] **POP QUIZ 15.5**

An adult patient reports drinking a half pint of antifreeze about an hour before arriving in the ED. The nurse administers fluid resuscitation and fomepizole. Repeat laboratory tests reveal that the patient is in metabolic acidosis with an elevated blood urea nitrogen and creatine level. What is the most likely next intervention?

[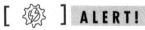] **ALERT!**

Patients who stop using opioids, like heroin, for a period of time and then restart often return to the same amount used prior to stopping, potentially leading to significant overdose, respiratory depression, and death.

Patient Education *(continued)*

- Keep toxic substances and medications in a locked area or otherwise away from and out of sight of children and teenagers.
- Learn proper use of prescribed medications.
- Learn the serious consequences of skittling, or polysubstance use.

SUBSTANCE USE

Overview

- Substance misuse changes the release of certain chemicals in the brain, altering feelings and thoughts while creating pleasure. This can lead to addiction.
- Patients who are addicted to drugs may need to keep increasing the dose to get the same reward or pleasure out of using, which risks overdose.
- Pregnant people who use substances increase the risk of fetal alcohol syndrome, miscarriage, low birth weight, neonatal abstinence syndrome, premature delivery, and stillbirth.
- Screening tools such as AUDIT-C (alcohol use disorders identification test), TAPS (tobacco, alcohol, prescription medication, and other substance use), and BSATD (brief screener for alcohol, tobacco, and other drugs) can help assess for substance use.

Signs and Symptoms

Table 15.4 shows signs, symptoms, and complications of substance use.

TABLE 15.4 Signs, Symptoms, and Complications of Substance Use		
SUBSTANCE	**SIGNS AND SYMPTOMS**	**COMPLICATIONS**
Alcohol	• Enhanced or altered social ability • Relaxation	• Arrhythmias • Blackout • Cancer • Depression • Hypertension • Liver cirrhosis
Cannabinoids (marijuana)	• Altered behavior • Analgesia • Increased appetite • Relaxation • Sensory distortion	• Anxiety • Erectile dysfunction • Depression • Poor concentration
Depressants (e.g., GHB, flunitrazepam)	• GHB • Amnesia • Euphoria • Flunitrazepam • Amnesia • Impaired reaction time • Muscle relaxation • Sedation	• GHB • Bradycardia • Coma • Death • Flunitrazepam • Bradycardia • Confusion • Hypoventilation
Dextromethorphan	• Blurry vision • Nausea and vomiting • Unsteady gait	• Brain damage (cognitive impairment) • Coma • Death • Respiratory depression

(continued)

TABLE 15.4	Signs, Symptoms, and Complications of Substance Use *(continued)*	
SUBSTANCE	SIGNS AND SYMPTOMS	COMPLICATIONS
Hallucinogens (e.g., ayahuasca, ecstasy, ketamine, LSD, MDMA, mushrooms, and PCP)	• Dilated pupils • Dizziness • Loss of memory • Nausea and vomiting • Tachycardia	• Cardiac arrest • Coma • Flashbacks • Memory problems • Seizures
Inhalants (e.g., glue, leather cleaner, nitrous oxide, spray paint, and whipped cream aerosols)	• Euphoria • Headaches • Lightheadedness	• Asphyxiation • Brain damage • Choking • Coma • Liver and kidney damage • Seizures
Narcotics (e.g., heroin, fentanyl, morphine, and oxycodone)	• Analgesia • Bradycardia • Bradypnea • Euphoria • Nausea and vomiting • Pinpoint pupils	• Death • Pericarditis • Sclerosed vasculature
Stimulants (e.g., cocaine and methamphetamine)	• Dilated pupils • Euphoria • Epistaxis • Insomnia • Psychosis • Restlessness • Tremors	• Agitation • AMI • Arrhythmias • Dental problems (methamphetamine) • Hypertension • Psychosis • Seizures • Stroke
Tobacco (e.g., cigarettes, hookah, and smokeless tobacco)	• Clothing smelling of cigarettes • Hypertension • Spitting more than usual (smokeless tobacco) • Tachycardia	• Cancer • Coronary heart disease • Gum disease

AMI, acute myocardial infarction; GHB, gamma hydroxybutyrate; LSD, lysergic acid diethylamide; MDMA, 3,4-methylenedioxy methamphetamine; PCP, phencyclidine.

Diagnosis

Labs

■ Cardiac enzymes
■ CBC
■ Creatine kinase
■ CMP
■ Hepatitis C and HIV tests, if applicable
■ Liver function tests
■ Pregnancy test
■ Serum drug screen
■ Troponin
■ Urine drug screen

Diagnostic Testing
- Chest x-ray
- CT scan of head
- EKG

Treatment
- Adequate airway, breathing, and circulation; possible intubation in patients with acute lung injury from overdose
- Fluid resuscitation
- Medications (see Table 15.1 and Table A.2): antiemetics; benzodiazepines such as lorazepam, diazepam, and clonazepam for alcohol withdrawal; clonidine for hypertension related to withdrawal syndrome; naloxone for opioid and dextromethorphan overdose; benzodiazepines and phenobarbital for seizure control in stimulant overdose
- Social worker consult

Nursing Interventions
- Administer medications to control withdrawal symptoms.
- Assess for suicidal ideations.
- Assist with management of airway, breathing, and circulation.
- Consult social worker for inpatient or outpatient treatment options.
- Establish IV access and draw blood for laboratory tests.
- Monitor for seizures and take seizure precautions such as padding bed rails.
- Monitor for signs of aggression and use de-escalation interventions.
- Perform Clinical Institute Withdrawal Assessment (CIWA) and give medication to prevent delirium tremens.
- Place the patient on cardiac monitoring, perform EKG, and treat arrhythmias.
- Provide suction for opioid overdose when patient is unable to maintain secretions.

[ ] NURSING PEARL

Patients should be monitored for 1 to 6 hours post naloxone based on the amount of medication that was required. Symptoms to monitor for are respiratory depression and decreased responsiveness.

[ ] COMPLICATIONS

Patients with opioid withdrawal may have other conditions that need to be considered when providing treatment, such as mental disorders and concurrent use of alcohol or other substances.

Patient Education
- Develop a safety plan with the family or others in the home, which may include having a rescue dose of naloxone available and calling 911.
- Follow prescribed outpatient plan, including taking medications for withdrawal and to prevent relapse.
- Obtain referrals for peer support groups.
- Seek help from support groups and outpatient counseling.

WITHDRAWAL SYNDROME
Overview
- Many patients may have withdrawal symptoms from various substances, most commonly alcohol and opioids, which are discussed in this section.
- Alcohol withdrawal symptoms, such as tremors, anxiety, and increased heart rate, can start as soon as 6 hours after the last drink and may continue to worsen over the following 2 to 3 days. ▶

Overview *(continued)*

- The worst form of alcohol withdrawal is known as delirium tremens, which includes hypertension, altered mental status, seizures, and hallucinations.
- The CIWA is a scale used to determine the severity of withdrawal and provides a protocol for treatment of symptoms.
- The clinical opioid withdrawal scale (COWS) is used to measure the severity of symptoms.
- Opioids cause physical dependence and subsequent drug tolerance, requiring an escalation in doses for desired effects.
- Opioid withdrawal can be life threatening as a result of abruptly stopping the drug or taking an opioid antagonist; symptoms are consistent with autonomic hyperactivity.

Signs and Symptoms

Table 15.5 shows withdrawal symptoms by substance.

Diagnosis

Labs

- CBC
- CMP
- Hepatitis C and HIV tests, if applicable
- Troponin
- Urine drug screen

Diagnostic Testing

- CT scan of head
- EKG
- EEG

Treatment

- Airway, breathing, and circulation management
- IV glucose support
- Medications (see Table 15.1 and Table A.2): Alcohol and opioid withdrawal: clonidine, methadone, naltrexone, and buprenorphine
- NPO during acute withdrawal to prevent aspiration

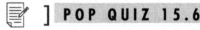 **POP QUIZ 15.6**

A young adult patient presents to the ED after vacationing with their parents. The patient states that they have drunk a bottle of wine every day for the past year. The patient states that while on vacation, they did not drink, and now their hands feel shaky. Upon assessment, the patient is tachycardic and hypertensive. The patient reports taking phenytoin and a multivitamin. What type of monitoring does this patient require?

TABLE 15.5	Withdrawal Symptoms by Substance	
SUBSTANCE	**WITHDRAWAL SYMPTOMS**	
Alcohol	• Agitation	• Headache
	• Anxiety	• Mood swings
	• Diaphoresis	• Sweating
	• Dilated pupils	• Tachycardia
Opioids	• Abdominal cramps	• Muscle aches
	• Chills	• Nausea/vomiting
	• Diaphoresis	• Runny nose
	• Dilated pupils	• Yawning
	• Goosebumps	

Nursing Interventions

- Administer prescribed medications.
- Establish IV access and draw blood for lab tests.
- Minimize noxious stimuli (e.g., bright lights, loud noises).
- Monitor for seizures.
- Perform COWS and CIWA assessments.
- Place patient on continuous cardiac monitoring.

Patient Education

- Learn about naloxone administration if an at-home prescription is provided.
- Obtain referrals to community addiction resources (e.g., Alcoholics Anonymous, Narcotics Anonymous).
- Seek medical care if withdrawing from alcohol or opioids.
- Seek outpatient counseling services.

RESOURCES

Centers for Disease Control and Prevention. (n.d.-a). *Carbon monoxide (CO) poisoning fact sheet*. U.S. Department of Health and Human Services. https://www.cdc.gov/co/pdfs/Flyer_Danger.pdf

Centers for Disease Control and Prevention. (n.d.-b). *Carbon monoxide poisoning: Frequently asked questions*. U.S. Department of Health and Human Services. https://www.cdc.gov/co/faqs.htm

Centers for Disease Control and Prevention. (n.d.-c). *Facts about cyanide*. U.S. Department of Health and Human Services. https://emergency.cdc.gov/agent/cyanide/basics/facts.asp

Centers for Disease Control and Prevention. (n.d.-d). *Prevent carbon monoxide poisoning on your boat*. U.S. Department of Health and Human Services. https://www.cdc.gov/co/boating.htm

Culnan, D. M., Craft-Coffman, B., Bitz, G. H., Capek, K. D., Tu, Y., Lineaweaver, W. C., & Kuhlmann-Capek, M. J. (2018). Carbon monoxide and cyanide poisoning in the burned pregnant patient: An indication for hyperbaric oxygen therapy. *Annals of Plastic Surgery*, *80*(3 Suppl 2), S106–S112. https://doi.org/10.1097/SAP.0000000000001351

de Laby, M. (2020a). Chemical, biological, radiologic, nuclear (CBRN) threats. In V. Sweet & A. Foley (Eds.), *Sheehy's emergency nursing: Principles and practice* (7th ed., pp. 178–179). Elsevier.

de Laby, M. (2020b). Toxicologic emergencies. In V. Sweet & A. Foley (Eds.), *Sheehy's emergency nursing: Principles and practice* (7th ed., pp. 340–352). Elsevier.

Graham, J., & Traylor, J. (2021). Cyanide toxicity. In *StatPearls*. StatPearls Publishing. https://www.ncbi.nlm.nih.gov/books/NBK507796

Hoffman, R. S., & Weinhouse, G. L. (2021, March 25). Management of moderate and severe alcohol withdrawal syndromes. *UpToDate*. https://www.uptodate.com/contents/management-of-moderate-and-severe-alcohol-withdrawal-syndromes

Leybell, I. (2021). Cyanide toxicity. *Medscape*. https://medscape.com/article/814287-overview

Lu, J. J., & Fernandez, R. (2018). Gastric lavage. In E.F. Reichman (Ed.), *Reichman's emergency medicine rocedures* (3rd ed.). McGraw-Hill. https://accessemergencymedicine.mhmedical.com/content.aspx?bookid=2498&sectionid=201310529

McKay, J. I. (2020). Substance use disorders. In V. Sweet & A. Foley (Eds.), *Sheehy's emergency nursing: Principles and practice* (7th ed., pp. 631–646). Elsevier.

MedlinePlus. (n.d.-a). *Alcohol withdrawal*. U.S. Department of Health and Human Services, National Institutes of Health, National Library of Medicine. https://medlineplus.gov/ency/article/000764.htm

MedlinePlus. (n.d.-b). *Delirium tremens*. U.S. Department of Health and Human Services, National Institutes of Health, National Library of Medicine. https://medlineplus.gov/ency/article/000766.htm

MedlinePlus. (n.d.-c). *Opiate and opioid withdrawal*. U.S. Department of Health and Human Services, National Institutes of Health, National Library of Medicine. https://medlineplus.gov/ency/article/000949.htm

National Center for Complementary and Integrative Health. (2021a). *Herb-drug interactions*. U.S. Department of Health and Human Services, National Institutes of Health. https://www.nccih.nih.gov/health/providers/digest/herb-drug-interactions

National Center for Complementary and Integrative Health. (2021b). *Herb-drug interactions: What the science says*. U.S. Department of Health and Human Services, National Institutes of Health. https://www.nccih.nih.gov/health/providers/digest/herb-drug-interactions-science#st-johns-wort

Park, K. S. (2014). Evaluation and management of caustic injuries from ingestion of acid or alkaline substances. *Clinical Endoscopy*, *47*(4), 301–307. https://doi.org/10.5946/ce.2014.47.4.301

Prescribers' Digital Reference. (n.d.-a). *Desferal (deferoxamine mesylate)* [Drug information]. https://www.pdr.net/drug-summary/Desferal-deferoxamine-mesylate-1993

Prescribers' Digital Reference. (n.d.-b). *DigiFab (digoxin immune fab (ovine))* [Drug information]. https://www.pdr.net/drug-summary/DigiFab-digoxin-immune-fab--ovine--2974

Prescribers' Digital Reference. (n.d.-c). *Flumazenil (flumazenil)* [Drug information]. https://www.pdr.net/drug-summary/Flumazenil-flumazenil-1729

Prescribers' Digital Reference. (n.d.-d). *Narcan (naloxone hydrochloride)* [Drug information]. https://www.pdr.net/drug-summary/Narcan-naloxone-hydrochloride-3837

Prescribers' Digital Reference. (n.d.-e). *Protopam chloride (pralidoxime chloride)* [Drug information]. https://www.pdr.net/drug-summary/Protopam-Chloride-pralidoxime-chloride-1131

Prescribers' Digital Reference. (n.d.-f). *Thiamine (thiamine hydrochloride)* [Drug information]. https://www.pdr.net/drug-summary/Thiamine-thiamine-hydrochloride-2546

U.S. Food and Drug Administration. (n.d.). *Drug interactions: What you should know*. U.S. Department of Health and Human Services. https://www.fda.gov/drugs/resources-you-drugs/drug-interactions-what-you-should-know

16 COMMUNICABLE DISEASES

CHILDHOOD DISEASES

Overview

- Childhood diseases can occur at any age; the diseases discussed in this section are more prevalent in children.
- *Measles*, or *rubeola*, is a highly contagious acute viral respiratory illness caused by a virus that lives in the nose and throat mucus of an infected person. It is spread to others by coughing and sneezing and can remain airborne for up to 2 hours after an infected person leaves an area.
- *Mumps*, or *parotitis*, is a viral infection that causes swelling of the salivary glands.
- *Pertussis*, or *whooping cough*, is a highly contagious respiratory disease caused by the bacterium *Bordetella pertussis*. Damage to the cilia causes the upper airway to swell.
- *Chickenpox*, or *varicella*, is a highly contagious infection caused by the varicella-zoster virus.
- *Diphtheria* is a bacterial infection (*Corynebacterium diphtheriae*) of the upper respiratory system that produces a toxin, affecting the nasal and throat mucous membranes. Diphtheria can also affect the skin, causing open sores or ulcers.

[ ] **COMPLICATIONS**

Complications of childhood disease include apnea, convulsions, ear infections, encephalitis, deafness, diarrhea, oophoritis, orchitis, mastitis, pancreatitis, pneumonia, permanent brain damage, and death.

Signs and Symptoms

Table 16.1 shows signs, symptoms, and treatment of childhood diseases.

Diagnosis

Labs

- Blood cultures (for pertussis)
- Complete blood count (CBC)
- Comprehensive metabolic panel (CMP)
- Indirect enzyme immunoassay (for measles)
- Nasopharyngeal culture (for identifying strains of *B. pertussis*)
- Polymerase chain reaction (for varicella, measles, mumps, and pertussis)
- Throat culture (for diphtheria)
- Serology
- Urinalysis (for measles)
- Wound culture

Diagnostic Testing

- Chest x-ray
- CT scan of the face to rule out differential diagnosis (e.g., in mumps)

[ ] **ALERTS!**

Children younger than 1 year with pertussis may have periods of life-threatening apnea and will most likely need to be hospitalized.

Treatment

- Implement isolation precautions.
- Administer medications specific to the disease (see Table 16.1).
- Provide supportive care, possibly including the following: intravenous (IV) fluids, rest.
- When treating diphtheria, avoid endotracheal intubation, if possible, to prevent introduction of upper respiratory bacteria to the lower respiratory tract.

Nursing Interventions

- Use standard precautions for isolation, along with the following: airborne precautions for chickenpox, which includes negative-pressure room; airborne and droplet precautions for measles; droplet precautions for mumps, pertussis, and respiratory diphtheria.
- Assess the airway and maintain patency, which may include suctioning.
- Administer supplemental oxygen therapy, if indicated.
- Administer medications as ordered.
- Monitor intake and output, which may include weighing diapers.
- Administer fluid therapy for rehydration.
- Monitor for signs of worsening infection and sepsis, such as confusion/irritability/inconsolability; fever; hypotension; tachycardia; tachypnea; sweaty or blotchy skin.
- Verify vaccination status and arrange boosters, if needed.
- Report communicable diseases to the health department per local protocol.

Patient Education

- Do not use aspirin for fever or pain to prevent Reye syndrome in children.
- Ensure vaccinations remain up to date, including varicella, Dtap (diphtheria and tetanus toxoids and acellular pertussis vaccine) for young children, and TdaP (tetanus, diphtheria, pertussis) for teenagers and adults. This can be done during routine checks with the provider.
- Follow isolation procedures at home, isolate from immunocompromised people, and do not return to school until cleared by the provider.
- If unvaccinated against varicella, avoid contact with people who have shingles with open blisters.
- Use a cool-mist humidifier for pertussis.
- Apply cool packs to swollen glands for mumps.
- Use creams for rashes and control itching with over-the-counter (OTC) antihistamines.
- Eat a soft diet for sore throat and ensure that adequate nutrition is consumed.
- Perform frequent hand hygiene.
- Practice coughing etiquette by coughing into the inside of the elbow.

 POP QUIZ 16.1

A patient presents to the ED with a chief complaint of new skin lesions. The patient states that they currently live in a group shelter. Upon assessment, an ulcer is noted that is coated with a gray membrane. The patient states that they do not remember if they received any vaccines as a child. What disease does the emergency nurse suspect?

CLOSTRIDIOIDES DIFFICILE

Overview

- *Clostridioides difficile* is a spore-forming, toxin-producing, gram-positive anaerobic bacterium. It colonizes the human intestinal tract and causes antibiotic-associated colitis after the normal gut flora has been disrupted.

 COMPLICATIONS

Complications of *C. difficile* infection include dehydration, severe diarrhea, colitis, toxic megacolon, sepsis, and death.

TABLE 16.1 Childhood Diseases: Signs and Symptoms and Treatment

DISEASE	SIGNS AND SYMPTOMS	TREATMENT
Varicella	• Blister-like rash - Appears on the chest, back, and face, then spreads out to the rest of the body • Fever • Fatigue • Headache • Itching • Loss of appetite	• Acetaminophen (see Table A.2) • Acyclovir (see Table 16.2) • Diphenhydramine
Diphtheria	• Fever • Difficulty breathing • Gray, thick pseudomembrane on the upper respiratory tract mucous membranes - Result of dead tissue from the toxins produced by the bacteria • Skin lesions (appear as ulcers with a pseuodomembrane on the base) • Sore throat • Swollen neck glands • Weakness	• Antibiotics based on cultures, such as penicillin or erythromycin (see Table A.1)
Measles	• Fever • Conjunctivitis • Coryza • Cough • Koplik spots (white spots inside the mouth) • Malaise • Red, teary eyes • Runny nose • Widespread maculopapular rash	• No specific treatment • Postexposure vaccination to nonimmunized patients within 72 hours • Immune serum globulin given within 6 days to infants or patients who are immunocompromised • Vitamin A (see Table 16.2)
Mumps	• Body aches • Difficulty breathing • Difficulty swallowing • Fatigue • Fever • Headache • Loss of appetite • Puffy cheeks • Tender jaw	• Control of pain and fever using acetaminophen or nonsteroidal anti-inflammatory drugs (see Table A.2) • Cold packs applied to swollen glands
Pertussis	• Apnea (in babies) • Cough - Ranges from mild to uncontrollable violent coughing fits, followed by deep breaths heard as a "whooping" sound • Exhaustion after coughing • Fever • Respiratory distress • Runny nose • Shortness of breath • Vomiting after coughing	• Antibiotics, such as azithromycin, clarithromycin, and erythromycin (see Table A.1)

TABLE 16.2 Medications for Communicable Diseases

INDICATIONS	MECHANISM OF ACTION	CONTRAINDICATIONS, PRECAUTIONS, AND ADVERSE EFFECTS
Antimycobacterial (rifampin and rifapentine)		
• Pulmonary TB	• Inhibits DNA-dependent RNA polymerase activity • Broad-spectrum and bactericidal	• Rare adverse effects are related to hematuria, acute kidney failure, psychoses, adrenal insufficiency, and lowered WBC count. • Negative interactions with other drugs (especially antivirals) are possible; consult pharmacist before administering. • Do not give live bacterial vaccines.
Antioxidant (vitamin A)		
• Supports immune system functioning	• Binds to retinol	• Too much vitamin A causes toxicity such as skin peeling and mental status changes.
Antitubercular agent (ethambutol, pyrazinamide, isoniazid)		
• TB prophylaxis • Treatment of TB	• Kills or stops the growth of bacteria that cause TB	• Use of ethambutol risks optic neuritis and hepatic toxicity.
Glycopeptide antibiotic (vancomycin)		
• Antibiotic to treat severe bacterial infections such as MRSA	• Bactericidal by inhibiting cell-wall biosynthesis • Used for gram-positive bacteria that are resistant to other antibiotics	• Common adverse effects include nausea, abdominal pain, and hypokalemia. • Monitor for nephrotoxicity higher in patients older than 65 years. • Ototoxicity (transient or permanent) may occur in patients who receive excessive doses. • Vancomycin has a narrow therapeutic index; trough levels should be 5–15 µg/mL and peak levels should be 20–40 µg/mL.
Guanine nucleoside antiviral (valaciclovir)		
• HSV-1 • HSV-2 • Varicella-zoster virus (chickenpox)	• Antiviral • Slows growth of herpes	• Nephrotoxic • Discontinue and follow up with provider for fever, easy bruising, red spots not related to chickenpox, bloody diarrhea, weakness, or fainting. • Can pass through breast milk and harm the fetus.
Nitroimidazole antibiotic (metronidazole)		
• Trichomoniasis • Rosacea • GI infections • Giardiasis • Postsurgical prophylactic	• Antibiotic • Antiparasitic properties	• Avoid alcohol for at least 3 days after final dose. • Avoid during the first trimester of pregnancy. • Consult provider if there is a history of Crohn's disease or blood, liver, or kidney disease. • Serious side effects are seizures, changes to sensation in hands and feet, flushing, joint pain, and confusion.

(continued)

TABLE 16.2 Medications for Communicable Diseases (continued)		
INDICATIONS	MECHANISM OF ACTION	CONTRAINDICATIONS, PRECAUTIONS, AND ADVERSE EFFECTS
Nucleoside analog (remdesivir, famciclovir)		
• Remdesivir for COVID-19 • Famciclovir for herpes zoster (shingles), cold sores, and genital herpes	• Antiviral	• Adverse effects to discuss with provider are mental or mood changes, decreased amount of urine, yellowing of eyes or skin, and easy bruising. • Use caution with preexisting conditions related to the liver or kidneys or if immunocompromised.

GI, gastrointestinal; HSV, herpes simplex virus; MRSA, methicillin-resistant *Staphylococcus aureus*; TB, tuberculosis; WBC, white blood cell.

Overview (continued)

▪ One of the most common healthcare-associated infections is *C. difficile,* which may cause significant morbidity and mortality. Patients may be asymptomatic, or the infection can progress to acute severe colitis and toxic megacolon.

▪ *C. difficile* spores can live on surfaces and soil for months—sometimes years.

Signs and Symptoms

▪ Abdominal distention

▪ Cramping

▪ Fever

▪ Lower abdominal pain

▪ Nausea

▪ Watery diarrhea (three or more loose stools in 24 hours)

Diagnosis
Labs

▪ CBC

▪ CMP

▪ Stool sample

Diagnostic Testing

▪ CT abdominal scan

Treatment

▪ Administer the following medications: analgesia (see Table A.2); antibiotics such as metronidazole and vancomycin (Table 16.2).

▪ Administer IV fluids.

▪ Discontinue the antibiotic that contributed to the development of the infection.

▪ Perform fecal microbiota transplantation to restore healthy bacteria to the colon; this is indicated for patients who have been admitted at least two times for infection. Immunocompromised patients are not appropriate candidates for this treatment.

▪ Initiate infection control practices and handwashing with soap; hand sanitizer is not effective against transmittal.

▪ Initiate prevention precautions for those at high risk.

▪ Perform surgery to remove the diseased part of the colon.

Nursing Interventions

- Administer ordered medications.
- Ensure proper contact isolation precautions are in place. Wear gowns and gloves; handwash with soap and water; do not use hand sanitizer because it is ineffective. Disinfect surfaces with appropriate sanitizer or bleach with a ratio of one part bleach to nine parts water. Remove any items in the patient's room that can be removed to avoid unnecessary contamination. Do not care for both a patient who is infected with C. *difficile* and a patient who is immunocompromised, if possible.
- Monitor intake and output.
- Perform good hygiene practices and perineal care, and watch for skin breakdown from excess watery stool.
- Provide rehydration as ordered.

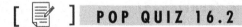

[⚡]   ALERTS!

Toxic megacolon can lead to septic shock. Treat it aggressively with fluid resuscitation and antibiotics.

Patient Education

- Take all antibiotics as prescribed to avoid antibiotic-resistant complications.
- Perform frequent hand hygiene with soap and water after using the bathroom.
- Disinfect high-touch surfaces in the home with a bleach solution of one part bleach to nine parts water.
- Return to the ED for increased diarrhea, diarrhea with blood, abdominal swelling, fever, rapid heart rate, and confusion.
- Use a separate bathroom from others in the household until you are no longer contagious (i.e., after two formed stools).

[📝]   POP QUIZ 16.2

The emergency nurse observes the patient who has an active C. *difficile* infection using alcohol-based sanitizer to perform hand hygiene. What should the emergency nurse do?

COVID-19

Overview

- SARS-CoV-2 (severe acute respiratory syndrome coronavirus 2) is the virus responsible for the coronavirus disease (COVID-19), including related atypical pneumonia, that reached pandemic status in 2020.
- "COVID pneumonia" has taken the lives of many patients because of acute respiratory distress syndrome (ARDS) and the inability of the lungs to exchange oxygen due to fluid buildup in the alveoli.
- COVID-19 is transmitted primarily by droplets but becomes aerosolized via coughing and sneezing and during some medical interventions, such as giving a nebulizer, applying bag mask ventilation, and intubating.
- The incubation period for COVID-19 is 2 to 7 days, and viral shedding can occur up to 7 days before symptom onset.

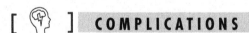

[🧠]   COMPLICATIONS

COVID-19 variants continue to evolve with various transmission rates and severity of illness.

Signs and Symptoms

- Abdominal pain
- Cough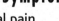

Signs and Symptoms *(continued)*

- Diarrhea
- Fatigue
- Fever
- Headache
- Hypoxia
- Loss of taste and/or smell
- Myalgia
- Shortness of breath
- Sore throat

Diagnosis

Labs

Laboratory tests are ordered based on acuity.

- Arterial blood gas (ABG)
- Antigen (rapid) to test for viral protein
- Basic metabolic panel
- CBC
- Coagulation panel
- D-dimer
- Nucleic acid amplification test (NAAT) to detect presence of viral RNA
- Serum antibody (may remain positive for 3 months)
- Serum lactate

Diagnostic Testing

- Chest x-ray
- EKG
- Chest CT to rule out pulmonary embolism (PE)
- Venous duplex ultrasound

Treatment

- Establish that airway is patent; intubation may be needed due to altered level of consciousness or respiratory fatigue.
- Administer oxygen via nasal cannula, mask, bilevel positive airway pressure (BIPAP), continuous positive airway pressure (CPAP), or high-flow nasal cannula.
- Monitor for arrhythmias.
- Treat thromboembolism with anticoagulants.
- Administer fluid resuscitation as needed.
- Give dexamethasone if indicated (see Table A.4).
- Give remdesivir if indicated (see Table 16.2).
- Monitor and treat multisystem organ failure with supportive treatment.
- Administer antibiotics for concurrent bacterial pneumonia (see Table A.1).
- Use prone positioning in awake and intubated patients for 12 to 16 hours per day.
- Admit patients based on severity of symptoms.

[ ]   **ALERTS!**

Extracorporeal membrane oxygenation may be indicated for patients with severe hypoxia that is refractory to other methods.

Nursing Interventions

- Use airborne and contact precautions, which include wearing an N95 mask or air-purifying device.
- Place the patient in a private room, if possible.
- Assist with establishing patent airway, which may include administering rapid sequence medications.
- Apply oxygen or assist with appropriate mask application.
- Establish two large-bore IV lines with laboratory draw and serial ABGs.
- Place patient on a cardiac monitor and observe for arrhythmias.
- Administer fluid resuscitation as ordered.
- Administer medications.
- Monitor for worsening of cardiac and respiratory complications, PE, and deep vein thrombosis (DVT).
- Use prone positioning for ARDS: suggested for 12 to 16 hours per day in both awake and intubated patients.

Patient Education

- Reduce risk of catching COVID by wearing a mask over the mouth and nose while in public or around others.
- Be tested for COVID if you suspect you were exposed or have symptoms of COVID.
- Self-isolate while sick and for 7 days after.
- Stay up to date on COVID vaccinations per Centers for Disease Control and Prevention (CDC) guidelines.
- Know that recovery from COVID can take weeks to months and may include complications for a lifetime.
- Let close contacts know when they may have been exposed and that they should take precautions to avoid spreading the virus.

HERPES ZOSTER

Overview

- Varicella-zoster virus infection causes two clinically distinct diseases: *Varicella* (chickenpox) results from primary infection, which is characterized by vesicular lesions concentrated on the face and trunk. *Herpes zoster*, also called *shingles*, results from reactivation of latent varicella-zoster virus that gained access to sensory ganglia during varicella. It is characterized by a painful, unilateral vesicular eruption in a specific dermatomal distribution.

 COMPLICATIONS

Complications of herpes zoster include postherpetic neuralgia, vision loss, encephalitis, skin infections, deafness, Ramsay Hunt syndrome, and another herpes zoster flare-up.

Signs and Symptoms

- Burning sensation on one side (commonly on the face, flank, or neck)
- Fever
- Fluid-filled blisters
- Headache
- Itching
- Pain (often a burning, throbbing, or stabbing sensation)
- Unilateral rash

Diagnosis

Labs

- Polymerase chain reaction test
- Direct fluorescent antibody testing on scrapings from vesicular skin lesions
- Viral culture

Diagnostic Testing

- Usually based on clinical presentation (unilateral, usually painful vesicular eruption with a well-defined dermal distribution)

Treatment

- Administer medications: antihistamines such as diphenhydramine; antivirals such as valaciclovir or famciclovir (see Table 16.2); corticosteroids such as prednisolone (see Table A.4).
- Goals of therapy are to promote rapid healing of skin lesions and lessen the severity and duration of pain associated with acute neuritis.

Nursing Interventions

- Administer prescribed medications to assist with itching. If necessary, the patient may be restrained, but this is not common.
- Place the patient in airborne and contact isolation precautions. Use a negative-pressure room, if available. Staff should wear an N95 mask or air-purifying device. The patient is contagious until the blisters are dry and crusted over.
- Pregnant staff may prefer not to care for patients with varicella due to the higher risk of complications for pregnant people and fetuses.
- Monitor for a rash near the eyes or ears.

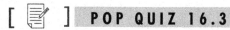

POP QUIZ 16.3

The emergency nurse is working in triage when two patients arrive with active herpes zoster infection. The patients are both hemodynamically stable and alert. The first patient has a rash on the left rib cage and complains of burning. The second patient has a rash on the right side of the face near the right eye. Which patient needs to be seen first?

Patient Education

- Stay up to date on vaccinations. The CDC suggests getting the vaccine even after exposure because patients can get shingles more than once.
- Stay away from immunocompromised people.
- Apply ice packs and cool compresses or take a cool bath with baking soda or uncooked oatmeal to relieve discomfort and itching.
- Use calamine lotion for itching.
- Keep fingernails trimmed and cover wounds to keep from shedding the virus.
- If you do scratch, wash hands for 20 seconds afterward.
- Take prescribed medications as ordered.
- Monitor and follow up with provider for signs of infection, such as wounds with moderate drainage, fever, or rash after treatment.
- See a provider right away if shingles progress to the eyes.

MONONUCLEOSIS

Overview

- *Infectious mononucleosis* is caused by a virus, most commonly the Epstein-Barr virus (EBV). Other viruses that can cause infectious mononucleosis include cytomegalovirus (CMV); toxoplasmosis; HIV; rubella; hepatitis A, B, or C; and adenovirus. ▶

COMPLICATIONS

Complications of mononucleosis include an enlarged spleen, hepatitis, jaundice, anemia, myocarditis, meningitis, Guillain-Barré syndrome, and possible upper airway obstruction related to swollen tonsils.

Overview *(continued)*

- Mononucleosis is spread primarily through saliva. It can also be spread through other bodily fluids, such as semen and blood products, or it can be contracted during organ transplantation.
- Symptoms do not typically arise until 4 to 6 weeks after the exposure.

Signs and Symptoms

- Fatigue
- Fever
- Rash
- Sore throat
- Swollen lymph nodes in the neck and armpits
- Swollen liver or spleen

Diagnosis

Labs

- CBC
- Viral capsid antigen (VCA): anti-VCA IgM (immunoglobulin M) appears in early infection; anti-VCA IgG (immunoglobulin G) appears in acute phase and peaks at 2 to 4 weeks.
- Early antigen: may be a sign of active infection
- EBV nuclear antigen: appears 2 to 4 months afterward and lasts for life
- Monospot test: may indicate infectious mononucleosis but does not confirm EBV
- Throat culture for streptococcus (strep)

Diagnostic Testing

There is no testing specific to diagnosing mononucleosis.

Treatment

- Monitor airway due to swelling.
- Administer antipyretics and analgesics (see Table A.2).
- Administer corticosteroids such as prednisolone (see Table A.4).
- Avoid antibiotic treatment unless strep throat is also present.
- Provide IV fluid resuscitation.
- Test the patient for strep throat.

Nursing Interventions

- Ensure that all utensils and cups are used only by the patient.
- Monitor the patient's airway.
- Monitor for sharp, sudden pain in the left upper abdomen because the patient is at higher risk for splenic rupture due to enlargement of the spleen.

Patient Education

- Avoid contact sports to prevent rupture of the enlarged spleen. Training can be restarted 3 weeks from symptom onset.
- Do not share drinking containers or utensils.
- Do not take penicillin-based antibiotics while infected with mononucleosis.
- Drink plenty of fluids.
- Know that fatigue in infectious mononucleosis can persist for 6 months or longer.
- Get plenty of rest. ▶

Patient Education *(continued)*

- Take OTC pain medication (e.g., acetaminophen, ibuprofen) as needed.
- Return to the ED if experiencing difficulty breathing or swallowing, neurologic symptoms, or severe abdominal pain.

MULTIDRUG-RESISTANT ORGANISMS

Overview

- Multidrug-resistant organisms (MDROs) are bacteria that have become resistant to an antibiotic; as a result, a stronger antibiotic is needed.
- Methicillin-resistant *Staphylococcus aureus* (MRSA) is found on skin and spread by contact with an infected wound or infected personal items. It is resistant to several antibiotics and, if left untreated, can lead to sepsis. It may be acquired in the hospital from bloodstream infections, pneumonia, or surgical site infections.
- *Vancomycin-resistant enterococcus (VRE)* is a type of bacteria that often lives in the intestines and vagina and can spread throughout the body. It is contagious by contact with urine, fecal material, and infected wounds.

[🧠] **COMPLICATIONS**

MDROs can result in an untreatable infection that may lead to sepsis and death.

- *Carbapenem-resistant Enterobacteriaceae (CRE)* are carbapenem-resistant bacteria such as *Klebsiella, Escherichia, Acinetobacter,* and *Pseudomonas* species. CRE infection is very difficult to treat because the bacteria are resistant to several other antibiotics, and carbapenem is a last-resort drug.
- Nosocomial infections are caused by MDROs that are acquired via invasive procedures or from failing to follow infection control policies. They are acquired after facility admission and may lead to sepsis and death.
- Two common preventable nosocomial infections are central line–associated bloodstream infection (CLABSI), which occurs because of pathogens entering the body during insertion of a central line; catheter-associated urinary tract infection (CAUTI), which is caused by pathogens entering the urethra and bladder from improper catheter insertion or maintenance.

Signs and Symptoms

Table 16.3 shows signs and symptoms of infections with MRSA, VRE, and CRE.

TABLE 16.3 Signs and Symptoms of MRSA, VRE, and CRE Infections

MRSA SKIN INFECTIONS	VRE	CRE
Bump on the skin with the following: • Drainage with pus • Fever • Pain • Redness • Swelling • Warmth to touch	• Body aches • Chills • Diarrhea • Fever • Nausea/vomiting • Redness, swelling, or pain in the body • Tachycardia • Tachypnea	• Abdominal pain (liver or spleen infection) • Chills • Dysuria (UTI) • Fatigue • Fever • Shortness of breath (pneumonia) • Skin infection • Stiff neck (meningitis)

CRE, carbapenem-resistant Enterobacteriaceae; MRSA, methicillin-resistant *Staphylococcus aureus*; UTI, urinary tract infection; VRE, vancomycin-resistant enterococcus.

Diagnosis

Labs

- Blood culture
- CBC
- CMP
- Lactate
- Nasal swab
- Stool culture
- Urine culture
- Wound sample

Diagnostic Testing

- CT abdominal scan

Treatment

- Administer antibiotics per laboratory culture, such as vancomycin (see Table 16.2).
- Remove central line as soon as it is not needed.
- Remove indwelling catheter as soon as it is not needed.
- Administer IV fluids.
- Drain the abscesses (for MRSA), if indicated.

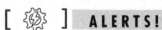 **ALERTS!**

MRSA can cause severe symptoms such as bloodstream infections, pneumonia, or surgical site infections that can lead to sepsis.

Nursing Interventions

- Monitor vital signs, watching for fever or changes that indicate sepsis, such as hypotension and tachycardia.
- Ensure that proper contact isolation precautions are in place: Place the patient in a private room. Wear a gown and gloves. Wear a mask and protective eyewear when performing activities that can cause splashing of body fluids.
- Interventions for CAUTI include the following: Remove indwelling catheter as soon as it is no longer needed. Use sterile procedure with catheter placement. Perform proper perineal area cleaning methods.
- Interventions for CLABSI include the following: Ensure sterile setup when placing central line. Access ports with aseptic techniques. Perform routine cleaning per hospital policy.
- Monitor intake and output.
- Perform frequent hand hygiene with soap and water.
- Wash surfaces frequently with proper sanitizing solution per facility policy.
- Perform wound care.

Patient Education

- Cover wounds with clean, dry bandages until healed. Avoid picking at sores, and perform frequent hand hygiene.
- Do not share personal items such as razors.
- Take antibiotics as prescribed. Do not stop taking prescribed antibiotics without checking with the provider.

TUBERCULOSIS

Overview

- *Tuberculosis (TB)* is an infection caused by *Mycobacterium tuberculosis* that typically affects the respiratory system; however, it can also infect the spine, kidneys, and brain. TB bacteria are spread through the air via coughing or speaking.
- Patients are not always sick when infected with TB bacteria. They can have either latent TB infection or TB disease.
- Latent TB can progress to TB disease if left untreated.

Signs and Symptoms

Table 16.4 shows the difference between latent and active TB with signs and symptoms.

Diagnosis

Labs

- CBC
- CMP
- Tuberculin skin test (Mantoux): intradermal skin test monitored 48 to 72 hours after administration; positive result is a bump with redness where the test was performed.
- TB blood test
- Sputum culture

Diagnostic Testing

- Bronchoscopy
- Chest x-ray
- Pulmonary function testing

[🧠]   **COMPLICATIONS**

Complications of TB include spine pain, damaged joints, meningitis, liver or kidney disease, and, rarely, cardiac tamponade.

TABLE 16.4 Difference Between Latent and Active TB With Signs and Symptoms

LATENT TB	ACTIVE TB
• Cannot spread to others	• Cough that lasts 3 weeks or longer
• Requires treatment for latent TB infection to prevent disease	• Chest pain
• Negative sputum smear	• Chills
• No symptoms	• Coughing up of blood or sputum
• Normal chest x-ray	• Decreased appetite
• Positive tuberculin skin test	• Fever
	• Possibly contagious
	• Requires treatment for active TB disease
	• Night sweats
	• Positive tuberculin skin test
	• Weakness or fatigue

TB, tuberculosis.

Treatment

- Antibiotics for latent TB, such as isoniazid and rifampin (see Table 16.2)
- Treatment for active TB: first-line antitubercular agents, such as isoniazid, rifampin, ethambutol, and pyrazinamide (see Table 16.2); second-line treatment with fluoroquinolone (see Table A.1)
- Supplemental oxygen therapy, if indicated
- IV fluids if indicated
- Bacillus Calmette-Guérin (BCG) vaccine in countries where TB infections are high

Nursing Interventions

- Ensure that proper airborne isolation precautions are in place. Use an N95 mask or air-purifying respirator. Place the patient in a negative-pressure isolation room if available.
- Promote airway clearance and apply oxygen, if needed.
- Monitor for liver complications.

Patient Education

- Avoid using acetaminophen and alcohol if taking medication to treat TB because these medications can be damaging to the liver.
- Know that directly observed therapy may be implemented if there are concerns about isolation and medication compliance. A local public health RN may follow up to ensure adherence to the medication schedule.
- If active TB disease is present, wear a mask around others, and, if possible, keep the windows in the house open and do not maintain close physical contact with others.
- Take the whole course of medication therapy as directed, even if symptoms improve.
- Know that the medication regimen for TB is around 6 to 9 months in length.

[✷] **ALERTS!**

Untreated TB can progress to respiratory failure, pneumothorax, and pneumonia.

[🌐] **NURSING PEARL**

A positive skin test reveals if the patient is a carrier of TB but not necessarily if they are contagious. The patient will need a negative chest x-ray and sputum test to be proved not contagious.

RESOURCES

Almeida, S.-L. (2020). Communicable disease and organisms in the health care setting. In V. Sweet & A. Foley (Eds.), *Sheehy's emergency nursing: Principles and practice* (7th ed., pp. 184–191). Elsevier.

American Academy of Family Physicians. (2020, April 17). *Mononucleosis.* familydoctor.org. https://familydoctor.org/condition/mononucleosis

Centers for Disease Control and Prevention. (n.d.-a). C. diff (Clostridioides difficile): *Prevent the spread of* C. diff. U.S. Department of Health and Human Services. https://www.cdc.gov/cdiff/prevent.html

Centers for Disease Control and Prevention. (n.d.-b). C. diff (Clostridioides difficile): *What is* C. diff? U.S. Department of Health and Human Services. https://www.cdc.gov/cdiff/what-is.html

Centers for Disease Control and Prevention. (n.d.-c). *Chickenpox (varicella): Collecting specimens for varicella zoster virus (VZV) testing.* U.S. Department of Health and Human Services. https://www.cdc.gov/chickenpox/lab-testing/collecting-specimens.html

Centers for Disease Control and Prevention. (n.d.-d). *Chickenpox (varicella): Prevention and treatment.* U.S. Department of Health and Human Services. https://www.cdc.gov/chickenpox/about/prevention-treatment.html

Centers for Disease Control and Prevention. (n.d.-e). *Chickenpox (varicella): Signs and symptoms.* U.S. Department of Health and Human Services. https://www.cdc.gov/chickenpox/about/symptoms.html

Centers for Disease Control and Prevention. (n.d.-f). *Chickenpox (varicella): Transmission.* U.S. Department of Health and Human Services. https://www.cdc.gov/chickenpox/about/transmission.html

Centers for Disease Control and Prevention. (n.d.-g). *Diphtheria: Diagnosis, treatment, and complications.* U.S. Department of Health and Human Services. https://www.cdc.gov/diphtheria/about/diagnosis-treatment.html

Centers for Disease Control and Prevention. (n.d.-h). Diphtheria: *Diphtheria antitoxin.* U.S. Department of Health and Human Services. https://www.cdc.gov/diphtheria/dat.html

Centers for Disease Control and Prevention. (n.d.-i). *Diphtheria: Symptoms and symptoms.* U.S. Department of Health and Human Services. https://www.cdc.gov/diphtheria/about/symptoms.html

Centers for Disease Control and Prevention. (n.d.-j). *Epstein-Barr virus and infectious mononucleosis: About infectious mononucleosis.* U.S. Department of Health and Human Services. https://www.cdc.gov/epstein-barr/about-mono.html

Centers for Disease Control and Prevention. (n.d.-k). *Epstein-Barr virus and infectious mononucleosis: Laboratory testing.* U.S. Department of Health and Human Services. https://www.cdc.gov/epstein-barr/laboratory-testing.html

Centers for Disease Control and Prevention. (n.d.-l). *Healthcare-associated infections (HAIs): Vancomycin-resistant enterococci (VRE) in healthcare settings.* U.S. Department of Health and Human Services. https://www.cdc.gov/hai/organisms/vre/vre.html

Centers for Disease Control and Prevention. (n.d.-m). *Measles (Rubeola): Complications of measles.* U.S. Department of Health and Human Services. https://www.cdc.gov/measles/symptoms/complications.html

Centers for Disease Control and Prevention. (n.d.-n). *Measles (Rubeola): For healthcare providers.* U.S. Department of Health and Human Services. https://www.cdc.gov/measles/hcp/index.html

Centers for Disease Control and Prevention. (n.d.-o). *Measles (Rubeola): Measles serology.* U.S. Department of Health and Human Services. https://www.cdc.gov/measles/lab-tools/serology.html

Centers for Disease Control and Prevention. (n.d.-p). *Measles (Rubeola): Signs and symptoms.* U.S. Department of Health and Human Services. https://www.cdc.gov/measles/symptoms/signs-symptoms.html

Centers for Disease Control and Prevention. (n.d.-q). *Methicillin-resistant* Staphylococcus aureus *(MRSA).* U.S. Department of Health and Human Services. https://www.cdc.gov/mrsa/index.html

Centers for Disease Control and Prevention. (n.d.-r). *Methicillin-resistant* Staphylococcus aureus *(MRSA): General information.* U.S. Department of Health and Human Services. https://www.cdc.gov/mrsa/community/index.html

Centers for Disease Control and Prevention. (n.d.-s). *Mumps: Complications of mumps.* U.S. Department of Health and Human Services. https://www.cdc.gov/mumps/about/complications.html

Centers for Disease Control and Prevention. (n.d.-t). *Mumps: Signs and symptoms of mumps.* U.S. Department of Health and Human Services. https://www.cdc.gov/mumps/about/signs-symptoms.html

Centers for Disease Control and Prevention. (n.d.-u). *Pertussis (whooping cough): Causes and how it spreads.* U.S. Department of Health and Human Services. https://www.cdc.gov/pertussis/about/causes-transmission.html

Centers for Disease Control and Prevention. (n.d.-v). *Pertussis (whooping cough): Diagnosis and treatment of whooping cough (pertussis).* U.S. Department of Health and Human Services. https://www.cdc.gov/pertussis/about/diagnosis-treatment.html

Centers for Disease Control and Prevention. (n.d.-w). *Pertussis (whooping cough): Prevention.* U.S. Department of Health and Human Services. https://www.cdc.gov/pertussis/about/prevention/index.html

Centers for Disease Control and Prevention. (n.d.-x). *Pertussis (whooping cough): Signs and symptoms.* U.S. Department of Health and Human Services. https://www.cdc.gov/pertussis/about/signs-symptoms.html

Centers for Disease Control and Prevention. (n.d.-y). *Pertussis (whooping cough): Specimen collection and diagnostic testing.* U.S. Department of Health and Human Services. https://www.cdc.gov/pertussis/clinical/diagnostic-testing/diagnosis-confirmation.html

Centers for Disease Control and Prevention. (n.d.-z). *Shingles (herpes zoster): Preventing varicella-zoster virus (VZV) transmission from herpes zoster in healthcare settings.* U.S. Department of Health and Human Services. https://www.cdc.gov/shingles/hcp/hc-settings.html

Centers for Disease Control and Prevention. (n.d.-aa). *Tuberculosis (TB): Latent TB infection and TB disease.* U.S. Department of Health and Human Services. https://www.cdc.gov/tb/topic/basics/tbinfectiondisease.htm

Centers for Disease Control and Prevention. (n.d.-bb). *Vaccines and preventable diseases: Shingles vaccine*. U.S. Department of Health and Human Services. https://www.cdc.gov/vaccines/vpd/shingles/public/shingrix/index .html

Centers for Disease Control and Prevention. (2022, August 30). *Testing for TB infection*. U.S. Department of Health and Human Services. https://www.cdc.gov/tb/topic/testing/tbtesttypes.htm

Healthwise Staff. (2020, September 23). *Vancomycin-resistant enterococci (VRE)*. Michigan Medicine. https://www .uofmhealth.org/health-library/tp23381spec

Lamont, J. T., Kelly, C. P., & Bakken, J. S. (2022). *Clostridioides difficile* infection in adults: Clinical manifestations and diagnosis. *UpToDate*. https://www.uptodate.com/contents/clostridioides-difficile-infection-in-adults-clinical -manifestations-and-diagnosis

Mayo Foundation for Medical Education and Research. (2020, December 1). *MRSA infection*. Mayo Clinic. https:// www.mayoclinic.org/diseases-conditions/mrsa/diagnosis-treatment/drc-20375340

Mayo Foundation for Medical Education and Research. (2020, December 22). *Mononucleosis*. Mayo Clinic. https:// www.mayoclinic.org/diseases-conditions/mononucleosis/diagnosis-treatment/drc-20350333

Mayo Foundation for Medical Education and Research. (2020, January 1). *Diphtheria*. Mayo Clinic. https://www .mayoclinic.org/diseases-conditions/diphtheria/symptoms-causes/syc-20351897

Mayo Foundation for Medical Education and Research. (2020, October 6). *Shingles*. Mayo Clinic. https://www .mayoclinic.org/diseases-conditions/shingles/symptoms-causes/syc-20353054

MedlinePlus. (2020, July 31). *Mononucleosis (mono) tests. U.S. Department of Health and Human Services, National Institutes of Health, National Library of Medicine.* https://medlineplus.gov/lab-tests/mononucleosis-mono-tests

MedlinePlus. (2020, September 29). *Infectious mononucleosis. U.S. Department of Health and Human Services, National Institutes of Health, National Library of Medicine.* https://medlineplus.gov/infectiousmononucleosis .html#cat_92

MedlinePlus. (2021, May 4). *U.S. Department of Health and Human Services, National Institutes of Health, National Library of Medicine.* https://medlineplus.gov/ency/article/000858.htm

Mohr, N. M., & Ellender, T. J. (2020). Coronavirus disease 2019 (covid-19). In J. E. Tintinalli, O. J. Ma, D. M. Yealy, G. D. Meckler, J. Stapczynski, D. M. Cline, & S. H. Thomas (Eds.), *Tintinalli's emergency medicine: A comprehensive study guide* (9th ed.). McGraw-Hill. https://accessemergencymedicine.mhmedical.com/content.aspx

Prescribers' Drug Reference. (n.d.-a). *Acyclovir (acyclovir sodium)* [Drug information]. https://www.pdr.net/drug -summary/Acyclovir-acyclovir-sodium-670

Prescribers' Drug Reference. (n.d.-b). *Azithromycin (azithromycin)* [Drug information]. https://www.pdr.net/drug -summary/Azithromycin-azithromycin-24249

Prescribers' Drug Reference. (n.d.-c). *Metronidazole injection (metronidazole)* [Drug information]. https://www.pdr .net/drug-summary/Metronidazole-Injection-metronidazole-1728

Prescribers' Drug Reference. (n.d.-d). *Penicillin G potassium (penicillin G potassium)* [Drug information]. https://www .pdr.net/drug-summary/Penicillin-G-Potassium-penicillin-G-potassium-1150

Prescribers' Drug Reference. (n.d.-e). *Rifadin (rifampin)* [Drug information]. https://www.pdr.net/drug-summary/Rifadin -rifampin-1036

Prescribers' Drug Reference. (n.d.-f). *Vancocin (vancomycin hydrochloride)* [Drug information]. https://www.pdr.net/drug -summary/Vancocin-vancomycin-hydrochloride-802

17 PROFESSIONAL ISSUES

DELEGATION OF TASKS

Overview

- Delegation of tasks allows the nurse to focus on nursing skills, such as assessment, planning, and treatments.
- The licensed or registered nurse as a delegator has the authority to delegate an appropriate task to a delegatee within the designated scope of practice.
- Individual state nurse practice acts determine what can be delegated. A delegatee is a person who accepts a task that they are competent to perform and may be an RN, LPN/LVN, or unlicensed assistive personnel (UAP). A delegator is a licensed professional, including an APRN, RN, or LPN/LVN, who may delegate appropriate tasks to a delegatee.
- Essential components of delegation include the following: Nurses have a professional duty and responsibility to perform tasks within the scope of practice that is governed by each state. Nurses have the authority or ability to complete duties within their specific role that is derived from nurse practice acts and organizational policies. Nurses are accountable legally for actions related to patient care. The nurse may delegate responsibility and authority to complete a task. However, the nurse remains accountable for the overall outcome. This is guided by state nurse practice acts.

Five Rights of Delegation

- The American Nurses Association (ANA) has developed the five rights of delegation: right circumstance; right directions and communication; right person; right supervision and evaluation; right task.

[ ]   **POP QUIZ 17.1**

The RN asks the UAP to assist a patient to the bathroom. The RN then states, "I left their aspirin in the medicine cup on the table. Can you make sure the patient takes this when you return?" Is the UAP able to complete this task? Why or why not?

DISASTER MANAGEMENT

Stages of Disaster Management

- Disasters are widespread and can overwhelm entire communities, including hospitals. Nurses need to be prepared for these unpredictable events.
- In general, disasters are classified into the following categories: biological, such as the COVID-19 pandemic; chemical; explosive; natural/environmental; radiologic/nuclear.
- Disaster management starts with preparation for potential mass casualty events, which includes the participation of businesses (hospitals), government entities, and volunteer services. Step 1 of disaster management is mitigation to reduce the risk of loss, which includes routine analysis of building codes and fire alarms. Step 2 is preparation, which includes EDs, police, and local emergency medical services (EMS) working together to practice for mass casualty incidents (MCIs) that may be likely to occur in the area. Step 3 is the response effort that occurs immediately after the incident, such as search and rescue. Step 4 is the recovery period, in which the community is returned to normal.

Mass Casualty Incidents

- MCIs are inherently chaotic, but adequate training for a wide range of situations is key to gaining control of the situation.
- MCIs require a command system, which includes police, firefighters, EMS, and hospital administration, to facilitate communication between the scene and the hospital. This information is used to mobilize resources, call in staff, and expedite discharges in the ED to make more beds available.
- During an MCI, the following should happen: Assign staff a clear role and require wearing of proper identification. Have a way to track and identify patients upon arrival (often on paper). Establish a staging area and set up hazmat if needed. Triage and sort patients.
- The most widely used triage process during an MCI is summed up by the acronym SALT, which stands for sort, assess, lifesaving interventions, and treatment/transport. Sort patients based on the severity of the injury and assign them a color status that prehospital and hospital professionals recognize universally. Tags are physically tied or attached to a patient.

DISCHARGE PLANNING

Discharge Goals

- A well-organized discharge assists the patient with transition to another level of care.
- Adequate and efficient discharge planning will help. Maintain the patient's quality of life and continuity of care. Reduce unplanned readmissions. Decrease the financial burden to hospitals that is caused by readmission of patients with complex medical conditions.

Discharge Process

- Upon the arrival of a patient to the ED, the discharge process should be started.
- Assess for barriers to discharge planning, which may include low literacy level, lack of financial and/ or psychosocial resources, lack of health insurance, and language barriers. Ensure that the discharge paperwork is written at a level the patient can understand (often an eighth-grade reading level is average). Use a translator phone or program as needed to ensure discharge instructions are understood properly. Consult social work to coordinate community resources for the patient as needed.
- Discharge instructions should be individualized and patient centered.
- Discharge planning should include patient education, post-ED interventions (e.g., home care, medications), coordination of referrals, and any other follow-up services.
- The patient should verbalize understanding and provide return demonstrations when appropriate.

END-OF-LIFE CARE

Advance Directives

- Emergency care staff often provide interventions that are lifesaving but that may not be in the best interest of the patient. In a patient with advanced age and chronic medical conditions, there may no longer be a desire for invasive procedures or prolonged attempts at resuscitation. Advance directives are legal documents that provide the following information.

Palliative Care

- Palliative care provides support and treatment while allowing the natural process of death. The goal is to provide comfort and emotional support in the following ways: pain control to ease discomfort and assist with breathing distress (large doses may be ordered); positioning for comfort with an elevated head of bed, humidified air, or a fan; emotional and spiritual support from family and clergy. ▶

Palliative Care *(continued)*

◼ Complications to providing end-of-life care in the ED include lack of space for family, time constraints of having multiple patients requiring different levels of care, and insufficient training related to palliative care orders.

Death in the ED

◼ Consider inviting the family members to observe prolonged resuscitation efforts such as CPR. Knowing staff did everything they could may help the family start the grieving process.

◼ Document the time the patient expired and the name of the provider who declared the death. The final cardiac rhythm should be recorded.

◼ Contact the donor network for all deaths, including patients on ventilators who are considered to be brain dead.

◼ When delivering a death notification, avoid euphemisms. Be direct (e.g., "The patient has died") to prevent ambiguity or confusion.

◼ Postmortem care is done per policy. The family needs to be contacted and should be allowed to spend time with the deceased if time allows. Personal belongings and valuables should be offered to the family unless the death is being investigated as part of a crime scene. In that case, the belongings should be given to the police following the chain-of-custody protocol.

◼ Autopsies may be required by a medical examiner or requested by a family member. Suspicious, unusual, or unexpected deaths may require an autopsy by the medical examiner. Some states require an autopsy if the death is suspected to be a result of a public health threat, such as a rapidly spreading disease or foodborne illness. Autopsies are best performed within 24 hours of death. The body should be kept cool in a morgue, if possible. Some states have laws that honor religious objections. Medical examiners may change the way they do autopsies to abide by the patient's or family's religious objections.

ORGAN AND TISSUE DONATION

Overview

◼ Nurses are in a unique position to communicate openly about the donation process as well as to provide education and information to the patient and family to make an informed decision.

◼ The Organ Procurement and Transplant Network oversees and connects all providers in the United States to the donor registry network.

◼ Early recognition of potential donors will make the most favorable conditions to harvest organs.

◼ Patients from infancy to advanced age should be considered as potential donors. Age, race, ethnicity, religion, and health (in most cases) do not prevent patients from becoming donors.

◼ Many people can donate tissue and eyes despite chronic health conditions.

◼ Organs of children will most likely go to another child of the same size.

Donation Process

◼ Early recognition of death and notification of the donor network are the first steps. Brainstem death is an irreversible loss of function of all brain activity. The patient is considered clinically dead. Reflexes are absent, and the patient is apneic when the ventilator is paused. Transplant of Human Organs Act of 1994 states that brain death must be certified by four medical experts not connected to the transplant team. Ventilated patients who will be donating heart, lungs, liver, or kidneys will be admitted to the ICU, and measures will be taken to support blood and oxygen circulation until a transplant can occur. The patient will be taken to the operating room to complete the transplant into a live person. Alternatively, organs may be shipped by ground or flight by trained personnel. ▶

Donation Process *(continued)*

- Consulting with the family should be done by a trained social worker or donor network representative, if available.

ETHICAL DILEMMAS

Ethical Decision-Making

- Nurses frequently face very complex ethical dilemmas that require moral courage to assist in making decisions that ultimately affect the patient and the community. Nurses are expected to advocate for patients with patients' best interests in mind. An ethical dilemma may occur when a decision needs to be made between two different courses of action. Significant distress can occur when a nurse feels a moral obligation to the patient but is constricted by an outlying circumstance. An example of a current dilemma among healthcare providers involves vaccination against COVID-19. Some nurses may have personal or religious beliefs against vaccination; however, hospital systems require vaccination for the protection of patients and staff. Nurses must decide to either receive the vaccine and continue to provide care or leave the profession.
- The nurse must protect patient rights. Autonomy versus beneficence must be weighed in decision-making. Nonmaleficence, or the duty to do no harm, speaks to avoiding injury or harm to the patient.

FEDERAL REGULATIONS

Mandatory Reporting

- Federal law identifies nurses as mandatory reporters of abuse; individual states determine vulnerable populations and when mistreatment or abuse may be suspected. In general, vulnerable populations are children, people with disabilities, and older adults. Abuse between intimate partners also requires mandatory reporting. These laws typically cover neglect, as well as physical, sexual, emotional, and financial abuse.

Emergency Medical Treatment and Labor Law

- Emergency Medical Treatment and Labor Act (EMTALA) ensures public access to emergency services, including a medical screening examination, stabilizing treatment for emergency conditions, and labor within the capacity of the hospital. Patients cannot be turned away if they are unable to pay or lack insurance.
- Violating this act can incur fines, penalties, and exclusion from the Medicare program.
- If stabilization of a patient cannot be completed (e.g., due to lack of specialty resources) or if a patient requests to be transported to another facility, a transfer must be implemented to an appropriate facility.

Health Insurance Portability and Accountability Act

- Health Insurance Portability and Accountability Act (HIPAA) is the federal law requiring that all protected health information (PHI) be protected from disclosure and that access to PHI be limited to authorized users only. Consent must be received from the patient prior to sharing personal information, whether it is electronic, written, or oral. Patients have a right to access their own medical information.

[📝]   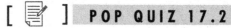 **POP QUIZ 17.2**

An ED technician posts a video to social media of themself and their coworkers in the patient hallway singing "Happy Birthday" to one of their managers. Patients are visible in the video. What federal regulation is the technician in violation of?

Occupational Safety and Health Administration

- Occupational Safety and Health Administration (OSHA) provides resources and assesses workplace safety, health management systems, and safe patient handling.
- OSHA monitors healthcare workers' exposure to hazards such as bloodborne pathogens, chemicals, poor body mechanics related to lifting and repetitive tasks, workplace violence, radioactive material, x-rays, and more.
- OSHA provides healthcare workers with education and training.

FORENSIC EVIDENCE

Overview

- The nurse identifies when evidence collection is required and follows hospital policy for collection, documentation, and chain-of-custody procedures.
- The nurse maintains patient privacy at all times.
- Statements from the patient should be documented in the patient's own words and placed in quotation marks. If paper charting, write legibly. Include specifics (name, place, time); when these are disclosed by the patient, use quotation marks. Remain objective during the interview process and when charting the history of events. Remember that there is a possibility that medical staff will be called to testify in court.
- Document injuries on a body diagram. Evidence that may be collected includes blood, clothing, debris, projectiles, saliva, stains, and urine. Collect debris (e.g., hair, leaves) by using a piece of clean paper and a cotton swab, then seal it in a labeled envelope. Handle all metal projectiles (e.g., arrows, bullets) with rubber-tipped forceps. Do not use metal forceps to avoid scratching the surface of the projectile. When removing clothes, do not cut through a hole or rip because it may be significant to the investigation. Instead, cut around it.
- Ensure a safe environment for the patient. Assist with planning for safe discharge, including providing resources for the patient to contact.
- Ensure the chain of custody is maintained during the investigation. Document who has the evidence with a name and date and describe where it is stored.

Sexual Assault Evidence Collection

- A sexual assault nurse examiner (SANE) should be used if available. These nurses have specialized training in establishing a report, collecting evidence, documenting, and providing emotional support.
- The nurse should follow hospital policies and procedures when a patient arrives with a suspected sexual assault. Preservation of evidence and careful documentation are key in caring for patients who have experienced sexual assault. The nurse must obtain consent for sexual assault kit collection. If the patient is stable, the nurse should have the patient remove clothing while standing on a hospital bed sheet or paper sheet and then place all clothing and shoes in individual paper bags. Plastic bags, which allow the development of moisture and can cause evidence to break down, should not be used. Transfer sheets from EMS or the hospital should also be stored in paper bags as evidence. The nurse should seal all bags with tape, placing a description of the contents on the outside of the bag; The nurse should inform law enforcement if any item inside a bag is wet. It is law enforcement's responsibility to take these items to the crime laboratory promptly.
- The nurse must provide privacy when conducting an interview.
- The nurse should wear gloves at all times and change them frequently when working with potential evidence.

PATIENT CONSENT

Overview

- Patients have the ethical and legal right to make informed decisions about what happens to them and their bodies.
- Patients need to have the risks, benefits, and alternatives to particular interventions explained to them.
- Frequently in the ED, patients present unconscious and require lifesaving interventions. In this situation, providers have the duty to treat or to make a decision to treat based on implied consent. The medical team would assume that a patient would want the intervention, that harm would result without the intervention, and that no next of kin is available to obtain permission.
- The patient has the right to make an informed decision; proper documentation needs to be recorded. In both informed consent and refusal, a nurse may be a witness.
- Three elements must be present to have informed consent: decisional capacity, delivery of information, and voluntary consent from the patient.
- Shared decision-making should be promoted between the provider and the patient.
- Implied consent is realized by the patient's actions (e.g., opening their mouth for a temperature check).
- Decision-making capacity is crucial to determine when obtaining consent and when a patient would like to leave against medical advice (AMA). The nurse and the provider should collaborate to determine if the patient is fully aware and educated on the risks of leaving AMA. The provider is ultimately responsible for determining decision-making capacity. Examples of impaired capacity are cognitive disorders, psychosis, intoxication, and unconsciousness.
- Some barriers to informed consent are language, education level, orientation level, and influence of drugs or alcohol.

Special Considerations

- Obtain phone consent. In the event that a minor or incapacitated patient cannot give consent, then the responsible party must be contacted by phone for the consent. Two witnesses are required to hear and document the conversation. The responsible person, such as the parent, guardian, power of attorney, or next of kin, should state their name, the patient's name, and their relationship to the patient when giving consent for treatment.
- Patients younger than 18 years require consent from their parent or guardian, which may also be received over the phone. Some states allow minors to be seen for sex-related complaints, such as sexually transmitted infections, without parental consent.
- Pregnant patients of any age, including younger than 18 years, can make decisions for themselves and their fetus.
- A patient in custody has the right to make their own decisions except in an emergency or as directed by the court.
- A patient may give verbal consent, which should be documented by two witnesses.
- Per hospital policy, consent may be required for blood transfusions.

 POP QUIZ 17.3

A patient who is alert, oriented, and fully competent arrives at the ED with complaints of numbness and tingling in the leg. Upon assessment, the leg is cool, and there is difficulty obtaining a dorsalis pedal or posterior tibial pulse. There is a concern for arterial occlusion. The patient is terrified of possible surgical intervention and requests to leave. The patient wants to leave AMA and would like to sign the appropriate paperwork. The patient understands the possible complications, including death. Which nursing ethical principle is involved in this scenario?

PROCEDURAL SEDATION

- Situations that frequently occur in the ED and require procedural sedation include the following: dislocation reduction; fracture reduction; head injury requiring imaging; lumbar puncture.
- Informed consent needs to be obtained before the procedure unless the patient is not decisional or it is an emergency situation.
- Goals of sedation are as follows: Ensure patient safety at all times. Perform a presedation checklist that includes a documented history, immediate access to advanced life support, and reversal drugs. Provide adequate analgesia, anxiolysis, and sedation. Continuously monitor the patient throughout and after the procedure. Have an adequate postprocedural observation period and a discharge plan. Keep patients without oral intake (NPO) prior to the procedure to prevent vomiting and aspiration.
- Procedural sedation requires capnography; continuous cardiac monitoring including heart rate, blood pressure, and respiratory rate; physical observation; and pulse oximetry.
- Sedation levels are classified based on consciousness (Table 17.1). In the ED, the goal for most procedures is conscious or moderate sedation, also referred to as "twilight sleep." Deep sedation is unsafe in the ED and should be done only in the operating room with an anesthesiologist. A hospital-approved provider must be at the bedside while sedation is being administered.
- A sedation scale should be used during the procedure. The Ramsey Sedation Scale provides a numeric score from 1 to 6 based on the level of responsiveness. The Richmond Agitation Sedation Scale allows providers to gauge the level of sedation and should be recorded throughout the procedure.

SYMPTOM SURVEILLANCE

- EDs see patients at the onset of symptoms and are critical in the reporting of possible outbreaks related to infectious or biological events.
- Impending outbreaks, such as influenza and COVID-19, are tested for and reported to authorities and public health officials so prevention efforts can be initiated. ▶

TABLE 17.1 Sedation Continuum				
	MINIMAL SEDATION	MODERATE SEDATION/ CONSCIOUS SEDATION	DEEP SEDATION	GENERAL ANESTHESIA
Airway	Unaffected	Intervention not needed	May require airway adjuncts intervention	May require intubation or other airway adjuncts intervention
Alertness	Responds to verbal stimuli	Responds to verbal or tactile stimuli	Responds purposefully after repeated painful stimuli	Unarousable
Cardiovascular function	Unaffected	Typically maintained	Typically maintained	May be affected
Spontaneous ventilation	Unaffected	Typically adequate	May be affected	Frequently affected

SYMPTOM SURVEILLANCE *(continued)*

- Nurses and providers watch for clusters of symptoms and take immediate steps on the front lines to stop the spread of illness, such as patient isolation, wearing masks, and reporting to public health officials within the local community. Public health authorities may request identifying information in certain situations, such as when a tuberculosis patient is in the community and there is a concern for noncompliance with the therapeutic regimen, possibly putting others at risk. Unidentifiable patient information (e.g., chief complaint, diagnostic codes) is sent from the ED to local and state health departments to monitor for public health concerns (e.g., influenza-like illness, opioid overdoses).
- The National Syndromic Surveillance Program collaborates with the Community of Practice to share unidentifiable electronic health information through the BioSense platform.
- Federal partners (e.g., the CDC), local and state health departments, and those who work in academics and the private sector form the Community of Practice and share information regarding outbreaks.

Transfers

- Any possible imaging studies or paperwork should travel with the patient to the accepting facility.
- Patients need to sign a document stating that they have been informed of the purpose, risks, and benefits of being transferred.
- Per EMTALA, all patients need a medical screening examination and stabilization prior to transferring to another facility.
- Transportation methods can include an ambulance, helicopter, or private conveyance.

TRANSITION OF CARE

Overview

- A smooth transition of care is the result of optimal communication and a patient-centered plan that is realistic and attainable.
- Transition of care occurs a few times in the ED: first when EMS delivers a patient, next if there is a nurse handoff, and finally when the patient is admitted or discharged.
- During any transition there is potential for communication breakdown. The most common reason for this is the pressure to do a quick handoff given the nature of the department. To avoid communication breakdown, limit distractions and interventions.
- Provide an organized handoff, such as by using the SBAR (situation, background, assessment, recommendations) technique. Provide the situation that brought the patient to the ED; provide background information, such as the medical history; use the patient's chart for this; provide assessment findings; provide recommendations for anticipated orders and important precautions, such as fall risk or need for seizure pads, isolation, or a sitter to remain at the bedside.
- Ideally, reports should be given over the phone, in person, or at the bedside.
- If a patient is being transferred back to a nursing home or community-based facility, the report should be called to the facility before calling for transport. This ensures that a bed is still available and that the facility is still able to meet the patient's level of needs.
- If the patient is returning home, ensure that they will be able to get into the house. If they require assistance with home care, this arrangement should be in place before discharge.

TRIAGE

Triage Severity

- Triage is a high-risk area, but using the Emergency Severity Index (ESI) algorithm consistently allows patients to be triaged and seen in the appropriate order.
- Every triage starts with an across-the-room observation assessing level of consciousness, work of breathing, and skin condition (e.g., diaphoretic, pale).
- The nurse considers a series of questions to assign an ESI level to the patient based on the severity of symptoms and the number of resources that will be needed. The scale is from 1 to 5; level 1 indicates the sickest patient who requires immediate lifesaving interventions. whereas level 5 indicates a patient who is considered to have minor complaints and requires no significant resources. A patient should be assigned ESI level 1 if they will require lifesaving interventions. If the patient does not require immediate lifesaving treatment, then the nurse should consider if the patient is an ESI level 2. If the patient does not qualify for ESI level 2, then the nurse should determine how many anticipated resources the patient will need.

Triage Assessments

- All triage assessments should include the following: Confirm patient identity. Obtain the chief complaint. Obtain the medical history, current medications, and allergies. Perform a focused assessment regarding the chief complaint. Obtain a full set of vital signs, including blood sugar for patients with diabetes or for anyone with an altered level of consciousness.
- Triage considerations include the following: For language barriers, an interpreter should be used. Infectious disease prevention should be considered, a mask should be provided, and the patient should be isolated as much as possible while waiting for a treatment room. Pediatric assessment should include a documented weight. Caution should be used with psychiatric patients and safety kept in mind. Obstetric and laboring patients should be assessed in the ED per policy; emergent delivery or hemorrhaging may need to remain in the ED for care. EKGs, CT scans, or point-of-care glucose testing should be obtained as needed.
- Patients who are in the waiting area for extended periods of time to see a provider should routinely be checked for changes in condition. The triage nurse should reassess vital signs and bring the patient to a room sooner if indicated.
- Some EDs have predesigned protocol orders, called advance nursing interventions, that nurses place based on their assessment. This allows laboratory results and x-rays to be received sooner, so action can be taken for abnormal results.

Crowding in Triage

- Crowding and overcapacity in the ED create a backup in the waiting room, which can lead to unsafe conditions for patients waiting to see a provider. This is often a hospital-wide problem resulting from a lack of inpatient beds available ▶

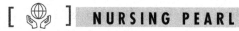

NURSING PEARL

The experienced triage nurse will draw on past experiences and anticipate potential complications.

ALERTS!

If a patient presents to the triage area in significant distress and needs immediate intervention, they should be taken directly to a treatment room to initiate resuscitation. There are generally more resources available in a treatment room than in a triage room.

POP QUIZ 17.4

A stable patient arrives via EMS for a complaint of uncomplicated atraumatic knee pain. The average wait to be seen by a provider is 2 hours. Another patient presents with suspected stroke and is taken emergently to the CT scanner. The patient with knee pain asks, "Why are they going before me? I came by ambulance." How should the nurse respond to this?

Crowding in Triage *(continued)*

for admissions. It can lead to boarding in the ED, which puts strain on nurses by reducing their ability to provide adequate care. It is both unethical and illegal to turn patients away for any reason. It does not matter if the ED is at capacity or if the patient has no health insurance. The federal EMTALA was put in place to protect patients from being turned away. Crowding leads to a delay in treatment of emergent conditions, increased acuity levels, increased nurse-patient ratios, increased mortality, and an increase in patients who leave without being seen.

RESOURCES

Agency for Healthcare Research and Quality. (2019). *Handoffs and signouts.* U. S. Department of Health & Human Services. https://psnet.ahrq.gov/primer/handoffs-and-signouts

American College of Emergency Physicians. (n.d.). *Understanding EMTALA.* https://www.acep.org/life-as-a-physician/ethics--legal/emtala/emtala-fact-sheet

American College of Emergency Physicians. (2016). *Appropriate interfacility patient transfer.* https://www.acep.org/patient-care/policy-statements/appropriate-interfacility-patient-transfer

American College of Emergency Physicians. (2017, July). *Procedural sedation in the emergency department.* https://www.acep.org/patient-care/policy-statements/procedural-sedation-in-the-emergency-department

American Society of Anesthesiologists. (2019, October 13). *Continuum of depth of sedation: Definition of general anesthesia and levels of sedation/analgesia.* https://www.asahq.org/standards-and-guidelines/continuum-of-depth-of-sedation-definition-of-general-anesthesia-and-levels-of-sedationanalgesia

Barrow, J. M., & Sharma, S. (2022). Five rights of nursing delegation. In *StatPearls.* StatPearls Publishing. https://www.ncbi.nlm.nih.gov/books/NBK519519

Bonalumi, N. (2020). Organ and tissue donation. In V. Sweet & A. Foley (Eds.), *Sheehy's emergency nursing: Principles and practices* (7th ed., pp. 142–148). Elsevier.

Centers for Disease Control and Prevention. (n.d.-a). *How we conduct syndromic surveillance.* U.S. Department of Health and Human Services. https://www.cdc.gov/nssp/how-sys.html

Centers for Disease Control and Prevention. (n.d.-b). *New to syndromic surveillance?* U.S. Department of Health and Human Services. https://www.cdc.gov/nssp/new-users.html

Centers for Disease Control and Prevention. (n.d.-c). *Surveillance strategy report—Syndromic reporting.* U.S. Department of Health and Human Services. https://www.cdc.gov/surveillance/initiatives/symptoms-signal.html

Centers for Disease Control and Prevention. (n.d.-d). *What is syndromic surveillance?* U.S. Department of Health and Human Services. https://www.cdc.gov/nssp/overview.htm

Centers for Disease Control and Prevention. (2022, October 5). *FAQ: COVID-19 data and surveillance.* U.S. Department of Health and Human Services. https://www.cdc.gov/coronavirus/2019-ncov/covid-data/faq-surveillance.html

Centers for Medicare & Medicaid Services. (2021, March 4). *Emergency Medical Treatment and Labor Act (EMTALA).* Department of Health and Human Services. https://www.cms.gov/Regulations-and-Guidance/Legislation/EMTALA

Chan, G. K., & Vega, C. (2020). Palliative and end-of-life care in the emergency department. In V. Sweet & A. Foley (Eds.), *Sheehy's emergency nursing: Principles and practices* (7th ed., pp. 131–140). Elsevier.

Dorvil, B. (2018). The secrets to successful nurse bedside shift report implementation and sustainability. *Nursing Management, 49*(6), 20–25. https://doi.org/10.1097/01.NUMA.0000533770.12758.44

Emergency Nurses Association. (2012). *Patient transfers and handoffs.* Author. https://www.ena.org/docs/default-source/resource-library/practice-resources/position-statements/patienthandofftransfer.pdf?sfvrsn=e2c42cb6_22

Emergency Nurses Association. (2013, June). *Safe discharge from the emergency department.* Author. https://www.ena.org/docs/default-source/resource-library/practice-resources/position-statements/safedischargefromed.pdf?sfvrsn=998ee45f_12

Emergency Nurses Association. (2018). *Resuscitative decisions in the emergency care setting.* Author. https://www
.ena.org/docs/default-source/resource-library/practice-resources/position-statements/resuscitativedecisions
.df?sfvrsn=76de2555_18

Emergency Nurses Association. (2019). *Clinical practice guideline: Synopsis the use of capnography during procedural
sedation/analgesia.* Author. https://www.ena.org/docs/default-source/resource-library/practice-resources/cpg/
non-mbr-synopsis/capnography-procedural-sedation-synopsis.pdf?sfvrsn=f870cc5_2

Federal Emergency Management Agency. (n.d.). *Emergency management in the United States.* U.S. Department of
Homeland Security. https://training.fema.gov/emiweb/downloads/is111_unit%204.pdf

Howard, P. K. (2020). Family presence during resuscitation and invasive procedures. In V. Sweet & A. Foley (Eds.),
Sheehy's emergency nursing: Principles and practices (7th ed., pp. 112–113). Elsevier.

Isaacs E. (2018). Informed consent. In E. F. Reichman (Ed.), *Reichman's emergency medicine procedures* (3rd ed.).
McGraw-Hill. https://accessemergencymedicine.mhmedical.com/content.aspx?bookid=2498&sectionid=201304450

The Joint Commission. (2016, February). *Informed consent: More than getting a signature.* Quick Safety. https://www
.jointcommission.org/-/media/tjc/documents/newsletters/quick_safety_issue_twenty-one_february_2016pdf

Lin, Y.-K., Liu, K.-T., Chen, C.-W., Lee, W.-C., Lin, C.-J., Shi, L., & Tien, Y.-C. (2019, January 23). How to effectively
obtain informed consent in trauma patients: A systematic review. *BMC Medical Ethics, 20*(1), Article 8. https://doi
.org/10.1186/s12910-019-0347-0

Matamoros, L. (2020). Ethical considerations. In V. Sweet & A. Foley (Eds.), *Sheehy's emergency nursing: Principles
and practice* (7th ed., pp. 43–45). Elsevier.

McConnell, T. C. (2020). Legal and regulatory constructs. In V. Sweet & A. Foley (Eds.), *Sheehy's emergency nursing:
Principles and practice* (7th ed., p. 17). Elsevier.

National Council of State Boards of Nursing. (2016). National guidelines for nursing delegation. *Journal of Nursing
Regulation, 7*(1), 5–14. https://doi.org/10.1016/s2155-8256(16)31035-3

National Institute on Aging. (2021). *End of life: Providing care and comfort at the end of life.* U.S. Department of Health
and Human Services, National Institutes of Health. https://www.nia.nih.gov/health/providing-comfort-end-life

Patel, P. R., & Bechmann, S. (2021). Discharge planning. In *StatPearls.* StatPearls Publishing. https://www.ncbi.nlm
.nih.gov/books/NBK557819

U.S. Department of Health and Human Services. (2021). *SALT mass casualty triage algorithm (sort, assess, lifesaving
interventions, treatment/transport).* Chemical Hazards Emergency Medical Management. https://chemm.hhs.gov/
salttriage.htm

U.S. Department of Health and Human Services. (2021, March 8). *START adult triage algorithm—CHEMM.* https://
chemm.nlm.nih.gov/startadult.htm

Yancey, C. C., & O'Rourke, M. C. (2022). Emergency department triage. In *StatPearls.* StatPearls Publishing. https://
www.ncbi.nlm.nih.gov/books/NBK557583

1. The ED nurse is teaching a new graduate nurse how to assess for jugular vein distention, explaining that the patient should be positioned:

   A. Left lateral decubitus with the head of the bed at 0°

   B. Supine with the head of the bed at 45°

   C. Supine with the head of the bed in Fowler's position

   D. Prone with the neck rotated 40° to the right

2. The nurse is treating a patient who thinks he has the flu. He reports fever and chills and states that his chest hurts when he breathes. He has no medical problems he is aware of but does admit to occasional recreational intravenous drug use. While performing the assessment, the nurse auscultates heart sounds and detects a murmur. The nurse anticipates that all the following tests will be performed EXCEPT:

   A. Blood cultures

   B. Chest x-ray

   C. EKG

   D. Cardiac catheterization

3. The nurse is assessing a patient with constant, sharp chest pain in the center of the chest. The nurse attempts to obtain a 12-lead EKG, but the patient refuses to lie down because it makes the pain worse. The patient is most comfortable leaning forward while sitting on the edge of the stretcher. Based on these findings, what condition should the nurse suspect?

   A. Endocarditis

   B. Pericarditis

   C. Myocarditis

   D. Congestive heart failure

4. Which of the following medications is the best option for a patient complaining of chest pain who has a pericardial friction rub and is unable to lie flat?

   A. Hydromorphone

   B. Morphine

   C. Ibuprofen

   D. Acetaminophen

5. Which of the following patients should be treated the most urgently? A patient with a blood pressure of:

   A. 200/100 mmHg who has run out of blood pressure medication

   B. 190/120 mmHg with an elevated creatinine

   C. 220/140 mmHg with normal lab results

   D. 170/90 mmHg who recently stopped drinking alcohol

6. The emergency nurse is treating a passenger in a motor vehicle collision who is intubated and on the ventilator. A portable chest x-ray performed to confirm the endotracheal tube placement indicates that the patient has a widened mediastinum. What immediate intervention is indicated?

   A. Adjust the ventilation rate and volume settings.

   B. Follow up with a chest CT scan.

   C. Prepare for chest tube insertion.

   D. Initiate a crystalloid fluid bolus.

7. The nurse is assessing the legs of a patient with a history of peripheral vascular disease. Which of the following signs indicate that an emergent condition is present?

   A. Lower leg pain that improves with rest.

   B. Thickened skin and hair loss bilaterally.

   C. Sudden onset of pain and pallor in one leg.

   D. Nonhealing skin ulcers.

8. The nurse is treating a patient who has been diagnosed with a lower-leg deep vein thrombosis. The nurse is explaining to the patient what to expect with treatment. Which of the following statements by the patient indicates that they understand the nurse's instructions?

   A. "I will try to stay seated as much as possible to keep off my leg."

   B. "I need to take this blood-thinning medication as prescribed for several months."

   C. "I will cut back to a half a pack per day of cigarettes."

   D. "I don't have any support hose, but I do have control-top hose I can wear."

9. All the following findings indicate improvement in a patient with cardiogenic shock EXCEPT:

   A. Decreased chest pain

   B. Improved mental status

   C. Increased urine output

   D. Increased heart rate

10. The nurse is preparing a patient with acute myocardial infarction for emergent percutaneous coronary intervention (PCI). The patient asks the nurse how this procedure will help her. The nurse explains that the primary goal of PCI is to:

    A. Reestablish blood flow through an occluded coronary artery

    B. Convert the patient to normal sinus rhythm

    C. Measure how well the heart is working to pump blood

    D. Insert an implanted defibrillator

11. When preparing to discharge a patient treated for epistaxis, the nurse needs to instruct the patient with which of the following?

   A. "Continue to use a nasal decongestant as needed for seasonal allergies."

   B. "Continue taking warfarin as prescribed."

   C. "If the bleeding recurs, try blowing your nose to clear it."

   D. "If the bleeding recurs, pinch your nose closed and hold pressure for at least 10 minutes."

12. An older patient reports vertigo, nausea/vomiting, and hearing loss in one ear. The symptoms have occurred before, the patient states, and lasted several hours each time. These symptoms are consistent with which condition?

   A. Vestibular neuritis

   B. Ménière's disease

   C. Benign positional vertigo

   D. Otitis media

13. A patient presents to the ED after accidentally splashing an ammonia-based cleaning solution in his eye. After irrigating the eye with normal saline, the pH is 7.4. What should the nurse do next?

   A. Irrigate the eye with a normal saline/sodium bicarbonate solution.

   B. Irrigate the eye for an additional 15 minutes, then recheck the pH.

   C. Stop irrigating and inform the provider.

   D. Irrigate the eye with a normal saline/boric acid solution.

14. The ambulance is transporting a patient from a manufacturing plant for possible cyanide exposure. What is the priority intervention for this patient?

   A. Supplemental oxygen

   B. A rapid crystalloid fluid bolus

   C. Amyl nitrite administration

   D. Sodium bicarbonate administration

15. Which of the following medications is the most appropriate for chest pain caused by a cocaine overdose?

   A. Labetalol

   B. Nitroprusside

   C. Nitroglycerin

   D. Thrombolytic therapy

16. A 16-year-old-male patient presents to the ED with a sudden onset of severe pain and swelling of one side of his scrotum. The patient denies any difficulty urinating or any discharge. What condition should the nurse suspect?

   A. Acute epididymitis

   B. Testicular torsion

   C. Testicular tumor

   D. Priapism

17. An 83-year-old man presents with urination problems. He reports frequency, nocturia, and a weak urine stream. He has been unable to void more than a few drops since early this morning. A bladder scan detects 500 mL of urine. The nurse is unable to insert a urinary catheter because of resistance. What should the nurse do next?

    A. Have the patient attempt to void again.

    B. Repeat the bladder scan.

    C. Insert a different size urinary catheter.

    D. Insert a curved-tipped Coudé catheter.

18. All the following interventions are appropriate for a patient with renal calculi EXCEPT:

    A. Urinary catheter insertion

    B. Crystalloid fluid bolus

    C. Ketorolac 15 mg intravenously

    D. Promethazine 25 mg intravenously

19. In which patient is it appropriate to insert an indwelling urinary catheter?

    A. A patient with urinary retention to check postvoid residual

    B. A patient with CHF who received a dose of furosemide intravenously

    C. A patient in septic shock receiving vasopressors

    D. A confused patient who is incontinent

20. A patient with preeclampsia is on a magnesium sulfate infusion. The nurse evaluates the patient and determines the medication is effective by what finding?

    A. The patient becomes flushed and feels weak.

    B. The blood pressure is 85/60 mmHg.

    C. Deep tendon reflexes are +1 bilaterally.

    D. No seizures occur.

21. A patient is being worked up for acute renal failure. To determine the patient's acuity, which of the following tests is the priority to obtain?

    A. CT scan of the abdomen with contrast

    B. Basic metabolic profile

    C. Urinalysis

    D. Renal ultrasound

22. What types of medications are used to treat myasthenia gravis?

    A. Antibiotics

    B. Anticholinesterases

    C. Psychotropics

    D. Antidysrhythmics

23. The nurse is treating a patient with multiple sclerosis who is experiencing blurred vision and profound weakness. Which of the following medications should the nurse anticipate administering?

   A. Cyclobenzaprine
   B. Venlafaxine
   C. Methylprednisolone
   D. Dextroamphetamine

24. The nurse is treating a patient who has a migraine headache. Which initial medication order should the nurse question?

   A. Ketorolac
   B. Hydromorphone
   C. Dihydroergotamine
   D. Promethazine

25. The nurse is preparing a patient for admission to the hospital for viral meningitis. Which of the following statements by the patient's family indicates the need for additional instruction?

   A. "We need to let the staff know if the patient's headache gets worse."
   B. "There won't be any antibiotics administered since it is viral meningitis."
   C. "We need to put on gowns and gloves each time we go into the patient's room."
   D. "The patient can have anything to eat or drink."

26. A patient with an ankle sprain is demonstrating crutch-walking in preparation for discharge. The nurse determines the client is knowledgeable about safe crutch-walking based on which observation?

   A. The top of the crutch fits tightly under the patient's armpits.
   B. The patient's elbows are slightly bent when holding the handgrips.
   C. The patient looks down while walking.
   D. The patient stands up straight and keeps the crutches aligned with the body.

27. What is the most common cause of osteomyelitis?

   A. *Clostridium tetani*
   B. *Clostridioides difficile*
   C. *Escherichia coli*
   D. *Staphylococcus aureus*

28. The nurse understands that a patient undergoing procedural sedation must be continually monitored throughout the procedure and recovery period. Which of the following actions does NOT support this monitoring?

   A. Placing the patient on a cardiac monitor and pulse oximeter
   B. Periodically assessing the patient's level of sedation
   C. Placing the patient in a room close to the nurses' station.
   D. Measuring the patient's vital signs frequently

29. While triaging a patient, the nurse asks about the patient's past medical history. The patient denies any health problems except for hypertension. All of the following findings would lead the nurse to suspect that the patient has chronic obstructive pulmonary disease EXCEPT:

    A. Pursed-lip breathing
    B. Nail clubbing
    C. Hyperresonance in the lung fields
    D. Crackles in the lung fields

30. Which of the following puncture wounds has the highest risk of infection?

    A. Nail in the thumb
    B. Piece of glass in the arm
    C. Metal sliver in the hand
    D. Piece of wood in the leg

31. A patient experiences return of spontaneous circulation after an overdose of opioid medications. The patient has been placed on a ventilator and is responsive to painful stimuli. In caring for this patient, the nurse would question implementing which of the following orders?

    A. Targeted temperature management
    B. Naloxone infusion protocol
    C. Social work consultation
    D. Ventilator-associated infection prevention bundle

32. When examining a patient for signs of right-sided heart failure, the emergency nurse knows to assess for:

    A. Jugular vein distention, hepatomegaly, and peripheral edema
    B. Crackles, shortness of breath, and fatigue
    C. Narrow pulse pressure, muffled heart sounds, and jugular vein distention
    D. Right-sided tracheal deviation, jugular vein distention, and diminished breath sounds on the left side

33. The nurse is evaluating a patient who has just received 150 mg of intravenous amiodarone over 10 minutes. How does the nurse determine whether the patient has had a positive response to this medication?

    A. Lowered blood pressure
    B. Lowered heart rate
    C. Increased oxygen saturation
    D. Improved level of consciousness

34. A patient presents to the ED with tearing, light sensitivity, and the sensation that something is in his right eye, although he does not recall anything coming in contact with his eye. When preparing the patient for the eye exam, what intervention does the nurse anticipate?

    A. Oral antibiotic administration
    B. Oral analgesic administration
    C. Instillation of fluorescein dye
    D. Eye patch application

35. Which eye assessment finding differentiates uveitis from conjunctivitis?

   A. Pain
   B. Redness
   C. Tearing
   D. Pupil size

36. Which of the following is the best indicator that treatment for a tricyclic antidepressant overdose has been effective?

   A. Pulse oximetry reading greater than 95%
   B. Normal QRS complex
   C. Lower blood pressure
   D. Elevated mood

37. A 22-year-old female patient arrives to the ED reporting intentional ingestion of 100 tablets of acetaminophen. The nurse should expect to:

   A. Administer N-acetylcysteine (acetate)
   B. Place a nasogastric tube and lavage with sterile water
   C. Administer an adult dose of activated charcoal
   D. Place the patient in the low-acuity section for monitoring

38. What does bruising around the umbilicus indicate in the patient with blunt abdominal trauma?

   A. Peritoneal irritation
   B. Intra-abdominal bleeding
   C. Retroperitoneal bleeding
   D. Gastrointestinal bleeding

39. The nurse is treating a patient diagnosed with pancreatitis. After administering intravenous fluids and pain medications, the nurse is most concerned about which of the following findings?

   A. Tachypnea
   B. Continued nausea
   C. Elevated amylase
   D. Elevated lipase

40. The nurse is giving discharge instructions to a patient diagnosed with an inevitable abortion. The nurse's teaching is effective if the patient states:

   A. "If I start bleeding like I'm having a heavy period, I need to be rechecked."
   B. "I can use a tampon for the bleeding."
   C. "I should expect to run a fever."
   D. "I can return to my regular activities tomorrow."

41. A patient who is 36 weeks pregnant is involved in a motor vehicle collision. She is fully immobilized with a cervical collar on a long backboard. What is one of the nurse's first interventions?

    A. Elevate the right side of the backboard.

    B. Elevate the left side of the backboard.

    C. Elevate the head of the backboard.

    D. Remove the cervical collar and backboard.

42. The nurse is treating a patient diagnosed with a thyroid storm. Which of the following medication orders should the nurse anticipate?

    A. Acetaminophen

    B. Atropine

    C. Hydromorphone

    D. Furosemide

43. Which condition of electrolyte imbalance causes hyperactive reflexes and tremors?

    A. Hypermagnesemia

    B. Hyponatremia

    C. Hyperkalemia

    D. Hypocalcemia

44. The nurse triages a patient who is being treated for leukemia and has a fever. What should the nurse do first?

    A. Administer acetaminophen.

    B. Obtain blood cultures.

    C. Place the patient in a private treatment room.

    D. Start an intravenous infusion.

45. While triaging a patient, the nurse reviews the patient's home medications. The presence of what medication would indicate that the patient's history recall might be limited because of dementia?

    A. Fluoxetine

    B. Warfarin

    C. Diazepam

    D. Donepezil

46. A nurse is assessing a patient who has sustained a neck injury from an all-terrain vehicle accident. The patient is bradycardic and hypotensive. What condition is most likely present in this situation?

    A. Hypovolemic shock

    B. Distributive shock

    C. Cardiogenic shock

    D. Obstructive shock

47. The emergency nurse is treating a patient who was stabbed in the back. While performing a neurologic assessment, the nurse observes that the patient has no motor function below the level of injury on one side of his body. On the other side of his body, the patient is unable to detect pain below the level of the injury. These findings are consistent with what condition?

    A. Anterior cord syndrome
    B. Central cord syndrome
    C. Cauda equina syndrome
    D. Brown-Séquard syndrome

48. A patient presents to the ED with a red, painful, swollen first toe. Which of the following elevated lab values is consistent with the diagnosis of acute gout?

    A. Uric acid levels in the blood
    B. White blood cell count
    C. Uric acid levels in the joint aspirate
    D. Sedimentation rate

49. An unresponsive patient who has overdosed on drugs is receiving treatment based on which type of consent?

    A. Involuntary
    B. Implied
    C. Informed
    D. Express

50. Administering a medication that causes a decreased level of consciousness but allows the patient to have a purposeful response to commands, breathe normally, and maintain his airway is a form of what type of sedation?

    A. Minimal
    B. Moderate
    C. Deep
    D. Dissociative

51. A visitor yells to the triage nurse that there is a person just outside the entrance slumped over the steering wheel of his car. What should the nurse do?

    A. Let the visitor know the nurse cannot leave the building.
    B. Ask the visitor to get the patient out of the car.
    C. Call 911 to have an ambulance respond.
    D. Go to the car to begin treating the patient.

52. The ED nurse is treating a patient who was shot with a rifle "by accident" while hunting. What is the nurse required to do?

    A. Document the name of the shooter in the patient's chart.
    B. Notify the health department.
    C. Notify the police department.
    D. Nothing is required, because the shooting was accidental.

53. What distinguishes major depression from normal sadness or a grief reaction?

    A. Difficulty sleeping at night
    B. Decreased ability to concentrate
    C. Symptoms that occur daily over a long period of time
    D. Feelings of guilt

54. An unrestrained driver in a high-speed motor vehicle collision arrives with hoarseness, signs of airway obstruction, and subcutaneous emphysema in the neck. What type of injury is suspected?

    A. Tracheobronchial disruption
    B. Pneumothorax
    C. Cardiac tamponade
    D. Diaphragm rupture

55. The nurse is preparing a patient with aspiration pneumonia for hospital admission. Which of the following statements by the patient indicates that the patient needs additional teaching?

    A. "I will receive intravenous antibiotics to clear up the infection."
    B. "I know I need to keep this tube in my nose to get oxygen."
    C. "I should only eat what is on the hospital meal tray."
    D. "I can eat anything as long as it is soft."

56. The nurse administers furosemide to a patient in pulmonary edema. How does the nurse assess the patient's response to this medication?

    A. By measuring the patient's urine output
    B. By monitoring the patient's oxygen saturation
    C. By assessing the patient's pain level
    D. By assessing the patient's skin color

57. A patient diagnosed with severe sepsis from pneumonia develops acute respiratory distress syndrome necessitating endotracheal intubation. The nurse evaluates the patient's response to this intervention and recognizes improvement in the patient's condition by:

    A. Decreasing fever
    B. Arterial blood gas results: PaO_2 84 mmHg
    C. Pulse oximetry reading: SpO_2 84%
    D. Decreasing white blood cell count

58. After an intubated patient is repositioned, the ventilator alarm sounds. What is the priority intervention?

    A. Suction the patient.
    B. Increase the oxygen concentration.
    C. Silence the alarm.
    D. Assess placement of the tube.

59. A patient is undergoing suture repair of a laceration to the lower leg. What time frame should the nurse instruct the patient to expect until the sutures are removed?

   A. 3 to 5 days
   B. 5 to 7 days
   C. 7 to 10 days
   D. 10 to 14 days

60. The nurse is treating an older patient who has a sacral pressure injury. The nurse should perform all of the following interventions EXCEPT:

   A. Insert a urinary catheter to prevent wound contamination
   B. Alert other staff caring for the patient to the presence of the wound
   C. Use a draw sheet when repositioning the patient
   D. Measure/document the wound and its appearance

61. A patient who presents to the ED states that he cannot catch his breath, and he feels like his heart is racing. The nurse performs a quick assessment and places the patient on the cardiac monitor. The patient's heart rate is 160 beats/min with no discernible P waves, and the rhythm is irregularly irregular. The nurse anticipates that which medication will be ordered?

   A. Diltiazem
   B. Lidocaine
   C. Adenosine
   D. Magnesium

62. A patient presents to the ED stating that she "just doesn't feel right." The patient complains of a pain in her chest, nausea, and vomiting. The cardiac monitor shows a heart rate of 200 beats/min. The patient's respiratory rate is 18 breaths/min and blood pressure is 112/60 mmHg. The decision is made to cardiovert the patient. The initial cardioversion attempt is unsuccessful, but the patient tolerated it without any adverse change in her condition. What should the nurse prepare to do next?

   A. Select a lower joule setting to be used for the next attempt.
   B. Administer intravenous analgesia and sedation.
   C. Prepare to switch to unsynchronized cardioversion.
   D. Resynchronize in preparation for the next attempt.

63. The patient's visual acuity should be measured before starting treatment in all the following situations EXCEPT:

   A. Acute retinal detachment
   B. Foreign body removal
   C. Uveitis
   D. Ocular burn

64. A patient presents with coughing and vomiting after attempting to siphon gas from a car. The patient's oxygen saturation on room air is 90%. What complication is this patient at risk for developing?

    A. Hematochezia
    B. Bradycardia
    C. Gastritis
    D. Pneumonitis

65. Which of the following assessment findings is expected in a case of suspected opioid overdose?

    A. Teardrop-shaped pupils
    B. Reactive, dilated pupils
    C. Fixed, pinpoint pupils
    D. Fixed, dilated pupils

66. The nurse prepares a patient with hepatitis for discharge. The nurse determines that the patient understood the discharge instructions when the patient states:

    A. "I will use a condom when I have sex with my spouse."
    B. "I will try to exercise several times a week."
    C. "I will eat several servings of fruits and vegetables daily."
    D. "I will limit myself to a glass of wine every couple of days."

67. A 24-year-old female patient presents with a sudden onset of right-sided pain. Her vitals are temperature 98.4°F (36.9°C), pulse 130 beats/min, respiration 20 breaths/min, and blood pressure 95/66 mmHg. The provider determines that the patient has a ruptured ovarian cyst. What is the most serious complication the nurse should anticipate for this patient?

    A. Infection
    B. Pain
    C. Hypovolemia
    D. Infertility

68. Which lab finding is expected in a patient with adrenal insufficiency?

    A. Low hemoglobin
    B. Hypernatremia
    C. Hyperkalemia
    D. Hyperglycemia

69. A normally active 70-year-old female patient presents to the ED with profound weakness and a decreased level of consciousness. Lab work drawn on arrival reports a serum osmolality of 400 mmol/kg, glucose of 1,238 mg/dL, blood urea nitrogen of 32 mg/dL, and creatinine of 1.1 mg/dL. An arterial blood gas shows pH of 7.41, HCO_3 25.0 nmol/L, Po_2 98 mmHg, and PCO_2 42 mmHg. What condition should the nurse suspect?

    A. Syndrome of inappropriate antidiuretic hormone secretion
    B. Diabetes insipidus
    C. Diabetic ketoacidosis
    D. Hyperosmolar hyperglycemic syndrome

70. The nurse is treating a patient who has received multiple medications as well as a crystalloid intravenous fluid infusion. After several hours, the nurse realizes that the patient has not voided since arrival and appears to be more confused. For what underlying condition should the patient be assessed?

    A. Dehydration
    B. Acute kidney injury
    C. Urinary obstruction
    D. Delirium

71. Signs that administering tissue plasminogen activator (tPA) to a patient with a cerebrovascular accident has been effective include:

    A. National Institutes of Health Stroke Scale score decreases to 4.
    B. National Institutes of Health Stroke Scale score increases to 40.
    C. Systolic blood pressure increases.
    D. Bleeding is controlled at all puncture sites.

72. How does the nurse differentiate between delirium and dementia?

    A. Assess the symptom duration, because dementia develops gradually.
    B. Assess the symptom duration, because delirium develops gradually.
    C. Assess the patient's ability to focus, because dementia affects attention span.
    D. Assess the patient's ability to recall past events, because delirium causes memory loss.

73. A patient was a front-seat passenger in a car that was struck from behind in a motor vehicle collision. The patient presents to the ED complaining of neck pain and says he has "whiplash." What is the mechanism of injury for this patient?

    A. Rotational
    B. Hyperflexion
    C. Hyperextension
    D. Axial loading

74. A patient is transported to the ED by ambulance with signs and symptoms of a stroke. The ambulance technicians initially screened the patient and calculated a National Institutes of Health Stroke Scale (NIHSS) score of 10. The nurse evaluates the patient after arrival, and the patient's condition has improved to an NIHSS score of 2 without the patient receiving any intervention. What condition does the nurse suspect?

    A. Transient cerebral edema
    B. Cerebrovascular accident
    C. Hypoglycemia
    D. Transient ischemic attack

75. A nurse is evaluating a patient treated for chest pain. After the medical workup, the patient is diagnosed with costochondritis. The nurse determines the patient's condition has improved by all the following indicators EXCEPT:

    A. Decreased respiratory distress
    B. A return to normal sinus rhythm
    C. Less coughing
    D. Good range of motion in the torso

76. The nurse is treating a patient who reports lower back pain for the past 2 weeks. The patient denies urinary symptoms, and there are no circulatory or neurologic deficits in either leg. Which of the following interventions should the nurse anticipate for this patient?

    A. Administering NSAID medication.

    B. Administering narcotic analgesia.

    C. Applying a lumbar back brace.

    D. Preparing the patient for a lumbar spine CT scan.

77. A patient was playing basketball and felt a pop in his calf muscle, followed by intense pain. He is unable to walk normally because he cannot bend the affected foot downward to push off from the ground. Which of the following interventions is appropriate for this patient?

    A. Apply an ankle stirrup splint.

    B. Apply a posterior full-leg splint.

    C. Perform the Thompson test.

    D. Ice and elevate the affected leg.

78. A visitor keeps standing outside the patient's doorway near the nurses' station. Which of the following is the most appropriate intervention?

    A. Ask the visitor to return to the patient's room.

    B. Allow the visitor to stay there because he is not disruptive.

    C. Cover any patient care documents on the desk.

    D. Speak quietly on the phone so the visitor cannot hear.

79. Which of the following is NOT an essential component of informed consent?

    A. Explanation of the procedure or care to be provided

    B. Explanation of the risks and benefits

    C. Documentation of a patient's ability to understand the situation

    D. Documentation of a legal mandate for the patient's treatment

80. A patient with a possible ankle fracture presents to the ED unable to bear weight on the affected leg. Circulation and neurologic checks to the foot are within normal limits. Using the Emergency Severity Index (ESI) five-level triage framework, how should this patient be triaged?

    A. ESI Level 2

    B. ESI Level 3

    C. ESI Level 4

    D. ESI Level 5

81. The nurse is treating a patient diagnosed with a sexually transmitted disease. As the nurse is giving the patient his discharge instructions, the patient asks if anyone will find out about his disease. How should the nurse respond?

    A. "We are required to report your demographic information along with your lab results to the local health department."

    B. "The HIPAA does not allow us to release this information without your permission."

    C. "We will follow up with you to verify that you have informed your sexual partner of your diagnosis."

    D. "We can only give this information to your spouse if she asks."

82. The nurse is triaging a patient who complains of feeling very overwhelmed and sad. Additionally, the patient reports difficulty sleeping, loss of appetite, and weight loss. What is the priority assessment for this patient?

    A. Presence of suicidal thoughts

    B. How much sleep the patient is getting

    C. Nutritional intake

    D. Amount of weight loss

83. The emergency nurse is reassessing a patient who has been treated for acute anxiety. All of the following indicators should be reassessed EXCEPT:

    A. Telemetry readings

    B. The patient's perceived anxiety level

    C. The patient's ability to manage stress

    D. Respiratory status

84. The nurse is treating a patient who took an overdose of prescription medication. The patient is somnolent and difficult to arouse. The nurse expects to perform all of the following interventions, but based on the assessment findings, which one is the MOST important?

    A. Measure vital signs, obtain intravenous access, and initiate cardiac monitoring.

    B. Clear the room of all objects that could be used for self-harm.

    C. Initiate one-on-one observation.

    D. Secure the patient's airway and administer supplemental oxygen.

85. Which of the following factors puts a patient with rib fractures at higher risk for complications?

    A. Advanced age

    B. Tobacco use

    C. Use of pain medication

    D. Productive cough

86. Emergency medical services intubates a patient prior to arrival at the ED . The nurse auscultates breath sounds and determines that they are present only on the right. What does this finding indicate about the endotracheal tube?

    A. It is in the proper position.

    B. It is inserted too far.

    C. It should be inserted further.

    D. It should be removed and replaced.

87. A nursing home resident left the facility and went out to eat at a restaurant with family members. By the next day, the patient had gained 5 pounds and developed respiratory distress. The patient arrived with labored respirations and bilateral crackles in both bases, and is unable to lie flat comfortably. What condition does the nurse suspect?

    A. Community-acquired pneumonia

    B. Pulmonary edema

    C. Healthcare-associated pneumonia

    D. Pleural effusion

88. What does the nurse need to consider when performing a head-to-toe assessment on a patient who sustained a gunshot wound?

    A. The nurse should clean off the gunpowder residue to prevent infection.
    B. The bullet can enter one area of the body and exit from another area.
    C. The patient's clothing should be removed and discarded.
    D. Documenting a general description of the wound is sufficient.

89. A patient was brought into the ED after being stabbed with a knife during an altercation. When assessing this patient, what does the nurse need to consider about the wound?

    A. In a stab wound, the weapon is usually inserted and withdrawn at the same angle.
    B. If it is still in the wound, the weapon should be removed to allow for a more thorough exam.
    C. The size of the wound opening does not correspond to the amount of internal damage.
    D. The depth of the wound usually corresponds to the length of the weapon.

90. A trauma patient is being treated in the ED. During the head-to-toe assessment, the patient's pants are removed and the nurse notices a soft red mass protruding from an open wound in the lower abdomen. What is the appropriate next step?

    A. Cover the area with a dry, sterile dressing.
    B. Cover the area with a moist, sterile dressing.
    C. Administer intravenous narcotic pain medication.
    D. Immobilize the patient on a backboard.

91. A patient with congestive heart failure has evidence of pitting edema in her lower extremities that takes approximately 10 seconds to rebound. How is this edema classified?

    A. 1+ pitting edema
    B. 2+ pitting edema
    C. 3+ pitting edema
    D. 4+ pitting edema

92. An older patient complaining of sudden abdominal and back pain suddenly becomes unresponsive. Which of the following is a priority nursing intervention for this patient?

    A. Administer naloxone.
    B. Establish two large-bore intravenous sites.
    C. Perform a fingerstick blood glucose test.
    D. Prepare the patient for a head CT scan.

93. A patient presents to the ED with a sudden onset of painless loss of vision in one eye. These are signs of what condition?

    A. Acute angle-closure glaucoma
    B. Central retinal artery occlusion
    C. Corneal ulcer
    D. Ocular foreign body

94. Which of the following interventions is appropriate for the treatment of acute angle-closure glaucoma?

    A. Irrigate the eye until the eye pH is 7.0 to 7.5.
    B. Place the patient supine on the stretcher.
    C. Administer antiemetic medication.
    D. Apply cold compresses to the affected eye.

95. What is the appropriate treatment for organophosphate poisoning?

    A. Induce vomiting
    B. Administer activated charcoal
    C. Intramuscular injection of atropine
    D. Intravenous injection of epinephrine

96. A patient is brought to the ED with shortness of breath, dizziness, and chest pain after a diving trip with friends. Which condition should the nurse suspect?

    A. Air embolism
    B. Decompression illness
    C. Nitrogen narcosis
    D. Carbon monoxide poisoning

97. Herpes zoster is characterized by what type of rash?

    A. Diffuse red rash over the torso
    B. Red, pruritic rash with burrow channels
    C. Scaly, crusty rash
    D. Red blisters in a unilateral pattern

98. A patient with deep partial-thickness burns should receive all the following medications EXCEPT:

    A. Antibiotics
    B. Analgesics
    C. Tetanus prophylaxis
    D. Silver sulfadiazine

99. Which finding is most concerning in a patient with a bowel obstruction?

    A. Abdominal pain
    B. Abdominal swelling
    C. Vomiting
    D. Fever

100. A patient is referred to the ED by his personal physician because "his blood count is low." The patient complains of weakness and shortness of breath and reports having dark stools. The nurse anticipates all of the following tests to be performed EXCEPT:

  A. EKG

  B. Arterial blood gas

  C. Complete blood count

  D. Blood type and crossmatch

101. The nurse is preparing to administer a vitamin K injection to a patient with cirrhosis. What is the primary reason for this medication in this situation?

  A. To improve bone health

  B. To improve nutritional status

  C. To decrease the risk of bleeding

  D. To correct low potassium levels

102. The nurse gives discharge instructions to a patient diagnosed with pelvic inflammatory disease. The nurse recognizes that the patient needs additional teaching when the patient states:

  A. "I will avoid sexual intercourse until after I follow up with my physician."

  B. "I will take the antibiotic until my fever is gone."

  C. "I will call my doctor if I develop a high fever."

  D. "I will get rechecked if I notice more vaginal discharge."

103. The nurse is assessing a patient with vaginal bleeding that the patient describes as "heavier than a normal period." The nurse can best estimate and quantify the amount of blood lost by:

  A. The duration of the bleeding

  B. The number of sanitary pads the patient has used

  C. The number of clots the patient has observed

  D. The patient's ranking of the amount of bleeding on a 1 to 10 scale

104. An older patient with chronic obstructive pulmonary disease presents to the ED with shortness of breath, weakness, and anorexia. Vital signs are temperature 98.2°F (36.8°C), pulse 88 beats/min, respiration 26 breaths/min, and blood pressure 87/59 mmHg. The patient states he ran out of his medications a week ago. The unexpected discontinuation of which of these medications is consistent with this patient's clinical presentation?

  A. Prednisone

  B. Levofloxacin

  C. Theophylline

  D. Albuterol

105. A patient presents to the ED with a fever and chills. Which of the following factors would prompt the nurse to triage this patient at a higher urgency level?

  A. The patient is an insulin-dependent diabetic.

  B. The patient is undergoing chemotherapy for breast cancer.

  C. The patient's temperature is 104°F (40°C).

  D. The patient's pulse is 116 beats/min.

106. Which lab value indicates that the treatment for a patient with thrombocytopenia was successful?

    A. D-dimer of 20 ng/mL
    B. International normalized ratio (INR) of 1.0
    C. Hemoglobin of 12 g/dL
    D. Platelet count of 200,000 cells/mm^3

107. What is the most severe complication of hypoglycemia?

    A. Neurologic changes
    B. Blurred vision
    C. Tachycardia
    D. Renal failure

108. The nurse is caring for a patient with an intracerebral hemorrhage. The nurse knows that the priority intervention for improving outcome will be:

    A. Administration of antiplatelet medications
    B. Blood glucose regulation
    C. Early tissue plasminogen activator (tPA) administration
    D. Blood pressure regulation

109. An older adult patient arrives to the ED complaining of a sudden headache. The patient states, "This is the worst headache of my life." The patient has an NIH Stroke Scale score of 0. The nurse has a high index of suspicion for:

    A. Acute ischemic stroke
    B. Epidural hematoma
    C. Subarachnoid hemorrhage
    D. Bacterial meningitis

110. While performing a neurologic exam on a patient, the nurse asks the patient to shrug her shoulders. Which cranial nerve does this assess?

    A. II
    B. V
    C. IX
    D. XI

111. A pedestrian struck by a car is transported to the ED. The patient has sustained visible bilateral lower extremity fractures and suspected pelvic fractures. What is the immediate intervention for this patient?

    A. Immobilizing the legs
    B. Initiating a crystalloid fluid bolus
    C. Administering narcotic pain medication
    D. Administering oxygen

112. A nurse preparing a patient for transfer to an outside facility documents the patient's problems, allergies, and all medications administered in the ED in a one-page summary. What type of communication does this represent?

    A. Bedside shift report

    B. Triage summary

    C. Handoff communication

    D. SBAR report

113. A restrained driver in a high-speed motor vehicle collision is brought in by ambulance. The patient is awake and complaining of chest pain. The patient's vital signs are pulse 96 beats/min, respiration 18 breaths/min, and blood pressure 149/72 mmHg. Using the Emergency Severity Index (ESI) five-level triage framework, how should this patient be triaged?

    A. ESI Level 1

    B. ESI Level 2

    C. ESI Level 3

    D. ESI Level 4

114. A patient presents with a throbbing headache, photophobia, nausea, and vomiting. The patient has a history of migraine headaches and states that this headache is similar to past headaches. Based on the Emergency Severity Index (ESI) five-level triage framework, how should this patient be triaged?

    A. ESI Level 2

    B. ESI Level 3

    C. ESI Level 4

    D. ESI Level 5

115. The nurse administered haloperidol 5 mg intramuscularly to an agitated patient experiencing acute psychotic symptoms. When reevaluating the patient, which finding would be the most concerning?

    A. Drowsiness

    B. Muscle spasms

    C. Fever and tachycardia

    D. Decreased agitation

116. During triage, an upset patient states he is so mad at his boss he wants to kill her. All of the following are appropriate assessment questions to ask this patient EXCEPT:

    A. "How often do you think about doing this?"

    B. "If you had the chance, how would you kill your boss?"

    C. "Have you ever hurt someone before?"

    D. "What has your boss done to you?"

117. Someone who just found out a close family member has died starts moaning, crying, and verbalizing feelings of shock and despair. All of these actions are symptoms of what condition?

    A. Depression

    B. Acute grief reaction

    C. Anxiety attack

    D. Psychosis

118. Which of the following assessment findings indicates a flail chest?

    A. Subcutaneous emphysema

    B. Paradoxical chest wall movement

    C. Respiratory distress

    D. Severe chest wall pain

119. In a trauma patient, tracheal deviation to the right indicates what condition?

    A. Pneumothorax

    B. Cardiac tamponade

    C. Tension pneumothorax on the right side

    D. Tension pneumothorax on the left side

120. A patient with a gunshot wound to the chest has decreased breath sounds on the left side, accompanied by a sucking sound from the wound when the patient takes a breath. What should the nurse do first?

    A. Apply an occlusive dressing over the wound secured on three sides.

    B. Apply an occlusive dressing over the wound secured on all sides.

    C. Prepare for chest tube placement.

    D. Prepare for intubation.

121. The patient arrives via emergency medical services with complaints of epigastric pain, dyspnea, and aching in his jaw. Prehospital EKG shows an ST-elevated myocardial infarction. The most important factor in this patient's outcome will be:

    A. Prompt administration of 4 mg morphine sulfate

    B. Minimizing the time to revascularization of the occluded coronary vessels

    C. Minimizing the time to administration of antiplatelet drugs

    D. The presence of atrioventricular blocks on the patient's rhythm strip

122. The nurse is caring for a patient experiencing a ST-elevated myocardial infarction. When reviewing his telemetry strip, the nurse finds that the Q wave duration is 0.30 second. The nurse recognizes that this Q wave duration:

    A. Indicates an impending ventricular tachycardia

    B. Indicates injury affecting the myocardium

    C. Indicates that this is a non-acute ST-elevated myocardial infarction

    D. Will improve once the patient has been treated with nitroglycerin

123. The nurse is caring for a patient with severe angina. The nurse knows that the effectiveness of nitroglycerin on angina can best be assessed by:

    A. A decrease in systolic blood pressure of at least 20 mmHg

    B. A decrease in serum troponin levels

    C. A decrease in the patient's chest pain score

    D. An increased level of exhaled nitric oxide

124. X-rays of a patient hit in the face by a baseball bat show an orbital fracture. What additional findings should the emergency nurse look for to assess the patient for a ruptured globe?

    A. Pupil shape
    B. Eye pain
    C. Photophobia
    D. Blurred vision

125. Which of the following statements indicates the need for additional discharge instructions for a patient diagnosed with mononucleosis?

    A. "I will not share any food or drink with anyone else."
    B. "I will rest as much as possible."
    C. "I can gargle with warm salt water to help the throat pain."
    D. "I should expect to bruise easily while I am recovering."

126. A parent brings a child to the ED because the child has had diarrhea for a couple of weeks. During the interview, the nurse learns that the patient has been swimming in a pond behind the neighbor's house. Based on this information, what condition should the nurse suspect?

    A. *Clostridioides difficile* colitis
    B. Giardiasis
    C. Salmonella infection
    D. Viral infection

127. A patient is suspected of contracting hepatitis A after eating at a local restaurant. Which of the following treatments is most appropriate?

    A. Antibiotic administration
    B. Antidiarrheal medications
    C. Vaccine administration
    D. Aggressive fluid resuscitation

128. A parent brings an unvaccinated child to the ED with a fever, runny nose, and white spots with blue centers on the inside of the cheeks. These spots are a characteristic sign of which childhood illness?

    A. Pertussis
    B. Mumps
    C. Chickenpox
    D. Measles

129. All of the following interventions are appropriate for the initial management of a patient with right upper quadrant pain, fever, nausea, and vomiting, EXCEPT:

    A. Nasogastric tube placement
    B. 1 L normal saline IV fluid bolus
    C. Ceftriaxone 1 g IV
    D. Ondansetron 4 mg IV

130. When preparing a patient with ascites for a paracentesis, the nurse should do all of the following EXCEPT:

   A. Confirm that the patient's bladder is empty.

   B. Position the patient supine on the stretcher.

   C. Assess the patient's vital signs.

   D. Insert a nasogastric tube.

131. The nurse is preparing the patient for a pelvic exam to assess for a retained foreign body. All of the following interventions are appropriate EXCEPT:

   A. Have the patient void before the exam.

   B. Verify that all needed equipment and supplies are ready.

   C. Start an intravenous infusion and obtain lab work.

   D. Explain the procedure to the patient.

132. A patient asks to be checked for what she thinks is a sexually transmitted disease. The patient's significant other insists on staying in the treatment room with the patient and tries to answer all the assessment questions. What should the nurse be concerned about for the patient?

   A. Sexual or other types of abuse

   B. Incompetence to make healthcare decisions

   C. Lack of knowledge regarding her health

   D. Low self-esteem

133. When preparing for an emergent delivery, what should the nurse do first?

   A. Check the mother's vital signs.

   B. Offer verbal support and reassurance to the mother.

   C. Put on sterile gloves and gown.

   D. Call for qualified personnel from the obstetric unit to assist.

134. A patient with diabetes is unresponsive with a fingerstick blood glucose reading of 37 mg/dL. Multiple attempts to obtain intravenous access are unsuccessful. What is the priority intervention for this patient?

   A. Oxygen

   B. Naloxone

   C. Glucagon

   D. Oral glucose

135. Soon after arrival to the ED , a patient develops ventricular fibrillation. Lab work shows a potassium of 8 mEq/L. The nurse can anticipate administering any of the following medications EXCEPT:

   A. Sodium polysterene

   B. Albuterol

   C. Insulin

   D. Calcium gluconate

136. The nurse receives notification that a patient has a critically low sodium of 110 mEq/L. What is the priority indicator to assess in this patient?

    A. Heart rate
    B. Urinary output
    C. Mental status
    D. Muscle strength

137. A 68-year-old woman presents with decreased responsiveness. Vital signs are temperature 95.2°F (35.1°C), pulse 56 beats/min, respiration 10 breaths/min, and blood pressure 90/50 mmHg. These initial findings are consistent with which of the following conditions?

    A. Syndrome of inappropriate antidiuretic hormone secretion
    B. Pheochromocytoma
    C. Thyroiditis
    D. Myxedema coma

138. The nurse administered mannitol to a patient with a closed head injury. Which of the following intracranial pressure readings indicates a positive response to the medication?

    A. 45 mmHg
    B. 35 mmHg
    C. 25 mmHg
    D. 15 mmHg

139. The nurse is monitoring a patient with cerebral edema. Which of the following is an early sign that the patient may be experiencing brain herniation?

    A. Restlessness
    B. Bradycardia
    C. Fixed pupils
    D. Posturing

140. Which of the following is an example of an action that occurs during the preparedness phase of emergency management?

    A. Pulling out additional supplies based on the projected number of patients expected
    B. Conducting an annual disaster drill to practice decontamination techniques
    C. Implementing a disaster triage system
    D. Undergoing critical incident stress debriefing

141. The nurse is preparing to bring the family into the treatment area to be with their mother as she is resuscitated. One of the family members stops before entering the room and says he is not sure he wants to watch this. How should the nurse respond?

    A. "This can be stressful to watch, but other people find it helps them manage their feelings in the long run."

    B. "I understand your hesitation, but the family has already agreed this is what they want to do."

    C. "I know this is stressful, but if you do not watch, you may always wonder what really happened."

    D. "I know this is a difficult time for you. If you want to observe, I will stand with you and explain what is going on."

142. An older patient experienced the return of spontaneous circulation (ROSC) in the ED after being resuscitated, and is intubated and on the ventilator. Family members have now arrived and state that the patient would not want to be kept alive on "life support." What is the most appropriate response?

    A. "Let's find out more about the patient's condition and what the options are for his treatment."

    B. "We are going to leave him on it for a few hours to see what happens."

    C. "If only the patient had written this down, then we would know what he wanted."

    D. "I understand this is difficult for you to see."

143. The nurse triages a patient with a red, itchy rash that developed after working in the yard. Based on the Emergency Severity Index (ESI) five-level triage framework, how should this patient be triaged?

    A. ESI Level 1

    B. ESI Level 2

    C. ESI Level 4

    D. ESI Level 5

144. The nurse administers diphenhydramine to a patient experiencing a dystonic reaction from antipsychotic medication. The nurse re assesses the patient and determines that the medication was effective by noting:

    A. The patient denies any further suicidal thoughts.

    B. The patient's psychosis has improved.

    C. The patient's muscle spasms have decreased.

    D. The patient has become more alert.

145. When treating a patient with psychosis, what is the priority for the nurse?

    A. Maintain patient safety.

    B. Improve the patient's self-esteem.

    C. Reorient the person back to reality.

    D. Stop all hallucinations/delusions.

146. A patient who believes the people on television are broadcasting messages specifically for him is experiencing what?

   A. An auditory hallucination

   B. Anxious thoughts

   C. Disorganized thoughts

   D. A delusion

147. A parent arrives at the ED screaming that her 1-year-old child choked on a piece of food. The child is unresponsive. What is the initial intervention?

   A. Administer back blows.

   B. Administer abdominal thrusts.

   C. Perform a blind finger sweep of the mouth.

   D. Place the head in the sniffing position.

148. During triage, a patient reports night sweats and a productive cough with bloody sputum. The patient lives with a family member who was recently released from prison. What should the nurse do first?

   A. Place the patient in a negative pressure room.

   B. Collect a sputum sample.

   C. Place a mask on the patient.

   D. Place a purified protein derivative (PPD) skin test in the patient's arm.

149. A patient was brought in to the ED after being rescued from a house fire. Which of the following findings would cause the nurse to anticipate that the patient needs early endotracheal intubation?

   A. Tachypnea

   B. Hoarseness and stridor

   C. Unresponsiveness

   D. Clear, productive cough

150. A patient with a pleural effusion has undergone a thoracentesis. When evaluating the patient's response to the procedure, the nurse would expect to find all of the following EXCEPT:

   A. Blood or other fluid leaking from the puncture site

   B. Decreasing respiratory distress

   C. Several hundred milliliters of drainage

   D. Patient's ability to take a deep breath

1. B) Supine with the head of the bed at 45°

Jugular venous distention is best assessed with the patient supine and the head of the bed at 45°. This position allows for venous return to be unimpeded by body habitus or neck positioning. The other positions are not appropriate for jugular vein assessment.

2. D) Cardiac catheterization

With chest pain, signs of illness, and a history of intravenous drug use, this patient's presentation is concerning for endocarditis. Cardiac catheterization is not performed in cases of endocarditis. Blood cultures are indicated to identify the type of infection. A chest x-ray is performed to rule out a source of infection in the lungs, and an EKG is usually done to assess for any changes in the heart rhythm.

3. B) Pericarditis

Pericarditis is the inflammation of the sac surrounding the heart. The classic sign of this condition is the patient leaning forward while sitting to alleviate the chest pain; lying down makes the pain worse. Endocarditis is the inflammation of the innermost layer of the heart. It produces flu-like symptoms, but not usually chest pain. Myocarditis is the inflammation of the heart muscle. It causes chest pain, but not the characteristic positional chest pain of endocarditis. Congestive heart failure does not usually cause chest pain.

4. C) Ibuprofen

This patient has signs of pericarditis for which a nonsteroidal anti-inflammatory drug (NSAID) such as ibuprofen is indicated. Hydromorphone and morphine are both narcotic analgesics that do not have anti-inflammatory properties. They may be used if the patient has severe pain persisting after taking the NSAID. Acetaminophen has no anti-inflammatory properties and will not be as effective as ibuprofen.

5. B) 190/120 mmHg with an elevated creatinine

A hypertensive emergency is evident in a patient with an elevated blood pressure reading and signs of impending organ damage. The level of the blood pressure reading is less significant than the risk of organ dysfunction. The patient with an elevated creatinine has evidence of kidney injury. The patient who ran out of medication should be able to lower the blood pressure by restarting medication. The patient with the highest blood pressure reading has no evidence of organ dysfunction in this case. Alcohol withdrawal causes elevated blood pressure, which can be treated with medication.

6. D) Initiate a crystalloid fluid bolus

A widened mediastinum in a trauma patient is caused by a transecting aorta, which leads to rapid exsanguination and death in many cases. This patient's airway is secure, so the immediate priority is to begin fluid resuscitation. Adjusting the ventilator is not indicated because the widened mediastinum is not respiratory in origin. A CT scan may be performed if the patient is stable, but it is not the initial priority. A chest tube is inserted for a hemothorax or a pneumothorax, not for an aortic injury.

7. **C) Sudden onset of pain and pallor in one leg**

   The sudden onset of pain and pallor in an extremity should be treated emergently to prevent loss of circulation. Claudication—pain that occurs with activity and is relieved by rest—is a sign of peripheral vascular disease. Thickened skin and hair loss are signs of chronic peripheral vascular disease and not an emergent finding. Nonhealing skin ulcers are a sign of chronic peripheral vascular disease, not a new condition.

8. **B) "I need to take this blood-thinning medication as prescribed for several months."**

   Patients with a deep vein thrombosis (DVT) are prescribed anticoagulant medications to decrease the risk of additional clotting. Patients with a DVT should not sit for a prolonged period, which could increase the risk of additional clotting. Patients should not smoke at all, because smoking increases the risk of clots. Patients should wear support hose but avoid wearing anything that constricts and blocks the return of blood to the heart, such as control-top hose.

9. **D) Increased heart rate**

   Increased heart rate is a sign of cardiogenic shock, and if still present, does not indicate improvement. Decreased chest pain, improved mental status, and increased urine output each indicate that treatment of the cardiogenic shock was effective.

10. **A) Reestablish blood flow through an occluded coronary artery**

    The primary goal of percutaneous coronary intervention (PCI) therapy is to reopen occluded coronary arteries. A PCI will not convert a patient to normal sinus rhythm. An echocardiogram measures how well the heart is working to pump blood. The purpose of PCI is not to insert an implanted defibrillator.

11. **D) "If the bleeding recurs, pinch your nose closed and hold pressure for at least 10 minutes."**

    Basic interventions a patient can do at home to manage a nosebleed include leaning forward with the nose pinched shut with direct pressure. The patient should not continue using a nasal decongestant; this can cause the nosebleed to recur. Nosebleeds in patients on anticoagulants indicate that the dosage should be adjusted. Blowing the nose will worsen a nosebleed by disrupting any clot that has formed.

12. **B) Ménière's disease**

    Ménière's disease is characterized by vertigo, nausea/vomiting, and unilateral hearing loss. It is episodic, with attacks lasting for a few hours at most but occurring repeatedly over time. Vestibular neuritis has similar symptoms (vertigo and nausea/vomiting), but it is short term and resolves within days instead of recurring intermittently. Benign positional vertigo causes dizziness with a change in head position, but not hearing loss. Otitis media is an inner ear infection that does not usually cause these symptoms.

13. **C) Stop irrigating and inform the provider.**

    An ammonia-based cleaner is an alkaline solution. The correct way to treat this is to irrigate the eye with normal saline until the eye's pH reaches a normal level of 7.2 to 7.4. Adding sodium bicarbonate, also an alkali, to the normal saline will worsen the damage. It is not necessary to irrigate the eye any longer, 7.4 is a normal pH. Irrigating the eye with boric acid solution is not recommended for alkali burns.

14. **A) Supplemental oxygen**

    Cyanide poisoning causes rapidly progressing symptoms for which securing the airway and oxygen administration are the top priority. Intravenous fluids are indicated but are not the top priority. Amyl nitrite is one of the antidotes for cyanide poisoning. It will be administered, but the initial priority is to administer oxygen. Cyanide poisoning causes severe lactic acidosis, so sodium bicarbonate may be administered, but it is not the initial intervention.

15. **C) Nitroglycerin**
Nitroglycerin counteracts cocaine-induced vasoconstriction, improving blood flow and decreasing chest pain. Labetalol is a beta-blocker that may be given, but it is not the best choice for a cocaine overdose. Nitroprusside lowers blood pressure but does not relieve chest pain. Thrombolytic therapy is not usually indicated for cocaine-induced chest pain.

16. **B) Testicular torsion**
Testicular torsion is a urologic emergency characterized by the sudden onset of severe pain and swelling to one side of the scrotum. Acute epididymitis is an infection that develops gradually and causes ureteral discharge. Patients with a testicular tumor present with a change in testicular size over time, but not necessarily with pain. Priapism is also a urologic emergency. It is a prolonged, painful erection without scrotal pain or swelling.

17. **D) Insert a curved-tipped Coudé catheter.**
An older man who cannot void is likely experiencing urinary retention secondary to an enlarged or inflamed prostate. A curved-tipped Coudé catheter is specially designed to fit around an enlarged prostate. A patient with urinary retention is not going to be able to void more than a small amount. The bladder scan is performed initially to detect urinary retention and need not be repeated. Inserting a different size urinary catheter could be successful, but using a curved-tipped catheter is less painful for these patients.

18. **A) Urinary catheter insertion**
A patient with renal calculi (kidney stones) does not need a urinary catheter. Dehydration can contribute to the development of renal calculi, so crystalloid fluids are appropriate. Renal calculi are typically very painful. If the patient's kidney function is sufficient, ketorolac is an effective pain medication. Nausea and vomiting frequently occur with this condition, so administering promethazine is appropriate.

19. **C) A patient in septic shock receiving vasopressors**
An indwelling urinary catheter is appropriate to measure urinary output in a critically ill patient. A bladder scan is used to check postvoid residual, not a urinary catheter. A patient with congestive heart failure can have urine measured from a urinal or bedside commode; a urinary catheter is not required unless the patient is critically ill. Incontinence is not sufficient to necessitate the use of an indwelling urinary catheter.

20. **D) No seizures occur.**
Magnesium sulfate is administered to patients with preeclampsia to prevent seizures. Becoming flushed and feeling weak are side effects of the medication. Patients with preeclampsia are hypertensive, but lowering the blood pressure too much results in hypotension, so a blood pressure reading of 85/60 mmHg may be too low. Deep tendon reflexes should be assessed regularly in this patient because overmedication depresses reflexes (normal reflexes are rated +2 and depressed reflexes are rated +1).

21. **B) Basic metabolic profile**
Obtaining a basic metabolic profile is the priority. This lab test measures several blood components that can indicate the acuity of a patient's renal failure, including potassium and creatinine levels. Giving a patient with acute renal failure contrast agent to perform an abdominal CT is contraindicated. A urinalysis will be obtained, but that result does not help determine the severity of the patient's renal failure. A renal ultrasound identifies masses and other structural abnormalities in the kidneys but does not measure renal output, the most immediate indicator of the patient's acuity.

22. B) Anticholinesterases

Myasthenia gravis is an autoimmune disorder that affects neuromuscular transmission. Anticholinesterase medications, including pyridostigmine bromide and neostigmine bromide, are used to treat it. Antibiotics are used to treat bacterial infections, not myasthenia gravis. Psychotropic medications are used for psychological issues, not for myasthenia gravis. Antidysrhythmics help regulate cardiac rhythm, not neuromuscular transmission.

23. C) Methylprednisolone

Steroid medications such as methylprednisolone are used to improve symptoms from acute flare-ups of multiple sclerosis, including blurred vision and weakness. Cyclobenzaprine is a muscle relaxant that does not improve muscle weakness or blurred vision. Venlafaxine is an antidepressant and does not treat muscle weakness or blurred vision. Dextroamphetamine is a stimulant but is not indicated for the treatment of multiple sclerosis exacerbations.

24. B) Hydromorphone

Hydromorphone is a narcotic analgesic that is not as effective for migraines as other medications. It may be used if the pain is unrelieved by the initial medications. Ketorolac is a nonsteroidal anti-inflammatory medication that is effective for treating migraine headaches. Dihydroergotamine is an analgesic indicated for migraine headaches. Promethazine is an antiemetic used to treat the nausea and vomiting that accompany migraine headaches.

25. C) "We need to put on gowns and gloves each time we go into the patient's room."

Patients with viral meningitis do not require isolation precautions (only patients with certain types of bacterial meningitis do), so this statement indicates the need for further teaching. Letting the staff know if the patient's symptoms are worsening is appropriate. Acknowledging that antibiotics are not indicated for viral conditions indicates understanding of the patient's condition. Patients with meningitis usually do not have any diet restrictions unless other complications are present, so this statement indicates comprehension of the instructions.

26. B) The patient's elbows are slightly bent when holding the handgrips.

Proper use of crutches has the elbows slightly bent when the patient holds the handgrips. The top of the crutch should not fit tightly under the armpits: there should be a space of 1 to 2 inches. The patient should look forward, not down, while walking. The patient should lean forward slightly with the crutches in front of the body instead of standing straight with the crutches even with the body.

27. D) *Staphylococcus aureus*

Osteomyelitis, a bone infection, is most commonly caused by *Staphylococcus aureus*, an organism found on the skin. *Clostridium tetani* causes tetanus, not osteomyelitis. *Clostridioides difficile* causes diarrhea and colitis, not osteomyelitis. *Escherichia coli* causes intestinal illnesses, not osteomyelitis.

28. C) Placing the patient in a room close to the nurses' station

Procedural sedation requires the patient to be continuously monitored throughout the procedure and during the recovery period. Placing the patient in a room close to the nurses' station does not indicate that the nurse will be able to continuously monitor the patient. Placing the patient on a cardiac monitor and pulse oximeter, assessing the patient's level of sedation, and measuring vital signs frequently all demonstrate that the nurse is monitoring the patient.

29. D) Crackles in the lung fields

Crackles in the lung fields are associated with fluid in the lungs, not with chronic obstructive pulmonary disease (COPD). Pursed-lip breathing by COPD patients helps with ventilation. Fingernail clubbing is associated with COPD and other lung disorders. Hyperresonance in the lung fields is associated with COPD and indicates that air is trapped in the lungs.

30. D) Piece of wood in the leg

Wounds containing organic materials such as wood are more likely to cause infection because these types of materials trigger a more significant inflammatory response. A nail, a piece of glass, and a metal sliver are all inert objects that usually do not cause much inflammatory response.

31. A) Targeted temperature management

Drug overdose, risk of bleeding, and preexisting coma are contraindications to utilization of targeted temperature management. All other protocols are appropriate.

32. A) Jugular vein distention, hepatomegaly, and peripheral edema

Right-sided heart failure impedes venous return, causing venous congestion in the venous circuit. This causes back pressure in the jugular veins, hepatic circulation, and peripheral tissues. Crackles, shortness of breath, and fatigue are classic findings in left-sided heart failure. Narrow pulse pressure, muffled heart sounds, and jugular vein distention are hallmarks of cardiac tamponade referred to as Beck's triad. Right-sided tracheal deviation, jugular vein distention, and diminished breath sounds on the left side of the chest indicate tension pneumothorax.

33. B) Lowered heart rate

Amiodarone is an antiarrhythmic medication administered for ventricular tachycardia. Reassessing the patient's heart rate to see that it is lower is the most appropriate action. Hypotension is a side effect of amiodarone, but this drug is not administered to lower blood pressure. A patient's oxygen saturation may improve as the patient's heart rate improves, but this is not a direct effect of amiodarone. Amiodarone does not affect the patient's level of consciousness.

34. C) Instillation of fluorescein dye

This patient has signs and symptoms of a corneal abrasion. Applying fluorescein dye to the surface of the eye helps the provider detect a corneal abrasion. Ophthalmic antibiotic drops may be administered but oral antibiotics are not indicated for corneal abrasions. Anesthetic ocular drops will be administered; oral analgesics are not indicated. Placing an eye patch over the affected eye is no longer recommended for corneal abrasions.

35. A) Pain

Unlike conjunctivitis, uveitis causes pain in the affected eye. Both uveitis and conjunctivitis cause redness and tearing. Pupil size is not affected by either condition.

36. B) Normal QRS complex

An overdose of tricyclic antidepressants can disrupt the electrical conduction in the heart, causing a prolonged QRS complex and making the patient prone to life-threatening arrhythmias. Although a pulse oximetry reading greater than 95% is a positive outcome, it is not the most specific outcome in this case. A tricyclic antidepressant overdose can cause hypotension, so lower blood pressure would not indicate an improvement. Elevated mood does not indicate that the treatment for a tricyclic antidepressant overdose has been effective.

37. A) Administer *N*-acetylcysteine (acetate)
N-Acetylcysteine protects the liver in acetaminophen overdose by restoring hepatic glutathione. Gastric lavage is no longer recommended for gastrointestinal decontamination and activated charcoal is not an appropriate therapy. This patient would be considered high acuity due to the risk for liver toxicity and cardiac dysrhythmia.

38. C) Retroperitoneal bleeding
Bruising around the abdomen is known as Cullen's sign and indicates retroperitoneal bleeding. Rebound tenderness, not bruising, indicates peritoneal irritation. Referred pain to the left shoulder, known as Kehr's sign, indicates intra-abdominal bleeding. Gastrointestinal bleeding does not cause bruising around the umbilicus.

39. A) Tachypnea
Tachypnea indicates the patient is beginning to experience respiratory complications from pancreatitis. Nausea is an expected symptom of the condition and can be treated with medication. Elevated serum amylase and lipase levels are expected in pancreatitis.

40. A) "If I start bleeding like I'm having a heavy period, I need to be rechecked."
With an inevitable abortion, the bleeding should get progressively lighter. Any heavy bleeding should be evaluated. The patient should not place anything in the vagina until cleared to do so by her follow-up provider. A fever is not normal: it is a sign of infection and should be evaluated. The patient should not return to normal activities until cleared to do so by her follow-up provider.

41. A) Elevate the right side of the backboard.
The right side of the backboard should be elevated to prevent the weight of the fetus from pressing against the vena cava and causing hypotension. Elevating the left side of the backboard does not alleviate the pressure on the vena cava. Elevating the head of the backboard does not alleviate the pressure on the vena cava. The cervical collar and backboard should not be removed unless the patient has been medically cleared for these actions to be done.

42. A) Acetaminophen
A thyroid storm is a hypermetabolic state secondary to hyperthyroidism. Elevated temperature is characteristic of this condition and is treated with acetaminophen. Tachycardia is present in a thyroid storm, so atropine is contraindicated. Pain is not typically present, so hydromorphone is not indicated. Excess fluid is not typically present, so furosemide is not administered.

43. D) Hypocalcemia
Hypocalcemia causes hyperactive reflexes and muscle tremors. Hypermagnesemia causes muscle weakness and decreased deep tendon reflexes. Hyponatremia does not affect muscle strength, and hyperkalemia causes muscle weakness.

44. C) Place the patient in a private treatment room.
A patient with leukemia is immunosuppressed and at high risk of contracting an illness. This patient should be placed in isolation as soon as possible for the patient's protection. Administering acetaminophen, obtaining blood cultures, and starting an intravenous infusion are all important interventions, but they are not the initial priority.

45. D) Donepezil

Donepezil is commonly prescribed to enhance cognition in dementia patients. Fluoxetine is an antidepressant; it does not improve cognitive function. Warfarin is an anticoagulant used to treat and prevent blood clots, not dementia. Diazepam is an antianxiety medication and is not prescribed for dementia.

46. B) Distributive shock

Bradycardia and hypotension are signs of neurogenic shock, which is a form of distributive shock that occurs when there is disruption in the sympathetic nervous system pathways secondary to injury. Hypovolemic shock, which occurs when there is extensive blood loss, causes tachycardia instead of bradycardia. Cardiogenic shock occurs secondary to problems with the heart, such as acute coronary syndrome or congestive heart failure. Obstructive shock occurs secondary to cardiac tamponade, tension pneumothorax, and similar conditions.

47. D) Brown-Séquard syndrome

Brown-Séquard syndrome is characterized by ipsilateral loss of motor function and contralateral loss of pain and temperature sensation below the level of the injury. Anterior cord syndrome causes the loss of motor function, pain, and temperature sensation below the level of the injury. Central cord syndrome causes loss of motor and sensory function below the level of the injury, with a greater loss of function in the upper extremities compared to the lower extremities. Cauda equina syndrome causes varying degrees of motor and sensory function loss in the lower extremities.

48. C) Uric acid levels in the joint aspirate

Aspirating fluid from the affected joint to test for uric acid levels is definitive for diagnosing an acute gout attack. Serum uric acid levels may be elevated in patients who are at high risk for gout without the patient experiencing an acute attack. An elevated white blood cell count indicates an infection, not gout. An elevated sedimentation rate indicates inflammation in the body but is not specific to gout.

49. B) Implied

Implied consent allows treatment in an emergency situation when the patient is unable to give consent. Involuntary consent is given by a physician or police officer in situations when the patient cannot make treatment decisions. Informed consent requires the patient to be awake, alert, and able to comprehend the situation. Express consent is a written or oral consent to treatment.

50. B) Moderate

Moderate sedation causes the patient to have a decreased level of consciousness, but keeps airway and respiratory functions intact, as well as purposeful response to verbal or touch commands. Minimal sedation allows normal cardiac and respiratory functions as well as normal response to verbal commands. Deep sedation depresses consciousness to the point that the patient is not easily aroused; assistance is required to maintain respiratory functioning. Dissociative sedation causes a catatonic state.

51. D) Go to the car to begin treating the patient.

The EMTALA (Emergency Medical Treatment and Labor Act) requires that anyone who presents for treatment within 250 yards of the main hospital building must receive a medical screening exam and stabilizing treatment. The hospital should have a policy on how nursing and medical staff respond to medical incidents outside the building. It is inappropriate to ask the visitor to help the patient. It is not necessary to call an ambulance to transport a patient who is just outside the ED.

52. **C) Notify the police department.**

EDs are required to report all gunshot wounds to the police, regardless of the circumstances. Documenting the name of the shooter and notifying the health department are not required in this situation.

53. **C) Symptoms that occur daily over a long period of time**

Sadness and grief reactions share many of the characteristics of major depression, including insomnia, poor concentration, and guilt. The critical difference is the duration and pervasiveness or severity of the symptoms. Patients who are depressed experience these symptoms daily over a longer period of time.

54. **A) Tracheobronchial disruption**

Blunt or penetrating trauma to the neck or upper chest can cause tracheobronchial disruption. A pneumothorax does not cause hoarseness or signs of airway obstruction. Cardiac tamponade is detected by auscultating for muffled heart sounds. A ruptured diaphragm is associated with diminished breath sounds as well as bowel sounds in the abdomen.

55. **D) "I can eat anything as long as it is soft."**

Patients with aspiration pneumonia either are not allowed to eat or drink anything or are placed on a special diet. The hospital tray will contain a prescribed diet. As part of the treatment, the patient will receive intravenous antibiotics and supplemental oxygen to maintain appropriate oxygen saturation. Depending on the patient's ability to swallow, soft foods may still be problematic for the patient.

56. **A) By measuring the patient's urine output**

Furosemide is a diuretic administered to cause excretion of excess fluid, so the patient's urine output should be closely monitored. Oxygen saturation should improve as the pulmonary edema is treated, but it is not directly affected by furosemide. Pain is not associated with pulmonary edema or treated with furosemide. Skin color reflects a patient's perfusion status but is not directly affected by furosemide.

57. **B) Arterial blood gas results: Pao_2 84 mmHg**

An arterial blood gas from a patient with acute respiratory distress syndrome will show significant hypoxemia. A Pao_2 of 84 is in the normal range and demonstrates an improvement. Intubation has no effect on fever. Pulse oximetry readings of oxygen saturation at 84% are below normal. White blood cell count is not affected by intubation.

58. **D) Assess placement of the tube.**

Tube placement should be assessed first. There is a risk of dislodging the endotracheal tube when repositioning an intubated patient. Suctioning the patient may be necessary, but in this situation, there is no indication that suctioning is necessary. Silencing the alarm does not address the underlying cause of the alarm.

59. **D) 10 to 14 days**

Sutures to the lower legs and feet should be removed in 10 to 14 days. Most sutures in the face are removed in 3 to 5 days. Some face sutures and scalp sutures are removed in 5 to 7 days. Sutures on the torso are removed in 7 to 10 days.

60. **A) Insert a urinary catheter to prevent wound contamination**

Routine urinary catheterization is not indicated for patients with sacral wounds because of the risk of developing a catheter-associated urinary tract infection. The wound's presence should be reported to other staff treating the patient so they can continue to monitor and treat the wound appropriately. A draw sheet should be used to decrease the risk of further damage from friction and shearing when repositioning the patient. The wound should be measured to obtain a baseline assessment for future comparison.

61. A) Diltiazem

This patient is in atrial fibrillation with a rapid ventricular response. Diltiazem, a calcium channel blocker, is indicated in this situation to slow the heart rate. Lidocaine is administered for ventricular tachycardia, not atrial fibrillation. Adenosine is contraindicated in this situation because the heart rhythm is irregular. Magnesium is used to treat polymorphic ventricular tachycardia, not atrial fibrillation.

62. D) Resynchronize in preparation for the next attempt.

This patient is considered stable for synchronized cardioversion. If more than one attempt is made, it is necessary to resynchronize after each cardioversion. The number of joules is increased, not decreased, for subsequent attempts. Analgesia and sedation should be administered before the first attempt, not after. There is no indication to switch to unsynchronized cardioversion, as the patient has not become unstable.

63. D) Ocular burn

An ocular burn is a true emergency for which eye irrigation should be initiated without delay. Acute retinal detachment is also a true emergency, but visual acuity should be checked as part of the diagnostic process. Visual acuity can be checked before removing a foreign body. Uveitis decreases visual acuity, so this will be checked as part of the diagnostic workup before treatment.

64. D) Pneumonitis

Pneumonitis is lung inflammation not caused by an infection. Patients with hydrocarbon poisoning (in this case, gas ingestion) are at risk for this complication. Hematochezia, or blood in the stools, is not an expected complication, as the patient is experiencing respiratory symptoms. Hydrocarbon poisoning can cause ventricular arrhythmias, not bradycardia. Gastritis does not cause a low oxygen saturation and is less likely to occur than pneumonitis in this case.

65. C) Fixed, pinpoint pupils

Pinpoint pupils that do not react to bright light occur with opioid overdose. Teardrop-shaped pupils occur with globe rupture secondary to eye trauma. Dilated pupils occur with cocaine overdoses. Fixed, dilated pupils are associated with brain injury.

66. A) "I will use a condom when I have sex with my spouse."

Hepatitis B is transmitted through sexual and other close contact with bodily fluids. Condoms should be worn to protect the sexual partner. Exercise is a benefit to overall health but does not specifically affect hepatitis. Eating fruits and vegetables daily is a healthy practice, but it does not directly affect hepatitis. Patients with hepatitis should avoid all alcohol. Consuming even a small amount of alcohol can adversely affect these patients.

67. C) Hypovolemia

Excessive bleeding from a ruptured ovarian cyst can lead to hypovolemic shock. This patient has tachycardia and hypotension—two signs of significant blood loss. The risk of infection is present, but the immediate life-threating concern is hypovolemia. Pain control is important, but replacing blood loss is the priority. Future fertility is a valid but not immediate concern.

68. **C) Hyperkalemia**

A patient with adrenal insufficiency has a decreased aldosterone level and is unable to regulate the amount of water excreted by the kidneys. This causes increased sodium and water excretion, which in turn causes hyperkalemia. Hemoglobin levels are not affected by aldosterone. Hyponatremia, not hypernatremia, occurs in these patients. Hypoglycemia, not hyperglycemia, develops in these patients.

69. **D) Hyperosmolar hyperglycemic syndrome**

Hyperosmolar hyperglycemic syndrome causes weakness and mental status changes characterized by elevated glucose and serum osmolality without acidosis. Syndrome of inappropriate antidiuretic hormone secretion causes mental status changes but decreased plasma osmolality and does not directly affect blood glucose levels. Diabetes insipidus shows elevated serum osmolality, but not elevated glucose levels or acidosis. Diabetic ketoacidosis shows elevated blood glucose levels, but is differentiated from hyperosmolar hyperglycemic syndrome by the presence of acidosis.

70. **B) Acute kidney injury**

Acute kidney injury typically causes decreased urine output and confusion and should be considered in this situation. Dehydration causes decreased urine output, but this patient is receiving intravenous fluids, so urine output should increase. The patient was able to void earlier, so a urinary obstruction is unlikely. Delirium is another term for confusion and does not describe an underlying condition.

71. **A) National Institutes of Health Stroke Scale score decreases to 4.**

If given shortly after the onset of symptoms, tPA can decrease stroke symptoms. A lower score on the NIH Stroke Scale indicates that fewer signs and symptoms of a stroke are present. Conversely, a higher score indicates more signs and symptoms of a stroke. Systolic blood pressure can be elevated during a cerebrovascular accident, but this does not indicate improvement. Bleeding is a side effect of this medication and does not indicate improvement.

72. **A) Assess the symptom duration, because dementia develops gradually.**

A key difference between delirium and dementia is that dementia develops over time, whereas delirium has a sudden onset caused by an illness or reaction to a medication. Dementia primarily affects memory, whereas delirium affects attention span.

73. **C) Hyperextension**

Hyperextension, or rapid backward movement of the head beyond the cervical column, is the mechanism of injury in this case. Rotational forces cause the head to flex and move laterally from the spinal column; they can occur if the car is struck from the side or is spun around. Hyperflexion is forward flexion of the cervical spine and would result in the head striking the windshield. Axial loading occurs when force is transmitted through the vertebral column vertically, for example, in a diving accident.

74. **D) Transient ischemic attack**

Transient ischemic attack causes stroke-like symptoms that do not last and is the most likely cause of this patient's symptoms. Cerebral edema is swelling of the brain tissue, a condition that is not typically transient. A cerebrovascular accident causes permanent damage; the symptoms do not spontaneously resolve without treatment. Hypoglycemia should be considered in a patient with stroke symptoms, but it does not spontaneously resolve without treatment.

75. **B) A return to normal sinus rhythm**

Costochondritis is an inflammation of the cartilage in the ribcage caused by coughing or a physical strain. It causes chest pain that mimics serious heart conditions, but it does not cause a change in heart rhythm. Decreased respiratory distress occurs when the chest pain is controlled and the patient can breathe normally. Less coughing will help minimize the pain of costochondritis. Good range of motion in the torso indicates that the pain has improved and the patient feels better able to move.

76. **A) Administering NSAID medication.**

First-line treatment for uncomplicated lower back pain includes NSAID (nonsteroidal anti-inflammatory drug) administration. Narcotic pain medications are not indicated unless the patient has severe pain uncontrolled by other interventions. A back brace is not indicated for emergency treatment of low back pain, although it may be prescribed later during the patient's follow-up care. Advanced imaging is not indicated for uncomplicated low back pain, so a lumbar CT scan would not be performed.

77. **D) Ice and elevate the affected leg.**

This patient has signs and symptoms of an Achilles tendon rupture. Ice and elevation of the affected leg are important interventions to reduce pain and swelling. An ankle stirrup splint applies support to the lateral sides of the ankles for ankle injuries, which is not the appropriate type of support for an Achilles tendon injury. The lower leg boot or splint is indicated, but not a posterior full-leg splint. The Thompson test (squeezing the gastrocnemius muscle to check for associated plantar flexion) aids in the diagnosis of a ruptured Achilles tendon, but it does not treat the injury.

78. **A) Ask the visitor to return to the patient's room.**

Asking the visitor to return to the room keeps the visitor from overhearing other patient information. Allowing the visitor to stand outside the door increases the risk that the visitor will hear or see confidential information about other patients. Covering patient care documents on the desk will prevent the visitor from reading them, but does not prevent the visitor from overhearing confidential information. Speaking quietly on the phone may not be practical and does not eliminate the risk that the visitor will hear confidential information.

79. **D) Documentation of a legal mandate for the patient's treatment**

Police- or court-mandated treatment represents involuntary consent. Explanation of the care and its risks and benefits and documentation of the patient's ability to understand the situation and make a decision are all required elements of informed consent.

80. **C) ESI Level 4**

This patient requires an x-ray to rule out a fracture—and is therefore ESI Level 4 (the patient requires one resource). Level 2 indicates that the patient needs to be seen as soon as possible after arrival, which is not the case for this patient. Levels 3 to 5 are based on the amount of resources the patients may need. Resources are services that are more complex than simple interventions the provider can perform at the bedside. A Level 3 patient requires two or more resources. Although this patient may ultimately need a splint and crutches, these are not considered resources. Level 5 patients do not require any resources.

81. **A) "We are required to report your demographic information along with your lab results to the local health department."**

By law, a patient's demographic information along with the diagnosis of a sexually transmitted disease must be reported to the health department—even if the patient does not give permission. The patient should inform his sexual partner of the diagnosis to decrease the risk of transmitting the illness, but the ED does not follow up on this. Medical information cannot be released to a spouse unless the patient gives permission.

82. A) Presence of suicidal thoughts

Assessing for suicidal ideations is the priority, as these ideations pose a risk to the patient's life. How much sleep the patient is getting, the patient's nutritional intake, and the amount of weight loss are all important questions to ask someone who is depressed, but they are not the top priority.

83. C) The patient's ability to manage stress

The patient's ability to manage stress can affect anxiety, but this should be addressed in the patient's follow-up care, not as part of emergency treatment. Patients with anxiety experience tachycardia and palpitations; reviewing the telemetry readings can determine whether the patient's heart rate has returned to baseline. Asking a patient whether she feels less anxious after treatment is essential. Because anxious patients typically feel short of breath or hyperventilate, assessing respiratory status is important.

84. D) Secure the patient's airway and administer supplemental oxygen.

Maintaining the patient's airway and supporting respiratory function comprise the top priority. After initially establishing and supporting the airway, the nurse should take vital signs, establish an intravenous line, and place the patient on cardiac monitoring. The room should be cleared of all objects, but the priority is to medically stabilize the patient. Continuous observation of the patient is important, but the initial priority is stabilizing the patient's airway.

85. A) Advanced age

Older patients with rib fractures are at higher risk for complications because of progressive decreases in lung capacity as they age. This decline, paired with the pain and inflammation from the injury, can limit pulmonary function, leading to atelectasis and other complications. Patients who smoke tobacco are at increased risk of developing other lung conditions, but not necessarily with rib fractures. The use of pain medication is appropriate for rib fractures to promote good ventilation and prevent atelectasis. Coughing is part of good pulmonary toilet and preventing atelectasis.

86. B) It is inserted too far.

If the endotracheal tube is inserted too far, it will enter the right mainstem bronchus, causing breath sounds to be diminished or absent on the left. Pulling back on the tube repositions it above the carina so both lungs will be ventilated. The tube is not in the proper position if lung sounds are only heard on one side of the chest. Advancing the tube further does not improve the position. There is no indication to remove the tube unless no breath sounds were heard on either side, which would indicate that the tube was in the esophagus.

87. B) Pulmonary edema

Pulmonary edema can be triggered by increased sodium intake. This resident ate at a restaurant and did not receive his usual prescribed diet. Labored respirations, crackles, and a sense of "suffocation" when lying flat collectively are signs of pulmonary edema. Sudden weight gain is a sign of the excess fluid retention that is present with pulmonary edema, but not with pneumonia or pleural effusions. Patients with pneumonia may have respiratory distress or crackles but can lie flat. A pleural effusion is usually associated with diminished breath sounds.

88. **B) The bullet can enter one area of the body and exit from another area.**

   A head-to-toe assessment of a patient with a gunshot wound is crucial to identify all the entry and exit wounds, which may not be near each other, indicating the possibility of more widespread internal injuries. The gunpowder residue should not be removed initially until the evidence collection is complete. The patient's clothing should be removed to facilitate a thorough assessment, but be preserved as evidence. Detailed descriptions of the wounds, including measurements, are important to document for patient care as well as legal purposes.

89. **C) The size of the wound opening does not correspond to the amount of internal damage.**

   The size of the wound opening does not correspond to the amount of internal damage. For example, the weapon may not fully enter the skin, or it may do so at an angle and create a long surface opening but a shallow wound. If the weapon is still in the wound, it should not be removed as part of the assessment because it will cause more damage. The wound depth does not necessarily correspond to the length of the weapon—the weapon could have been only partially inserted.

90. **B) Cover the area with a moist, sterile dressing.**

   The patient appears to have an evisceration of internal organs. This area should be covered with a moist, sterile dressing to prevent the tissue from drying out. A dry dressing protects the area but does not prevent it from drying out. This patient likely has pain, but the immediate concern is protecting the internal organs. Immobilizing the patient on a backboard does not treat the evisceration in any way.

91. **C) 3+ pitting edema**

   3+ pitting edema is characterized by 10- to 12-second rebound of the skin. 1+ is classified by barely detectable edema with instantaneous rebound. 2+ pitting edema typically takes less than 3 or 4 seconds to rebound. 4+ pitting edema is indicated by deep pitting that requires more than 20 seconds to rebound.

92. **B) Establish two large-bore intravenous sites.**

   The sudden onset of this pain combined with a decreased level of consciousness indicates that this patient is possibly experiencing an aortic dissection. Large-bore intravenous lines are needed to provide fluid resuscitation and blood products. Naloxone, an opioid antagonist, is administered for possible drug overdoses. Blood glucose levels are assessed in diabetic patients to rule out hypoglycemia, which does not cause abdominal or back pain. A head CT scan is ordered to diagnose neurologic conditions that affect the patient's level of consciousness.

93. **B) Central retinal artery occlusion**

   Central retinal artery occlusion causes sudden painless, unilateral blindness and is a medical emergency. Acute angle-closure glaucoma causes decreased peripheral vision and halos around lights, not blindness. Corneal ulcers cause photophobia, not blindness. An ocular foreign body can cause pain but does not usually cause blindness.

94. **C) Administer antiemetic medication.**

   In acute angle-closure glaucoma, the goal of treatment is to facilitate drainage of aqueous humor and decrease intraocular pressure. Administering antiemetic medication prevents nausea and vomiting, which are common symptoms of the condition which increases intraocular pressure. Eye irrigation is indicated for ocular burns, not acute angle-closure glaucoma. A patient with central retinal artery occlusion should be supine, but a patient with acute angle-closure glaucoma should always be positioned so the head is higher than the waist. Applying a cold compress is beneficial for allergic conjunctivitis, but not for acute angle-closure glaucoma.

95. **C) Intramuscular injection of atropine**

Atropine is the antidote for organophosphate poisoning. Inducing vomiting is not routinely recommended for any type of poisoning. Activated charcoal is administered as an antidote for many ingested poisons, but not organophosphates. Epinephrine is indicated for allergic reactions but not for organophosphate poisoning.

96. **A) Air embolism**

These signs and symptoms are consistent with an air embolism, which can occur when the diver does not exhale properly during ascent. Decompression illness causes joint pain, shortness of breath, and headache. Nitrogen narcosis causes mental status changes and impaired coordination. Carbon monoxide poisoning causes headache, confusion, and shortness of breath.

97. **D) Red blisters in a unilateral pattern**

Herpes zoster causes red blisters in a unilateral pattern that follow a dermatome. A diffuse red rash over the torso can have a variety of causes and is not specific to herpes zoster. Scabies causes a red, pruritic rash with burrow channels. A scaly, crusty rash occurs with ringworm.

98. **A) Antibiotics**

Prophylactic antibiotics are not indicated for deep partial-thickness burns. These patients should receive analgesics, tetanus prophylaxis, and have silver sulfadiazine applied to the burn.

99. **D) Fever**

Fever in patients with bowel obstructions can indicate a bowel perforation. Abdominal pain, swelling, and vomiting are all signs of an obstruction, but are not as concerning as fever.

100. **B) Arterial blood gas**

This patient likely has anemia secondary to lower gastrointestinal bleeding. The shortness of breath is likely secondary to anemia, so an arterial blood gas is not indicated at this point. An EKG is appropriate to assess for changes to the heart that are caused by low hemoglobin. A complete blood count will be done to check the patient's hemoglobin and hematocrit to assess for anemia. The patient's blood type should be identified to prepare for possible blood transfusion.

101. **C) To decrease the risk of bleeding**

Patients with cirrhosis are at high risk for bleeding related to coagulopathies that develop. Vitamin K increases the levels of prothrombin, a vital clotting factor. Vitamin K increases the levels of calcitonin, which in turn strengthens bones, but this is not the reason it is administered to someone with ascites. A vitamin K injection is not used as a nutritional supplement. Vitamin K does not affect potassium levels.

102. **B) "I will take the antibiotic until my fever is gone."**

It is important to take all the antibiotics and complete the course prescribed; incomplete treatment puts the patient at higher risk for a recurrence. Avoiding sexual intercourse until medically cleared is recommended. Following up for fever or worsening vaginal discharge is appropriate.

103. **B) The number of sanitary pads the patient has used**

Asking the patient how many sanitary pads she has saturated is the best way to estimate and quantify the amount of blood loss. The duration of the bleeding is not as reliable as an indicator because it does not consider the amount of flow each day. Clots can indicate heavy bleeding, but the number of clots does not necessarily correspond to the amount of blood loss. Having the patient rank the amount of bleeding on a scale relies on the patient's recall and judgment, as there is no standard scale for assessing bleeding.

104. A) Prednisone

The abrupt discontinuation of prednisone can precipitate an adrenal crisis characterized by weakness, hypotension, and anorexia. The discontinuation of levofloxacin should not cause these symptoms. Discontinuing theophylline or albuterol will cause worsening respiratory symptoms, but not the symptoms this patient is experiencing.

105. B) The patient is undergoing chemotherapy for breast cancer.

Patients receiving chemotherapy treatments are immunocompromised and are at high risk for developing sepsis. They should be evaluated and treated as soon as possible. Diabetic patients with a fever need to be evaluated, but not as urgently as someone who is immunocompromised. A high fever does not correlate to an increased risk level. Tachycardia is expected with a fever. It should be monitored, but does not increase the patient's acuity.

106. D) Platelet count of 200,000 cells/mm^3

Thrombocytopenia is a platelet deficiency that increases a patient's risk of bleeding. The normal range is 150,000 to 450,000 cells/mm^3. D-dimer, INR, and hemoglobin levels are not affected by treatment for thrombocytopenia.

107. A) Neurologic changes

Hypoglycemia, a blood glucose level less than 60 mg/dL, causes seizures, coma, and permanent neurologic damage if untreated. Blurred vision can occur but improves as the hypoglycemia is treated. Tachycardia is an early sign of hypoglycemia and resolves with treatment. Renal failure is not a complication of hypoglycemia.

108. D) Blood pressure regulation

Early blood pressure control with a systolic reading below 140 mmHg has been shown to help improve outcomes in hemorrhagic stroke. Antiplatelet medications and tPA are contraindicated in hemorrhagic stroke. Blood glucose regulation can affect outcomes, but is not the priority intervention for this patient.

109. C) Subarachnoid hemorrhage

Subarachnoid hemorrhage is most commonly caused by a nontraumatic aneurysm. The pain is often described as a thunderclap due to its sudden and intense nature. Acute ischemic stroke would present with neurologic deficits and an elevated NIH Stroke Scale score. Epidural hematomas are traumatic injuries that present with headache, trauma, and vomiting. Bacterial meningitis is infectious and presents with fever, irritability, headache, and nuchal rigidity.

110. D) XI

Cranial nerve XI (spinal accessory) is assessed by having the patient shrug the shoulders. Cranial nerve II (optic) is tested by having the patient read printed material. Cranial nerve V (trigeminal) is checked by having the patient simulate chewing. Cranial nerve IX (glossopharyngeal) is tested by checking the patient's ability to swallow.

111. B) Initiating a crystalloid fluid bolus

A patient with multiple lower extremity and pelvic fractures is at high risk for hypovolemic shock from blood loss. The priority is to insert two large-bore intravenous catheters and initiate a crystalloid fluid bolus. Immobilizing the legs is important, but not the first intervention performed. Controlling the patient's pain is crucial, but not the initial priority. Oxygen administration is important, but the immediate life-threatening concern is the risk of hypovolemic shock.

112. C) Handoff communication

Handoff communication occurs between nurses in the ED or with nurses from different units or facilities. Bedside shift report occurs among nurses in the same department and takes place in the patient's room. A triage summary includes the chief complaint and home medicines, not what treatment occurred during the ED visit. An SBAR (situation, background, assessment, recommendations) report includes more detailed information about the patient's history as well as the treatment recommendations going forward.

113. B) ESI Level 2

This patient is at high risk of having a serious injury requiring evaluation as soon as possible, so she is at ESI Level 2. This patient does not require an immediate lifesaving intervention (ESI Level 1). An ESI Level 3 patient requires two or more resources, and an ESI Level 4 patient requires one resource.

114. B) ESI Level 3

This patient will require two or more resources before the provider can decide on the patient's disposition, so should be triaged as Level 3. This patient has a history of migraine headaches and this headache does not appear to be unusual or high risk. In this case, resources will include intravenous (IV) fluids and medications to treat the headache, nausea, and vomiting. If the patient reported this was the worst headache ever or other high-risk symptoms, this patient would be a Level 2. A Level 4 patient requires only one resource; IV fluids and medications count as two separate resources. A Level 5 patient does not require any resources.

115. C) Fever and tachycardia

Fever and tachycardia are a sign of neuroleptic malignant syndrome, a serious side effect of antipsychotic medications. Drowsiness is an expected side effect of haloperidol and would not be concerning. Muscle spasms are a less serious side effect referred to as extrapyramidal symptoms or dystonic symptoms. Decreased agitation is an expected therapeutic effect of the medication.

116. D) "What has your boss done to you?"

Asking what the other person has done to the patient serves no therapeutic purpose and can agitate the patient even more. Asking how often the patient thinks about this can help the nurse determine how intense and pervasive the urge is. Asking how the patient would act on the desire assesses how well thought-out the plan is. Asking if the patient has hurt anyone before is important because people with a history of violence are more likely to be violent.

117. B) Acute grief reaction

A patient who is very emotional, appears to be in shock, and who feels sadness or guilt is experiencing an acute grief reaction—a normal response to the death of a loved one. Depression shares some of the same signs and symptoms but occurs over a longer period of time. Someone suffering an anxiety attack will feel panicked and have physical symptoms of excitement like tachycardia and shortness of breath, but will not usually feel sadness or guilt. Psychosis is an altered state of thinking involving delusions and hallucinations. There is no evidence of these conditions in this scenario.

118. B) Paradoxical chest wall movement

A flail chest occurs when part of the rib cage is detached and moves in the opposite direction of the rest of the chest wall. Subcutaneous emphysema is air trapped underneath the skin and can occur with other types of chest wall trauma. Respiratory distress typically accompanies most chest trauma. Severe chest wall pain is not specific to flail chest.

119. D) Tension pneumothorax on the left side

A tension pneumothorax develops when the air in the pleural space on one side of the chest pushes the contents of the chest, including the trachea, to the opposite side. The nurse will see tracheal deviation away from the affected side. Neither a simple pneumothorax nor a cardiac tamponade causes tracheal deviation.

120. A) Apply an occlusive dressing over the wound secured on three sides.

The patient has an open pneumothorax. The priority intervention is to apply a nonporous dressing with one side unsecured to allow air to escape when the patient exhales but not to reenter during inhalation. Securing the dressing on all sides does not allow air that has built up in the chest cavity to escape. A chest tube is placed if the patient develops a tension pneumothorax. Intubation may be required in this situation, but it is not the initial intervention.

121. B) Minimizing the time to revascularization of the occluded coronary vessels

The key indicator in the care of a myocardial infarction is the time to reperfusion of the obstructed coronary artery. Reperfusion will restore blood flow to the ischemic tissue and prevent further necrosis and functional loss. Morphine is a common treatment in myocardial infarction to decrease cardiac workload and relieve pain experienced by patients suffering from angina. Antiplatelets are often administered to prevent further platelet aggregation at the site of coronary obstruction. Atrioventricular block in concurrence with a myocardial infarction can indicate a higher mortality risk, but does not directly affect the patient outcome.

122. B) Indicates injury affecting the myocardium

A Q wave duration greater than 0.25 second or greater than 25% of the height of the R wave is indicative of damage to the myocardium and is associated with a permanent change in Q wave morphology. Although ventricular tachycardia can occur with an ST-elevated myocardial infarction, the Q wave alone is not an indicator of impending dysrhythmia. All ST-elevated infarctions are acute. Nitroglycerin will not affect the Q wave.

123. C) A decrease in the patient's chest pain score

Administration of nitroglycerin dilates coronary blood vessels to improve blood flow to the ischemic tissue. This should improve oxygenation to tissue and gradually lessen chest pain in patients. Although decreasing systolic blood pressure is an effect of nitroglycerin, it does not measure the drug's effectiveness in reducing coronary ischemia. Nitroglycerin will have no effect on a patient's troponin level. Exhaled nitric oxide does not indicate the effect of nitroglycerin.

124. A) Pupil shape

Patients with orbital fractures should be assessed for signs of globe rupture. A ruptured globe causes a teardrop shape to the pupil specific to this condition. Eye pain occurs with multiple ocular emergencies; it is not specific to a ruptured globe. Photophobia is typically associated with corneal abrasions and other eye conditions, not with a ruptured globe. Blurred vision is associated with other eye conditions; a ruptured globe usually causes diminished vision or vision loss.

125. **D) "I should expect to bruise easily while I am recovering."**

Mononucleosis can cause an enlarged spleen. The patient should be instructed to report any unusual symptoms such as unexplained bleeding or excessive bruising that would indicate that complications have occurred. Knowing not to share food and drink is essential to prevent spreading the disease to others. Rest is an important part of the treatment for mononucleosis. Gargling with warm salt water is appropriate to ease throat pain.

126. **B) Giardiasis**

Giardiasis is a gastrointestinal illness acquired from drinking improperly treated or untreated water from lakes, streams, or wells. *Clostridioides difficile* colitis develops in patients who are taking antibiotics. *Salmonella* infection is contracted from contaminated food, not from swimming in a pond. A viral infection can cause diarrhea, but it is not the most likely cause in this situation.

127. **B) Antidiarrheal medications**

Hepatitis A is a self-limiting condition contracted secondary to poor food preparation and other unsanitary practices. The treatment is directed toward managing the symptoms, which include fatigue, anorexia, and diarrhea. Antibiotics are not indicated for hepatitis A, which is a viral disease. Once a person has hepatitis A, they acquire lifelong immunity, so the vaccine is not effective or needed. Patients with hepatitis A are usually only mildly ill and should not require aggressive fluid resuscitation.

128. **D) Measles**

White spots on the inside of the cheek, referred to as Koplik's spots, occur during the beginning stages of measles. Pertussis presents with a fever and cough, but no spots or other lesions. Mumps cause fever and swollen salivary glands, but not Koplik's spots. Chickenpox causes a rash on the skin, not inside the cheeks.

129. **A) Nasogastric tube placement**

This patient has signs and symptoms of cholecystitis. A nasogastric tube is indicated if the vomiting is prolonged and continues after antiemetic medications are administered. Administration of intravenous fluids is necessary to treat any dehydration and fluid and electrolyte imbalances. Administering antibiotics (ceftriaxone) is important to prevent sepsis. Administering antiemetics (ondansetron) is necessary to decrease nausea and vomiting.

130. **D) Insert a nasogastric tube**

An NG tube is not necessary for a patient undergoing a paracentesis. Before the procedure, the patient should void, or a urinary catheter should be inserted to drain the bladder. The patient needs to be supine for the procedure. Measure vital signs before and after the procedure to assess the patient's condition.

131. **C) Start an intravenous infusion and obtain lab work.**

An intravenous infusion site and lab work are not required for a pelvic exam. The patient needs to empty her bladder before the exam to minimize discomfort from a full bladder. The nurse should verify that all the needed equipment and supplies are ready because once the pelvic exam starts, the nurse needs to stay in the room as a chaperone and cannot leave to get anything else. The procedure should be explained to the patient so she knows what to expect.

132. **A) Sexual or other types of abuse**

A significant other who will not leave the patient and tries to answer all the questions should raise the nurse's suspicion for the patient being in an abusive relationship. Someone answering questions on the patient's behalf does not necessarily mean the patient is not competent to make decisions or that the patient is not knowledgeable about her health. The significant other's interference does not indicate that the patient has low self-esteem.

133. **D) Call for qualified personnel from the obstetric unit to assist.**

The most important thing the nurse can do to prepare for an emergent delivery is to call for assistance from qualified labor and delivery staff. Assessing vital signs is not the top priority. Offering verbal support to the mother is important, but not the initial intervention. Sterile gloves and a gown can be used, but they are not the most critical intervention.

134. **C) Glucagon**

Glucagon 1 mg given intramuscularly is indicated for severe hypoglycemia if intravenous access is unavailable. Oxygen administration may be indicated later, but the immediate priority is correcting the hypoglycemia. Naloxone is administered to unresponsive patients for possible drug overdoses; it does not treat hypoglycemia. It is not safe to administer oral glucose to an unresponsive patient who is unable to swallow.

135. **A) Sodium polysterene**

Sodium polysterene is prescribed for hyperkalemia, but it has a slow onset of action and is not used for initial treatment in life-threatening situations. Nebulized albuterol can be administered to decrease potassium levels. Calcium gluconate lowers potassium rapidly and is particularly useful in this type of situation.

136. **C) Mental status**

Severe hyponatremia causes neurologic changes including confusion, coma, and seizures. A mental status assessment is the priority in this situation. Hyponatremia can cause tachycardia, but it is not the immediate concern. Hyponatremia causes increased urinary output, but this is not the most critical indicator to assess. Hyponatremia can cause weakness, but assessing the patient's mental status is the top priority.

137. **D) Myxedema coma**

A decreased level of consciousness accompanied by signs of decreased metabolism (hypothermia, bradycardia, hypoventilation, and hypotension) is consistent with myxedema coma, a severe form of hypothyroidism. Syndrome of inappropriate antidiuretic hormone secretion causes hypotension, but not these other symptoms. A pheochromocytoma is an adrenal tumor that causes tachyarrhythmias, not bradycardia. Thyroiditis is caused by an overstimulated thyroid and results in hyperthermia and tachycardia.

138. **D) 15 mmHg**

The normal intracranial pressure (ICP) range is 5 to 15 mmHg, so a reading in this range would indicate a positive response to the mannitol, which lowers the ICP. Any reading above 20 mmHg is treated for increased ICP, so readings between 25 and 45 mmHg are still elevated for the patient.

139. **A) Restlessness**

Restlessness is an early sign that brain tissue is beginning to shift downward within the skull toward the brainstem, also known as herniation. Bradycardia, fixed pupils, and posturing are all late signs of this condition.

140. B) Conducting an annual disaster drill to practice decontamination techniques

In the preparedness phase, conducting disaster drills is one way organizations prepare for disasters. Pulling out supplies to meet the patient demand is part of the response phase of a disaster. Implementing a disaster triage system is done during the response phase of a disaster. Undergoing critical incident stress debriefing is part of the recovery phase.

141. D) "I know this is a difficult time for you. If you want to observe, I will stand with you and explain what is going on."

Acknowledging the family member's feelings and offering support and open communication is the most appropriate response in these circumstances. Making a comparison with what others usually do is not helpful and can increase the family member's stress level. A family member should never be forced to observe a resuscitation because others are watching it. A family member's questions can be addressed even if the resuscitation is not observed.

142. A) "Let's find out more about the patient's condition and what the options are for his treatment."

Helping the family obtain more information and potentially make the decision to remove the patient from the ventilator is the best response. Informing the family that you are going to leave the patient on the ventilator to "see what happens" disregards their role in the end-of-life decision-making process. Criticizing the patient's lack of an advance directive is not beneficial in this situation. Acknowledging the family's difficult feelings is important, but simply expressing understanding does not indicate what should happen next.

143. D) ESI Level 5

The patient will be examined and receive prescriptions and discharge instructions—no resources will be used, making this patient an ESI Level 5. An ESI Level 1 patient requires an immediate lifesaving intervention. An ESI Level 2 patient does not require an immediate lifesaving intervention, but cannot wait to be seen. An ESI Level 4 patient requires one or more resources.

144. C) The patient's muscle spasms have decreased

Antipsychotic medications can cause muscle spasms, also referred to as a *dystonic reaction*. Diphenhydramine is administered to reverse these effects. Administering diphenhydramine does not change the patient's thoughts or affect psychosis. Diphenhydramine can make the patient drowsy, not more alert.

145. A) Maintain patient safety.

Patient safety is the top priority when treating a patient with psychosis. It is difficult to address self-esteem issues while the patient is having psychotic symptoms. Reorienting the person back to reality is important, but maintaining safety is the priority. The overall goal is to stop hallucinations and delusions, but this occurs over time as the treatment progresses—the immediate priority is patient safety.

146. D) A delusion

A delusion is a fixed, false belief. Thinking that the people on television are speaking directly to you is an example of a delusion. An auditory hallucination is hearing a sound that is not there. The patient is not expressing fear or apprehension related to the television, so there is no indication that this patient has anxious thoughts. Disorganized thoughts produce speech that makes no sense; there is no evidence that this patient's speech is disorganized.

147. **D) Place the head in the sniffing position.**

The patient is unresponsive so the nurse needs to initiate basic life support. The first step is to open the airway by tilting the head into the sniffing position. Back blows are appropriate for conscious infants. Abdominal thrusts are appropriate for conscious patients. Do not perform a blind finger sweep because it could push the foreign body farther back into the airway.

148. **C) Place a mask on the patient.**

Close contact with someone who is or has been in an institutional setting increases the risk of contracting tuberculosis, and night sweats and bloody sputum are symptoms of that disease. The initial priority in dealing with suspected tuberculosis is to minimize exposure to others. Thus, the initial intervention is to place a mask on the patient to immediately decrease the risk of exposing others. The patient will be placed in a negative-pressure room as part of respiratory isolation precautions, but until then is an exposure risk. A sputum sample will be collected to test for tuberculosis, but is not the initial priority. A PPD skin test is performed as part of the diagnostic workup, but is not the initial priority.

149. **B) Hoarseness and stridor**

Hoarseness and stridor indicate that swelling of the upper airway from smoke inhalation has already started to occur. Delaying intubation increases the risk of difficult intubation as the airways continue to swell. Tachypnea by itself does not indicate that the patient needs to be intubated. If the patient is unresponsive, this is no longer considered early intubation. A clear, productive cough in this patient is not as worrisome as the patient coughing up dark, burned secretions.

150. **A) Blood or other fluid leaking from the puncture site**

Blood or fluid should not leak from the site of the thoracentesis. Notify the provider if this occurs. Respiratory distress is expected to decrease as the fluid drains. The amount of drainage can vary, but it is not unusual for as much as several hundred milliliters of fluid to be removed during the procedure. After thoracentesis, the patient should be able to take a deep breath.

20 POP QUIZ ANSWERS

CHAPTER 2

POP QUIZ 2.1

The nurse suspects dissecting aortic aneurysm. The patient has a difference in systolic blood pressure of more than 20 mmHg. The patient also has Marfan syndrome, which places him at risk for a dissection.

POP QUIZ 2.2

In synchronized cardioversion, the delivery of electricity is synchronized with the R wave. If electricity is delivered during repolarization (T wave), this may induce ventricular fibrillation.

POP QUIZ 2.3

The nurse must palpate for a pulse for no more than 10 seconds. Patients in ventricular tachycardia may or may not have a pulse. If a pulse is not present, the nurse must begin CPR.

POP QUIZ 2.4

The mental status change is likely related to a decrease in cerebral blood flow and perfusion, which may occur if blood pressure is lowered too aggressively. In patients with hypertensive emergency, the nurse should aim to decrease the blood pressure by 25% in the first 2 hours of treatment.

POP QUIZ 2.5

The patient is demonstrating Beck's triad, as evidenced by muffled heart sounds, hypotension, and jugular vein distention these are symptoms associated with cardiac tamponade, likely related to pericardial effusion.

POP QUIZ 2.6

Chest pain that is worse when the patient is supine and improves when the patient sits up and forward is characteristic of pericarditis.

POP QUIZ 2.7

This patient appears to be experiencing intermittent claudication, lower extremity pain that occurs as a result of muscle ischemia during exercise and that improves with rest. It is often experienced by patients with atherosclerosis/peripheral vascular disease.

POP QUIZ 2.8

The nurse should suspect that the patient is experiencing cardiogenic shock secondary to the acute myocardial infarction. The patient will require judicious fluid administration and may require vasopressors to maintain blood pressure. Percutaneous coronary intervention or bypass grafting may be required to restore normal coronary circulation.

POP QUIZ 2.9

The nurse should suspect that this patient may have a deep vein thrombosis. The patient is at increased risk due to smoking history and venous stasis related to limited mobility while traveling by plane.

CHAPTER 3

POP QUIZ 3.1

The nurse should check for tube dislodgment, as this is a frequent complication of patients in the prone position.

POP QUIZ 3.2

The target oxygen saturation for the patient with chronic obstructive pulmonary disease is between 88% and 92% to promote adequate oxygenation while minimizing hyperoxia-induced hypercapnia.

POP QUIZ 3.3

The patient is at risk for aspiration pneumonia due to poor gag reflex secondary to cerebrovascular accident. The food or liquids may have entered airway and become stuck in the lungs, causing infection. This patient needs a swallow study and alterations in diet, such as pureed foods or thickened liquids.

POP QUIZ 3.4

The nurse should anticipate that the emergency provider may perform an emergent bedside cricothyrotomy to bypass the obstruction and facilitate ventilation.

POP QUIZ 3.5

The nurse should suspect that the patient may have developed a pneumothorax.

POP QUIZ 3.6

The nurse should first assess the dressing. It is possible that the dressing has become sealed on all four sides, not allowing air to escape from the chest cavity. If so, the nurse should remove the dressing, reapply a sterile three-sided occlusive dressing or a commercially prepared one-way valve dressing, and then reassess the patient.

POP QUIZ 3.7

Tobacco smoking, oral contraceptives, and recent air travel may all have contributed to the development of a pulmonary embolus.

CHAPTER 4

POP QUIZ 4.1

The nurse should suspect autonomic dysreflexia syndrome. This syndrome, usually occurring in spinal cord injury above T6, is a response to pain or irritation, which needs to be resolved. The nurse should assess for possible injuries such as burns or lacerations, bowel and bladder issues such as constipation or urinary retention, and other potential irritants such as restrictive clothing.

POP QUIZ 4.2

Combination therapy with carbidopa and levodopa is typically prescribed for patients with Parkinson disease.

POP QUIZ 4.3

The patient is displaying behavior that may indicate a subarachnoid hemorrhage.

POP QUIZ 4.4

The family should be informed that meningococcal meningitis is transmitted through respiratory droplets and that prophylactic antibiotics are indicated for all close contacts to prevent meningitis.

POP QUIZ 4.5

The nurse should assess the patient and score withdrawal symptoms using the Clinical Institute Withdrawal Assessment (CIWA) scale. The nurse should also institute seizure precautions for this patient, including padding side rails and limiting stimuli (such as bright lights) if possible.

POP QUIZ 4.6

Phytonadione (vitamin K), prothrombin complex concentrate, or fresh frozen plasma are indicated as emergency reversal agents for warfarin for life-threatening hemorrhage in adults.

CHAPTER 5

POP QUIZ 5.1

The patient most likely has hepatic encephalopathy secondary to elevated ammonia levels. The nurse should draw an ammonia level to confirm. The treatment for hepatic encephalopathy is to administer lactulose.

POP QUIZ 5.2

The nurse should anticipate that the patient will be discharged. Because the object has progressed to the stomach, it should pass naturally. The patient should monitor their stool for evidence that the screw has been expelled. The nurse should advise the patient to return for emergent treatment if rectal bleeding, uncontrolled or increased abdominal pain, and/or nausea and vomiting develop.

POP QUIZ 5.3

The nurse should immediately place two large-bore intravenous lines, draw blood for lab tests with type and screen, and get an order for a fluid bolus. A patient with a history of alcohol use who is vomiting blood should be suspected of having upper gastrointestinal bleeding from esophageal varices. The patient can lose a great amount of blood very quickly and requires close monitoring. Additionally, emergent transfusion or mass transfusion protocol may be indicated.

POP QUIZ 5.4

Patients with pancreatitis are at risk for respiratory complications from atelectasis, hypoxia, or pleural effusions due to the inflammatory chemicals secreted in the lungs. If untreated, these can progress to acute respiratory distress syndrome and multisystem organ failure. The nurse should reassess the patient's respiratory status frequently.

POP QUIZ 5.5

This patient has pain and bruising around the liver. Additionally, the patient has signs of hemodynamic instability. The nurse should suspect a liver injury with likely significant internal bleeding and hemorrhagic shock. The priority intervention is to initiate two large-bore IV lines begin fluid resuscitation with crystalloids, and be prepared to activate massive transfusion protocol. If the patient does not respond to fluid replacement, then vasopressors may be used.

CHAPTER 6

POP QUIZ 6.1

The patient may be experiencing symptoms related to a dislodged IUD. The nurse should anticipate that the ED provider will likely seek OB/GYN consultation and order radiographic imaging, such as x-ray or ultrasound, to confirm the location of the IUD. The nurse should also expect to collect blood for lab tests and a urine sample to investigate for infection and pregnancy.

POP QUIZ 6.2

The nurse should suspect that the patient has contracted syphilis during an unprotected sexual encounter. The nurse can expect that the provider will order antibiotics and swab the lesion for microscopy, as well as order serum testing to investigate for any other possible sexually transmitted infections (STIs). The nurse can also anticipate the need to educate the patient regarding follow-up, including appropriate notification of STI status to any recent sexual partners.

POP QUIZ 6.3

The nurse should notify the provider of the findings, indicating that the patient has sustained some type of genitourinary trauma. The catheter insertion should be delayed until further diagnostic testing is performed to rule out a urethral or bladder injury.

POP QUIZ 6.4

The patient appears to be experiencing an episode of ischemic priapism. Because permanent tissue damage begins within 6 hours, this patient must be prioritized for evaluation by the ED provider, and the nurse should expect orders to apply supplemental oxygen, draw blood for lab tests and initiate a peripheral IV in preparation for possible procedural sedation to facilitate aspiration of cavernosal blood and injection of an adrenergic agent, such as phenylephrine, by the ED provider.

POP QUIZ 6.5

The patient is experiencing signs of possible renal calculi. The nurse should expect orders for additional diagnostic testing including CT scan of the abdomen and pelvis or KUB x-ray, IV fluids, and pain medication.

POP QUIZ 6.6

The sudden onset of scrotal pain should prompt the nurse to suspect this patient has developed testicular torsion. *Testicular torsion* is the sudden twisting of the spermatic cord. It is a urologic emergency and requires prompt surgical intervention to prevent long-term complications.

POP QUIZ 6.7

The nurse should suspect that this patient has developed a complicated urinary tract infection. The nurse should collect a urine sample and urine culture with sensitivity testing from the catheter sampling port. Depending on institutional guidelines, remove and place a new catheter prior to collection. The nurse should expect further orders for laboratory studies such as a complete blood count, basic metabolic panel, lactate level, and blood cultures. Radiographic imaging such as an abdominal CT or renal ultrasound may be indicated to investigate flank pain. A head CT scan may also be indicated due to mental status changes.

CHAPTER 7

POP QUIZ 7.1

Some potential causes of abnormal vaginal bleeding include hormonal imbalance, gynecologic disorders, medication use, malnutrition, disordered eating, increased physiologic or psychological stress, or excessive weight loss or exercise.

POP QUIZ 7.2

Severe abdominal pain and vaginal bleeding should prompt the nurse to suspect placental abruption. Even patients who are initially stable may deteriorate rapidly if placental separation progresses. The nurse should initiate continuous cardiac monitoring, and the provider should consider consulting OB to initiate continuous fetal monitoring. The ED nurse should initiate two large-bore IV lines and prepare to administer crystalloid fluid boluses while closely monitoring maternal hemodynamic status.

POP QUIZ 7.3

The nurse should first administer oxygen before considering further interventions to treat this infant's low heart rate. Hypoxia is the most frequent cause of bradycardia in a newborn.

POP QUIZ 7.4

The patient is experiencing signs of ovarian cyst rupture with evidence of hypovolemia as indicated by active bleeding, tachycardia, and hypotension. Priority nursing interventions include placement of two large-bore IV lines, drawing blood to expedite processing of a complete blood count and type and screen, and administration of crystalloid fluids and blood products as ordered. The nurse should be prepared to contact the blood bank for possible emergent blood release.

POP QUIZ 7.5

The patient should be advised to complete the full course of antibiotics as prescribed, even if they are feeling better. If a sexually transmitted infection is identified, the patient should inform their sexual partner(s) of their diagnosis so the partner(s) can seek treatment as well. Additionally, the patient should be educated regarding methods of prevention of STIs.

POP QUIZ 7.6

The patient should be advised to continue feeding/pumping with the unaffected breast and to pump and discard milk from the affected breast. The nurse should reinforce the importance of completing the entire course of antibiotics as prescribed. The patient should also receive instruction regarding massage of inflamed areas and safe application of warm compresses to improve circulation and prevent milk stasis. The nurse should also inform the patient of reasons to return for further evaluation, such as fever or other signs of worsening infection.

POP QUIZ 7.7

The patient should stop exercising, drink fluids, and attempt to empty the bladder. The patient should then lie down to rest on the left side, monitoring onset and duration of contractions. The patient should seek evaluation if more than five contractions occur regularly within an hour, or if any bleeding, rupture of membranes, or severe pain occurs.

CHAPTER 8

POP QUIZ 8.1

The nurse should attempt to de-escalate the situation before the patient becomes more violent by remaining calm and speaking to the patient reassuringly. The nurse should first attempt to engage the patient in conversation and establish a therapeutic relationship. The nurse should incorporate nonverbal communication strategies to appear less threatening. If these techniques are unsuccessful, the nurse should administer medications or use restraints to protect the patient and staff.

POP QUIZ 8.2

The initial priority is to rule out a physiologic cause for the anxiety. The nurse should assess airway, breathing, and circulation as part of a complete physical examination, and then obtain other provider orders, such as an EKG and laboratory work. Supplemental oxygen may assist the patient. Once medical causes for the anxiety symptoms have been excluded, the nurse should administer any antianxiety medications ordered and use therapeutic communication techniques to establish rapport with the patient. This can help the patient identify concerns and feelings that they have and begin to work through their anxious feelings.

POP QUIZ 8.3

The nurse should assess the patient for suicidal thoughts. If present, the nurse should use a standard suicide risk assessment and implement appropriate interventions based on the scoring. These interventions can include placing the patient in a treatment room with potential hazards removed and keeping the patient on continuous 1:1 observation.

POP QUIZ 8.4

The patient's safety is the priority in this situation. The patient should be placed in a room that does not have any potentially dangerous objects. External stimuli should be minimized. The nurse should calmly speak to the patient using brief but direct instructions and keep the patient under close observation.

POP QUIZ 8.5

This may be an expression of suicidal ideation. The nurse should question the patient further to identify if the patient desires to end their life and has a specific plan to harm themself, and to assess the patient's level of intent to carry out that plan.

CHAPTER 9

POP QUIZ 9.1

The patient is most likely in diabetic ketoacidosis with a critical high blood sugar that is causing confusion and Kussmaul breathing, which are hallmark signs of acidosis.

POP QUIZ 9.2

The nurse should recognize that the patient is at increased risk for hyperkalemia. Spironolactone is a potassium-sparing diuretic that potentially causes hyperkalemia. The patient should be asked if they are still taking potassium supplements, because there could be a knowledge deficit regarding the recent medication change.

POP QUIZ 9.3

The patient is experiencing hypocalcemia. Multiple blood transfusions can cause hypocalcemia because the preservative in the transfused blood (citrate) binds with calcium.

CHAPTER 10

POP QUIZ 10.1

Dizziness, loss of balance or coordination, or trouble walking may be signs of stroke. Further evaluation of the patient's symptoms, physical assessment, and diagnostic testing are needed.

POP QUIZ 10.2

The patient may have Ludwig's angina, and airway management would be the priority.

POP QUIZ 10.3

The nurse suspects a ruptured tympanic membrane.

CHAPTER 11

POP QUIZ 11.1

Drain cleaner is an acidic solution. The nurse or provider will test the pH of the ocular fluid and then flush it with saline. Access to an eye wash station is ideal; otherwise, the nurse or provider will flush with saline until the pH is close to 7.5.

POP QUIZ 11.2

The emergency nurse suspects herpes zoster ophthalmicus.

POP QUIZ 11.3

The nurse suspects the patient is having central retinal artery occlusion. Head CT will be ordered to rule out a stroke.

CHAPTER 12

POP QUIZ 12.1

The nurse should assess the patient's hemodynamic status and control any bleeding. Patients with a traumatic amputation of an extremity are at high risk for significant blood loss.

POP QUIZ 12.2

The patient has signs of compartment syndrome. The priority intervention is to relieve pressure in the affected extremity. The patient's cast should be cut to allow the leg tissues to expand, and the provider should be notified immediately.

POP QUIZ 12.3

The nurse should not assume that the patient is experiencing musculoskeletal chest pain. Instead, the nurse should anticipate testing to rule out a myocardial infarction or other cardiac condition. Appropriate testing, including an EKG, cardiac enzymes, chest x-ray, and other relevant testing should be performed.

POP QUIZ 12.4

Before and after splinting and casting any injury, the nurse should assess the neurovascular status in the affected extremity. Pulses, capillary refill, and movement (not restricted by the splint) should be intact, and there should not be any numbness or tingling, which could indicate nerve impingement.

POP QUIZ 12.5

Patients who are unresponsive cannot report signs and symptoms, so a complete head-to-toe assessment must be done to identify any injuries not detected during the primary survey. The patient has a mechanism of injury that has likely caused orthopedic injuries.

CHAPTER 13

POP QUIZ 13.1

Irrigating a deep abrasion is essential to remove all foreign bodies, including dirt and debris. Any retained foreign bodies increase the risk of infection and can cause "tattooing" of the skin.

POP QUIZ 13.2

A degloving injury involves the avulsion of the skin circumferentially from an extremity. The nurse should assess the neurovascular status of the involved body part, both proximal and distal to the wound. Rapid assessment and treatment will improve the chance of successful tissue preservation.

POP QUIZ 13.3

Injection injuries usually have minimal exterior damage but significant interior tissue damage. The nurse should assign a high triage priority and alert the provider immediately. The nurse should monitor for signs and symptoms of compartment syndrome, clean and disinfect the entry wound, and prepare the patient for surgical exploration and wound debridement.

POP QUIZ 13.4

The patient should keep the wound clean and dry. No ointments, including antibiotic ointment, should be applied to the area. The adhesive will fall off within 5 to 10 days. Any signs and symptoms of infection (redness, swelling, drainage) should be evaluated.

POP QUIZ 13.5

A head-to-toe assessment must be performed on shooting victims to locate all potential injuries. External wounds may not correlate with internal damage. Gunshot wounds may follow an unpredictable path once they have penetrated the body.

CHAPTER 14

POP QUIZ 14.1

The nurse would remove the patient's clothing, if present, and determine the total body surface area affected. In this case, it would be approximately 22.5% following the rules of nines: 18% for the right leg and 4.5% for right arm involvement. An IV would be established on the left arm with blood drawn for lab tests and fluid resuscitation intitiated. The patient would receive 4,180 mL of IV lactated Ringer's solution, with 2 L given over the first 8 hours and the remaining given over the next 16 hours. The patient would be monitored for compartment syndrome with possible fasciotomy. The wound would be covered with a dry sterile dressing and the patient transferred emergently to a burn center.

POP QUIZ 14.2

The nurse should immediately flush the eyes for at least 20 minutes with normal saline or water; all tests such as pH and visual acuity should be done after flushing. Only immediate life-sustaining interventions would be done prior to flushing.

POP QUIZ 14.3

The nurse suspects that the car was electrified by the downed power wires touching the car. When the patient touched the car, it closed the circuit, causing current to pass through the patient's body, taking the internal path of least resistance. The nurse suspects internal damage to the heart, abdominal organs, and tissues of the arm and leg.

POP QUIZ 14.4

The nurse should immerse the site in hot water for 30 to 90 minutes and remove barbs. Antibiotics may be indicated.

POP QUIZ 14.5

Many conditions cause diarrhea, but swimming in a pond puts this patient at risk for contracting giardiasis. This is a gastrointestinal illness caused by the parasite *Giardia*, which is found in contaminated water, including lakes and ponds.

POP QUIZ 14.6

Patients with heat stroke have a higher core body temperature, greater than or equal to 104.0°F (40.0°C), and display signs and symptoms of central nervous system involvement, including ataxia, slurred speech, seizures, and coma.

POP QUIZ 14.7

Postexposure prophylaxis is initiated after an animal bite from a rabid animal to prevent the patient from contracting the disease. The nurse should instruct the patient on the importance of following up to receive all required dosages to prevent rabies, which is potentially fatal.

CHAPTER 15

POP QUIZ 15.1

The nurse will anticipate calling the poison control center for direction. The nurse will establish a large-bore IV and draw blood for lab tests with a toxicology screen. The nurse will monitor for altered metal status, respiratory distress, and cardiac arrhythmias. The nurse will anticipate IV fluid bolus, antiemetics, and admission and should ensure that the patient is referred to psychiatric services.

POP QUIZ 15.2

Pulse oximetry in carbon monoxide poisoning is unreliable because the sensor is unable to differentiate between carboxyhemoglobin and oxyhemoglobin. The patient may display confusion, so the nurse should continue to provide an explanation for supplemental oxygen. The patient should be treated with oxygen before carboxyhemoglobin and arterial blood gas testing and while awaiting results.

POP QUIZ 15.3

The priority intervention is decontamination. The patient should be decontaminated to decrease exposure and for safety of the staff.

POP QUIZ 15.4

A serious complication of taking St. John's wort and cyclosporine is decreased serum levels of cyclosporine that cause transplant rejection.

POP QUIZ 15.5

The patient will require hemodialysis and admission to the ICU.

POP QUIZ 15.6

The patient requires seizure precautions. The emergency nurse should follow up and question the purpose of the phenytoin prescription. It is possible that the patient is going through alcohol withdrawal and is at a higher risk of seizures.

CHAPTER 16

POP QUIZ 16.1

The nurse suspects cutaneous diphtheria.

POP QUIZ 16.2

The nurse should educate the patient that soap and water may be more effective than alcohol-based sanitizers in removing *C. difficile* spores, which are resistant to alcohol.

POP QUIZ 16.3

The patient with the rash on the face should be seen first, because untreated rash can cause vision loss.

CHAPTER 17

POP QUIZ 17.1

The unlicensed assistive personnel (UAP) should not complete this task. It is not within the UAP's scope of practice to administer medications.

POP QUIZ 17.2

The ED technician is in violation of Health Insurance Portability and Accountability Act. As the technician was using their phone in a patient care setting, patients were inadvertently video recorded and posted on social media without their consent.

POP QUIZ 17.3

The ethical principle of autonomy is involved in this scenario. The patient has the right to direct their care.

POP QUIZ 17.4

Patients are seen based on the severity of their condition and not necessarily in the order that they present to the ED. The nurse should reassure the patient that they will be seen by a provider.

APPENDIX A: COMMON MEDICATIONS FOR CERTIFIED EMERGENCY NURSING

TABLE A.1 Common Antibiotics and Antifungals for Certified Emergency Nursing

GENERAL INDICATIONS	GENERAL MECHANISM OF ACTION	GENERAL CONTRAINDICATIONS, PRECAUTIONS, AND ADVERSE EFFECTS
Aminoglycosides (e.g., gentamicin, streptomycin, neomycin)		
Common indications among aminoglycosides • Bacteremia and sepsis • Bone and joint infections • Community-acquired pneumonia • Empiric treatment for febrile neutropenia • Infective endocarditis • Intra-abdominal infections • Lower respiratory tract infections • Nosocomial pneumonia • Ophthalmic infections • Surgical infection prophylaxis Specific indications for gentamicin • Complicated UTIs • Meningitis and ventriculitis • PID • Pyelonephritis • Skin and skin structure infections Specific indications for streptomycin • Gram-negative bacillary bacteremia, meningitis, or lower respiratory tract infections in combination with other antimicrobials • UTI • Drug susceptible tuberculosis Specific indications for neomycin • Adjunctive therapy for hepatic encephalopathy • Infectious diarrhea	• Inhibit bacterial protein synthesis, causing bactericidal effect	• Medication is contraindicated in administration for organisms resistant to aminoglycosides. • Use caution in administering to patients with inflammatory bowel disease, as there is a high likelihood for developing pseudomembranous colitis or *Clostridioides difficile*. • Monitor closely for nephrotoxicity or neurotoxicity, including ototoxicity in all aminoglycoside medications. Nephrotoxicity or ototoxicity development requires dose adjustment or discontinuation. • Additional adverse effects include nausea, vomiting, auditory disturbances, headache, skin irritation, rash, anemia, and elevated liver enzymes.

(continued)

TABLE A.1 Common Antibiotics and Antifungals for Certified Emergency Nursing *(continued)*

GENERAL INDICATIONS	GENERAL MECHANISM OF ACTION	GENERAL CONTRAINDICATIONS, PRECAUTIONS, AND ADVERSE EFFECTS
Antibiotic, sulfonamide derivative (trimethoprim-sulfamethoxazole [TMP-SMX], also known as co-trimoxazole)		
• UTI • Pyelonephritis • Pneumocystic pneumonia • Otitis media • Acute bacterial exacerbations of chronic bronchitis	• Inhibits enzymes in folic acid synthesis pathway, causing bactericidal effects	• Medication is contraindicated in folate deficiency, megaloblastic anemia, G6PD deficiency, severe renal impairment, and hepatic disease. • Use caution in patients with hypothyroidism, colitis, GI disturbances, HIV/AIDS, cardiac disease, and arrhythmia. • Adverse effects include megaloblastic anemia, aplastic anemia, hemolytic anemia, TTP, angioedema, Stevens–Johnson syndrome, exfoliative dermatitis, anaphylactic reaction, anuria, hyperkalemia, rhabdomyolysis, seizures, hemolysis, leukopenia, QT prolongation, chest pain, dyspnea, nausea, vomiting, itching, fever, and chills.
Antiprotozoals, respiratory (pentamidine)		
• *Pneumocystis* pneumonia • Leishmaniasis • Oral inhalation antifungal agent used for various fungal infections	• Mechanism of action not clearly known; thought to interfere with fungal DNA and RNA replication	• Use caution if administering rapidly, as it can lead to hypotension. • Use caution in patients with renal, hepatic, or cardiac disease; asthma; or pregnancy. • Adverse effects include arrhythmia, bronchospasm, elevated AST/ALT, hypoglycemia, tremor, cough, fever, itching, diarrhea, headache, or night sweats.

(continued)

TABLE A.1	Common Antibiotics and Antifungals for Certified Emergency Nursing *(continued)*		
GENERAL INDICATIONS	**GENERAL MECHANISM OF ACTION**	**GENERAL CONTRAINDICATIONS, PRECAUTIONS, AND ADVERSE EFFECTS**	

Azoles (e.g., fluconazole)

GENERAL INDICATIONS	GENERAL MECHANISM OF ACTION	GENERAL CONTRAINDICATIONS, PRECAUTIONS, AND ADVERSE EFFECTS
• Cutaneous leishmaniasis • Cutaneous or lymphocutaneous sporotrichosis • Skin or skin structure *Candida* infection • Talaromycosis, coccidioidomycosis, or histoplasmosis prophylaxis in patients with HIV • Primary pulmonary histoplasmosis • Bacterial vaginosis • Treatment and prophylaxis treatment for recurrent vulvovaginal candidiasis infections • Osteomyelitis, bone and joint infection caused by *Candida* • Infective endocarditis caused by *Candida* • Infected pacemaker, ICD, or VAD caused by *Candida* • Treatment of meningitis due to *Histoplasma capsulatum* in patients with HIV • CNS infections due to *Coccidioides,* cryptococcus, or *Candida* • Organ transplant recipients • *Candida* prophylaxis in bone marrow transplant or high-risk cancer patients • Pyelonephritis caused by *Candida* • Urinary tract infection caused by *Candida* • Intra-abdominal infections caused by *Candida* • Pneumonia caused by *Candida* • Thrush	• Alter fungal cell membrane to inhibit fungal reproduction and growth through fungistatic action	• Use caution in cardiac, hepatic, or renal conditions. • Avoid use during pregnancy except in severe, life-threatening emergencies. • Adverse effects include dizziness, rash, diarrhea, nausea, and headache.

(continued)

TABLE A.1 Common Antibiotics and Antifungals for Certified Emergency Nursing (*continued*)

GENERAL INDICATIONS	GENERAL MECHANISM OF ACTION	GENERAL CONTRAINDICATIONS, PRECAUTIONS, AND ADVERSE EFFECTS
Carbapenems (e.g., ertapenem, meropenem)		
Indications for both ertapenem and meropenem • Bacterial encephalitis or meningitis • Intra-abdominal infections • Complicated skin and skin structure infections • Empiric treatment of febrile neutropenia • Bacteremia or sepsis • Pneumonia (CAP or nosocomial) Additional indications for ertapenem • Complicated UTI and pyelonephritis • Acute pelvic infection • Surgical prophylaxis	• Inhibit cell wall synthesis by binding to penicillin-binding proteins inside bacterial cell wall, resulting in cell death to prevent organism growth	• Use caution in patients receiving carbapenem treatment who undergo concurrent hematologic testing. A positive Coombs test has been reported in patients taking carbapenems (meropenem). • Use caution in patients with cephalosporin, penicillin, or other beta-lactam hypersensitivity, as cross sensitivity is possible. • Use caution in head injury or neurologic disease due to risk of seizure associated with carbapenem administration. • Use caution in renal failure, impairment, or dysfunction, as carbapenems are excreted by the kidneys and can result in further damage. • Use caution when administering to patients with inflammatory bowel disease due to high likelihood of developing pseudomembranous colitis and *C. difficile*. • Adverse effects include nausea, headache, diarrhea, rash, vomiting, confusion, delirium, hypoglycemia, pseudomembranous colitis, neutropenia, renal failure, and seizure.
Cephalosporins, first generation (cefazolin)		
• First-generation cephalosporins have coverage against most gram-positive cocci as well as gram-negative bacteria (e.g., *E. coli, Proteus mirabilis, Klebsiella pneumoniae*). • Upper respiratory tract infections • Skin and skin structure infections	• Inhibit cell wall synthesis by binding to penicillin-binding proteins inside bacterial cell wall, resulting in cell death to prevent organism growth, causing bactericidal effect.	• Do not administer in viral infections or organisms with antimicrobial resistance to cephalosporins. • Use caution in allergy to penicillin, as cross reaction is possible.

(continued)

TABLE A.1 **Common Antibiotics and Antifungals for Certified Emergency Nursing** *(continued)*

GENERAL INDICATIONS	GENERAL MECHANISM OF ACTION	GENERAL CONTRAINDICATIONS, PRECAUTIONS, AND ADVERSE EFFECTS
• Biliary tract infections • UTI • Infective endocarditis • Surgical infection prophylaxis • Lower respiratory tract infections (pneumococcal pneumonia and community-acquired pneumonia) • Bacteremia • Bone and joint infections • Mastitis • Bacterial encephalitis or meningitis		• Use caution in renal failure, impairment, or dysfunction. Cephalosporins are excreted by the kidneys and can result in further damage. • Adverse effects include headache, diarrhea, nausea, vomiting, maculopapular rash, fever, confusion, bleeding, seizures, azotemia, and renal failure. • Medication is contraindicated in cephalosporin-resistant organisms and viral infection.

Cephalosporins, second generation (cefuroxime)

• Second-generation cephalosporins have coverage against *Haemophilus, Moraxella catarrhalis,* and *Bacteroides* spp. • Chronic bronchitis • Skin and skin structure infections • UTI • Treatment of bone and joint infection • Pharyngitis • Gonorrhea • Lyme disease • Acute otitis media • Bacteremia • Meningitis • Surgical infection prophylaxis • Tonsillitis • Sinusitis • Intra-abdominal infections • Lower respiratory tract infections • Pneumonia (CAP and nosocomial)	• Inhibit bacterial cell wall synthesis by binding to specific penicillin-binding proteins within the cell wall, causing bactericidal effect	• Medication is contraindicated in penicillin allergy, viral infections, or bacteria with known drug resistance. • Use caution in renal failure/impairment, pseudomembranous colitis, and phenylketonuria. • Adverse effects include nausea, vomiting, flatulence, dyspepsia, dysuria, phlebitis, jaundice, Stevens–Johnson syndrome, and vasculitis.

(continued)

TABLE A.1   Common Antibiotics and Antifungals for Certified Emergency Nursing *(continued)*

GENERAL INDICATIONS	GENERAL MECHANISM OF ACTION	GENERAL CONTRAINDICATIONS, PRECAUTIONS, AND ADVERSE EFFECTS
Cephalosporins, third generation (ceftriaxone)		
• Third-generation cephalosporins have less coverage against most gram-positive organisms but increased coverage against Enterobacteriaceae, *Neisseria* spp., and *H. influenzae*. • Bacteremia and sepsis • UTI • Acute bacterial otitis media • Skin and skin structure infections • Surgical incision site infections • Necrotizing infections • Intra-abdominal infections • Surgical infection prophylaxis • PID • Bone and joint infections • Lower respiratory tract infection • Pneumonia (nosocomial and CAP) • Infective endocarditis • Meningitis and vasculitis • Gonorrhea infection • Lyme disease • Congenital syphilis • Bacterial sinusitis	• Inhibit bacterial cell wall synthesis by binding to specific penicillin-binding proteins within the cell wall, causing bactericidal effect	• Medication is contraindicated in penicillin allergy, jaundice, or hyperbilirubinemia in premature neonates; viral infection; or antimicrobial resistance. • Use caution in GI disease, as it may cause or worsen existing colitis. • Adverse effects include seizures, bronchospasm, pancreatitis, biliary obstruction, erythema multiforme, acute generalized exanthematous pustulosis, Stevens–Johnson syndrome, renal failure, thrombocytosis, elevated liver enzymes, anemia, thrombocytopenia, neutropenia, hypoprothrombinemia, jaundice, superinfection, edema, nausea, vomiting, headache, and itching.
Cephalosporins, fourth generation (cefepime)		
• Fourth-generation cephalosporins have similar coverage to third-generation cephalosporins but with additional coverage against gram-negative bacteria with antimicrobial resistance (e.g., beta-lactamase).	• Inhibit bacterial cell wall synthesis by binding to specific penicillin-binding proteins within the cell wall, causing bactericidal effect	• Medication is contraindicated in penicillin allergy and antimicrobial resistance. • Use caution in colitis, GI disturbances, and renal failure. Cefepime may worsen colitis, other GI issues, and kidney function.

(continued)

TABLE A.1   Common Antibiotics and Antifungals for Certified Emergency Nursing *(continued)*

GENERAL INDICATIONS	GENERAL MECHANISM OF ACTION	GENERAL CONTRAINDICATIONS, PRECAUTIONS, AND ADVERSE EFFECTS
• Monotherapy for febrile neutropenia • Complicated UTI and pyelonephritis • Intra-abdominal infections • Severe skin and skin structure infections • Pneumonia (CAP and nosocomial) • Bacterial meningitis • Infective endocarditis • Sepsis		• Adverse effects include seizure, anaphylactic shock, Stevens–Johnson syndrome, toxic epidermal necrolysis, erythema multiforme, agranulocytosis, pancytopenia, aplastic anemia, elevated liver enzymes, hypophosphatemia, hypoprothrombinemia, bleeding, colitis, vaginitis, pseudomembranous colitis, hypercalcemia, superinfection, confusion, hallucination, rash, vomiting, diarrhea, itching, nausea, headache, and fever.
Cephalosporins, fifth generation (ceftaroline fosamil)		
• Acute bacterial skin and skin structure infections • Community-acquired pneumonia • Sepsis • Coverage against methicillin-resistant staphylococci and penicillin-resistant pneumococci	• Inhibit bacterial cell wall synthesis by binding to specific penicillin-binding proteins within the cell wall, causing bactericidal effect.	• Medication is contraindicated in viral infection and antimicrobial resistance. • Use caution in patients with colitis, GI disturbances, or renal impairments/ failure. • Adverse effects include hyperkalemia or hypokalemia, bradycardia, seizure, renal failure, agranulocytosis, anaphylaxis, elevated liver enzymes, constipation, hepatitis, hyperglycemia, thrombocytopenia, pseudomembranous colitis, encephalopathy, diarrhea, rash, vomiting, abdominal pain, headache, and dizziness.
Fluoroquinolones (ciprofloxacin, delafloxacin, levofloxacin, moxifloxacin)		
• UTI, cystitis, and pyelonephritis • Lower respiratory tract infections, pneumonia (CAP and nosocomial) • Chronic bronchitis exacerbations • Skin and skin structure infections • Animal bite wounds • Enteric infections • Mild to moderate acute sinusitis	• Inhibit DNA synthesis, causing bactericidal effect	• Use caution in patients with cardiac disease, cardiac arrhythmias, or CNS disorders and in patients with history of myasthenia gravis, DM, renal impairments, or hepatic dysfunction.

(continued)

TABLE A.1 Common Antibiotics and Antifungals for Certified Emergency Nursing *(continued)*

GENERAL INDICATIONS	GENERAL MECHANISM OF ACTION	GENERAL CONTRAINDICATIONS, PRECAUTIONS, AND ADVERSE EFFECTS
<ul><li>Acute prostatitis</li><li>Febrile neutropenia</li><li>Bacterial conjunctivitis</li><li>Ophthalmic infections related to corneal ulcers</li><li>Acute otitis externa</li><li>Bone and joint infections</li><li>Meningococcal infection/prophylaxis</li><li>Intra-abdominal infections</li><li>Peritoneal dialysis infections</li><li>Dental infections</li><li>Surgical infection prophylaxis</li><li>Pulmonary infections in cystic fibrosis</li><li>Infective endocarditis</li><li>Sepsis</li><li>Traveler's diarrhea</li><li>Broad-spectrum antibiotics useful against gram-negative rods—*Escherichia coli, Klebsiella* spp., *Proteus* spp., *Pseudomonas* spp., *Pseudomonas aeruginosa, Providencia* spp. and *Serratia marcescens, Streptococcus pneumoniae*; also effective against *H. influenzae, Moraxella catarrhalis, Legionella* spp., *Mycoplasma* spp., *Chlamydia pneumoniae*</li><li>Effective against gram-positive organisms including *Staphylococcus aureus* and methicillin-resistant *S. aureus*</li><li>Effective against anaerobic bacteria, *Mycobacterium, Bacillus anthracis, Francisella tularensis*, and typhoid</li></ul>		<ul><li>Adverse effects include hepatotoxicity, phototoxicity, tendon rupture, neurotoxicity, hepatic dysfunction, hyper- or hypoglycemia, exacerbation of myasthenia gravis symptoms, worsening colitis or GI dysfunction, nausea, vomiting, or rash.</li><li>Discontinue immediately with any sign of tendon inflammation or tendon pain. These symptoms often present before tendon rupture.</li></ul>

(continued)

TABLE A.1 Common Antibiotics and Antifungals for Certified Emergency Nursing (*continued*)

GENERAL INDICATIONS	GENERAL MECHANISM OF ACTION	GENERAL CONTRAINDICATIONS, PRECAUTIONS, AND ADVERSE EFFECTS
Glycopeptides (vancomycin)		
• Infective endocarditis • Pseudomembranous colitis due to *C. difficile* infection • Enterocolitis • Sepsis and bacteremia • Serious gram-positive infections • Mastitis • Gram-positive lower respiratory infections (CAP and nosocomial pneumonia) • Pleural empyema • Surgical infection prophylaxis • Meningitis and other CNS infections • Bone and joint infections • Septic arthritis • Prosthetic joint infections • Febrile neutropenia • Intra-abdominal infections • Peritoneal dialysis-related peritonitis • Used to treat and prevent various bacterial infections caused by gram-positive bacteria, including MRSA • Effective for streptococci, enterococci, and MSSA infections	• Bind to parts of bacterial cell wall, preventing synthesis	• Medication is contraindicated in viral infection and vancomycin-resistant organisms • Use caution in renal disease, hearing impairment, and heart failure. • Adverse effects include rash, itching, nausea, abdominal pain, fever, diarrhea, and Stevens–Johnson syndrome.
Lincosamides (clindamycin)		
• Bacteremia • Lower respiratory tract infections, including CAP and nosocomial pneumonia • Intra-abdominal infections • Skin and skin structure infections • Animal bites • Diabetic foot ulcers • Gynecologic infections • Bacterial vaginosis • Acne • Mastitis • Bone and joint infections • Bacterial sinusitis • Acute otitis media • Surgical infection prophylaxis	• Bind to RNA of bacteria to inhibit protein synthesis	• Medication is contraindicated in patients with a history of enteritis, ulcerative colitis, and pseudomembranous colitis. • Use caution in patients with diarrhea or hepatic disease. • Adverse effects include toxic epidermal necrolysis, Stevens–Johnson syndrome, erythema multiforme, exfoliative dermatitis, proteinuria, oliguria, superinfection, fungal overgrowth, pseudomembranous colitis, edema, leukopenia, thrombocytopenia, elevated hepatic enzyme, fever, fatigue, dizziness, vomiting, nausea, headache, and itching.

(continued)

TABLE A.1   Common Antibiotics and Antifungals for Certified Emergency Nursing *(continued)*

GENERAL INDICATIONS	GENERAL MECHANISM OF ACTION	GENERAL CONTRAINDICATIONS, PRECAUTIONS, AND ADVERSE EFFECTS
Macrolides (azithromycin)		
• Mild to moderate bacterial exacerbations of chronic bronchitis in patients with COPD • Acute otitis media • Bacterial conjunctivitis • CAP • Skin and skin structure infections • PID • Gonorrhea • *Mycobacterium* infection • Acute bacterial sinusitis • Bacterial endocarditis prophylaxis	• Inhibit protein synthesis in bacterial cells, causing bacteriostatic effect • Bactericidal in high concentrations	• Medication is contraindicated in patients with a history of jaundice or hepatic dysfunction prior to macrolide use, viral infection, and drug-resistant bacteria. • Use caution in renal impairment, cardiovascular disease, colitis, or GI disease, and in patients with a history of myasthenia gravis. • Adverse effects include photosensitivity, arrhythmia and QT prolongation, renal failure, hyperkalemia, bronchospasm, seizures, elevated liver enzymes, hyperbilirubinemia, constipation, jaundice, superinfection, anemia, dermatitis, and hypo- or hyperglycemia.
Oxazolidinones (linezolid)		
• Lower respiratory tract infections • CAP and nosocomial pneumonia • Skin and skin structure infections • Sepsis and bacteremia caused by vancomycin-resistant enterococcus • MRSA bacteremia • MRSA-associated bone and joint infection • Septic arthritis • Prosthetic joint infections • Meningitis and other CNS infections • Febrile neutropenia • Intra-abdominal infections • Peritonitis	• Inhibit bacterial protein synthesis by preventing translation and protein production, thus preventing bacterial growth	• Medication is contraindicated in concurrent use of metrizamide or iohexol during procedures requiring radiographic contrast administration. • Use caution in uncontrolled hypertension, concurrent use with MAOIs, diarrhea, pseudomembranous colitis, history of seizures, and diabetes (may cause hypoglycemia). • Adverse effects include myelosuppression, short-term decreased fertility in male patients, hypoglycemia, pancytopenia, optic neuritis, seizures, anaphylaxis, angioedema, anemia, thrombocytopenia, elevated hepatic enzymes, hypertension, hypoglycemia, pseudomembranous colitis, diarrhea, vomiting, abdominal pain, rash, itching, and tooth discoloration.

(continued)

TABLE A.1 Common Antibiotics and Antifungals for Certified Emergency Nursing (continued)

GENERAL INDICATIONS	GENERAL MECHANISM OF ACTION	GENERAL CONTRAINDICATIONS, PRECAUTIONS, AND ADVERSE EFFECTS
Penicillins (ampicillin)		
• Severe infections including bacteremia • Infective endocarditis • Respiratory tract infections • Skin and skin structure infections • Genitourinary infections • UTI • Gastrointestinal infection	• Inhibit cell wall synthesis to produce a bactericidal effect, preventing organism growth	• Medication is contraindicated in penicillin-resistant organisms. • Use caution in renal impairments, cephalosporin and carbapenem hypersensitivity, colitis and other GI disturbances, and mononucleosis. • Adverse effects include antibiotic-associated colitis, anaphylaxis, exfoliative dermatitis, seizures, rash, nausea, vomiting, leukopenia, thrombocytopenia, platelet dysfunction, anemia, elevated hepatic enzymes, pseudomembranous colitis, superinfection, or diarrhea.
Tetracyclines (doxycycline)		
• Necrotizing ulcerative gingivitis • Treatment when penicillins are contraindicated • Uncomplicated gonorrhea • *Chlamydia* infection • Psittacosis • Respiratory tract infections • Skin and skin structure infection • Severe acne • Rocky mountain spotted fever • Cholera	• Bind to ribosomes of susceptible bacteria and inhibit protein synthesis • Bacteriostatic, bactericidal in high concentrations	• There are no direct contraindications. • Use caution in renal impairment/failure, hepatic disease, colitis, and GI disease. • Adverse effects include photosensitivity, exfoliative dermatitis, enterocolitis, hepatic failure, pericarditis, anaphylaxis, hemolytic anemia, azotemia, blurred vision, dysphagia, erythema, thrombocytopenia, neutropenia, nail discoloration, headache, vomiting, diarrhea, nausea, rash, and tooth discoloration.

Note: All agents are contraindicated in the presence of hypersensitivity to the medication or one of its components.

ALT, alanine aminotransferase; AST, aspartate aminotransferase; CAP, community-acquired pneumonia; CNS, central nervous system; COPD, chronic obstructive pulmonary disease; DM, diabetes mellitus; GI, gastrointestinal; ICD, implantable cardioverter-defibrillator; MAOIs, monoamine oxidase inhibitors; MRSA, methicillin-resistant *Staphylococcus aureus*; MSSA, methicillin-sensitive *Staphylococcus aureus*; PID, pelvic inflammatory disease; TTP, thrombotic thrombocytopenic purpura; UTI, urinary tract infection; VAD, ventricular assist device.

TABLE A.2   Common Pain and Sedation Medications for Certified Emergency Nursing

GENERAL INDICATIONS	GENERAL MECHANISM OF ACTION	GENERAL CONTRAINDICATIONS, PRECAUTIONS, AND ADVERSE EFFECTS
Analgesics with antipyretic activity: acetaminophen		
• Fever • Mild pain or temporary relief of headache, myalgia, back pain, musculoskeletal pain, dental pain, dysmenorrhea, arthralgia, and minor aches and pains with the common cold or flu • Moderate to severe pain with adjunctive opioid analgesics • Osteoarthritis pain • Acute migraine	• Increase pain threshold by inhibiting prostaglandin synthesis through the COX pathway	• Medication is contraindicated in severe hepatic impairment and severe active hepatic disease. • Use caution in renal disease and in patients with G6PD. • Adverse effects include elevated hepatic enzymes, rash, jaundice, hypoprothrombinemia, neutropenia, angioedema, hemolytic anemia, and rhabdomyolysis.
Barbiturates (phenobarbital)		
• Status epilepticus • Maintenance of all types of seizures • Short-term treatment of insomnia • Procedural sedation • Relief of preoperative anxiety • Sedation maintenance • Relief of anxiety, tension, and apprehension	• Nonselective CNS depressant with sedative hypnotic actions	• Medication is contraindicated in pulmonary disease in which obstruction or dyspnea is present, hepatic disease, hepatic encephalopathy, pregnancy, and porphyria. • Use caution in acute pain, as paradoxical reactions can occur. • Use caution during rapid IV administration, as this can cause bronchospasm. • Do not abruptly discontinue medication, as withdrawal can occur. • Adverse effects include suicidal ideation, megaloblastic anemia, bradycardia, depression, tolerance, impaired cognition, respiratory depression, confusion, elevated liver enzymes, hepatitis, jaundice, neutropenia, dependence, emotional lability, rash, nausea, vomiting, fatigue, decreased libido, and ptosis.
Gabapentinoids (gabapentin)		
• Adjunct treatment of partial seizures • Neuropathic pain • Moderate to severe restless leg syndrome • ALS • Tremor • Nystagmus • Spasticity due to MS • Pruritus • Fibromyalgia • Dysautonomia following sever TBI • Alcohol dependence	• Exact mechanism of action with GABA receptors unknown • Show a high affinity for binding sites throughout the brain correspondent to the presence of the voltage-gated calcium channels, especially alpha-2-delta-1, which seems to inhibit release of excitatory neurotransmitters in presynaptic areas that participate in epileptogenesis	• There are no contraindications to use. • Use caution in renal failure and pulmonary disease. Gabapentin is excreted in the kidneys; dose adjustments may be required for patients in renal failure or with renal impairments. • Do not abruptly discontinue, as withdrawal symptoms can occur. • Adverse effects include hyperglycemia, tolerance, depression, confusion and memory impairment, dehydration, jaundice, respiratory depression, dizziness, headache, fatigue, nausea and vomiting, tremor, decreased libido, back pain, emotional lability, skin irritation, diarrhea, and irritability.

(continued)

TABLE A.2 Common Pain and Sedation Medications for Certified Emergency Nursing *(continued)*

GENERAL INDICATIONS	GENERAL MECHANISM OF ACTION	GENERAL CONTRAINDICATIONS, PRECAUTIONS, AND ADVERSE EFFECTS
General anesthetics: etomidate		
• General anesthesia induction • Sedation during rapid sequence intubation • Procedural sedation	• Increase GABA transmission by increasing the number of GABA receptors available through displacement of natural binding of GABA inhibitors	• There are no true contraindications. • Avoid use, if possible, with sepsis or septic shock. • Use caution in older adult patients, as cardiac depression is possible. • Use caution in hepatic disease, as etomidate is metabolized in the liver. • Adverse effects include apnea, laryngospasm, bradycardia, arrhythmia, anaphylaxis, respiratory depression, hypoventilation, hypo- or hypertension, sinus tachycardia, nausea, and vomiting.
General anesthetics: ketamine		
• General anesthesia induction/maintenance • Preanesthetic sedation • Treatment of refractory bronchospasm in status asthmaticus • Treatment-resistant depression in adults • Moderate to severe pain • Induction agent during rapid sequence intubation	• Interrupt pathways in the brain prior to producing somesthetic sensory blockade; selectively depress the thalamo-neocortical system	• Medication is contraindicated in conditions for which additional blood pressure increase would be hazardous, including hypertension, hypertensive crisis, stroke, head trauma, intracranial mass, and intracranial bleeding. • Use caution in glaucoma and in patients with increased ICP, alcoholism, substance use disorder, or thyrotoxicosis. • Adverse effects include bradycardia, diabetes insipidus, arrhythmia, laryngospasm, apnea, ocular hypertension, increased ICP, hallucinations, delirium, hypertension, respiratory depression, confusion, withdrawal, psychosis, dysphoria, urinary incontinence, nightmares, nausea, vomiting, anxiety, and insomnia.
General anesthetics: propofol		
• General anesthesia • ICU sedation • Conscious sedation • Refractory status epilepticus • Refractory migraine • Postoperative nausea and vomiting prophylaxis • Agitation associated with alcohol withdrawal	• Inhibit NMDA receptors through channel gating modulation with agonistic activity at the GABA receptor	• Propofol is contraindicated when general anesthesia or sedation is contraindicated. • Use caution in cardiac disease, sepsis, and hypovolemia, as these patients will be more susceptible to propofol-induced hypotension. • Use caution in pancreatitis and hyperlipidemia; due to high lipid content, propofol can exacerbate or worsen these conditions. • Adverse effects include bradycardia, arrhythmia, laryngospasm, bronchospasm, hyperkalemia, ileus, hypotension, edema, hypoventilation, euphoria, wheezing, elevated hepatic enzymes, respiratory depression, hypertriglyceridemia, hepatomegaly, and drowsiness.

(continued)

TABLE A.2	Common Pain and Sedation Medications for Certified Emergency Nursing *(continued)*

GENERAL INDICATIONS	GENERAL MECHANISM OF ACTION	GENERAL CONTRAINDICATIONS, PRECAUTIONS, AND ADVERSE EFFECTS
Opioids: fentanyl		
• Control of moderate to severe pain • Intraoperative or procedural management of severe pain • Postoperative pain management • Management of chronic severe pain in opioid-tolerant patients requiring around-the-clock long-term opioid treatment • Management of severe breakthrough cancer pain in opioid-tolerant patients • Short-term management of acute postoperative pain • Adjunctive management of general anesthesia maintenance • Major surgery • Analgesia/sedation in mechanically ventilated ICU patients • Sedation and analgesia prior to rapid sequence intubation • Management of dyspnea in patients with end-stage cancer or lung disease • Procedural sedation	• Bind to pain receptors in the body to decrease pain pathways and alleviate pain	• Transdermal fentanyl patches are contraindicated in patients with known or suspected paralytic ileus or GI obstruction. • Nonparenteral fentanyl is contraindicated in status asthmaticus or severe respiratory depression. • Patients should not stop taking medication abruptly, as it may cause withdrawal symptoms. • Use caution in patients with history of alcoholism or substance use disorder, as there is a high risk for psychological dependence. • Use with caution in patients with respiratory disorders, as it may cause respiratory depression. • Use caution in head trauma and neurologic disorder, as it may increase drowsiness and decrease respirations • Adverse effects include GI obstruction, bradycardia, laryngospasm, respiratory depression, pneumothorax, apnea, chest wall rigidity, ileus, arrhythmia, constipation, hypokalemia, hypoventilation, dyspnea, confusion, hallucinations, dysphoria, blurred vision, psychologic and physiologic dependence, withdrawal, rash, vomiting, abnormal dreams, drowsiness, fatigue, paranoia, anxiety, agitation, emotional lability, and nausea.
Opioids: hydrocodone		
• Treatment of chronic severe pain requiring around-the-clock long-term opioid treatment • Treatment of refractory restless legs syndrome	• Agonistic activity at the mu receptors results in changes in the perception of pain at the spinal cord and into the CNS	• Medication is contraindicated in patients with significant respiratory depression, acute or severe asthma, known or suspected GI obstruction, or paralytic ileus. • Use caution in substance use disorder, depression, geriatric populations, CNS depression and/or head trauma, increased ICP, psychosis, opioid-naïve patients, seizures, cardiac disease, adrenal insufficiency, hypothyroidism, and myxedema. • Long-term use may increase risk of infertility. • Adverse reactions include GI obstructions, seizures, apnea, SIADH, respiratory arrest, constipation, depression, dyspnea, confusion, withdrawal if abruptly discontinued, respiratory depression, hypoxia, hypotension, psychological and physiologic dependence, infertility, nausea, tremor, anxiety, dizziness, and drowsiness.

(continued)

TABLE A.2 Common Pain and Sedation Medications for Certified Emergency Nursing *(continued)*

GENERAL INDICATIONS	GENERAL MECHANISM OF ACTION	GENERAL CONTRAINDICATIONS, PRECAUTIONS, AND ADVERSE EFFECTS
Opioids: hydromorphone		
• Relief of moderate to severe pain • Management of chronic severe pain in opioid-tolerant patients requiring around-the-clock long-term opioid treatment • Analgesia and/or sedation in mechanically ventilated ICU patients	• Act at the mu receptor causing changes in perception to pain at the spinal cord and into the CNS	• Medication is contraindicated in patients with respiratory depression, status asthmaticus (immediate-release tablets), paralytic ileus (extended-release tablets), and sulfite hypersensitivity. • Use caution in substance use disorder, opioid-naïve patients, head trauma or CNS depression, cardiac disease, geriatric populations, adrenal insufficiency, hypothyroidism, and myxedema. • Adverse reactions include bronchospasm, GI obstruction, bradycardia, anaphylaxis, laryngospasm, apnea, respiratory arrest, ileus, constipation, depression, dysphoria, hallucinations, confusion, euphoria, withdrawal if abruptly discontinued, urinary retention, nausea, drowsiness, vomiting, fatigue, dizziness, diarrhea, anxiety, tremor, paranoia, and lethargy.
Opioids: morphine		
• Acute and chronic moderate to severe pain • Management of chronic severe pain in patients who require around-the-clock long-term opioid treatment • Dyspnea in patients with end-stage cancer or pulmonary disease • Procedural sedation • Painful diabetic neuropathy • Refractory restless legs syndrome	• Act at the mu receptor, causing changes in perception to pain at the spinal cord and into the CNS	• Medication is contraindicated in significant respiratory depression in unmonitored settings, acute or severe bronchial asthma (oral solutions), respiratory depression or hypoxia, upper airway obstruction, acute alcoholism or delirium tremens (rectal route), known or suspected GI obstruction or paralytic ileus, hypovolemia, circulatory shock, cardiac arrhythmia or heart failure secondary to chronic lung disease, and concurrent use with MAOI therapy. • Use caution in substance use disorder, alcoholism, opioid-naïve patients, CNS depression, head trauma, seizures or increased ICP, cardiac disease, adrenal insufficiency, hypothyroidism, and myxedema. • Do not abruptly discontinue, as withdrawal symptoms can occur. • Adverse effects include ileus, bradycardia, arrhythmia, increased ICP, bronchospasm, GI obstruction, laryngospasm, depression, confusion, hypoxia, edema, euphoria, delirium, dysphagia, hallucinations, psychosis, physiologic dependence, adrenocortical insufficiency, drowsiness, diarrhea, constipation, headache, fever, nausea, restlessness, and vomiting.

(continued)

TABLE A.2 Common Pain and Sedation Medications for Certified Emergency Nursing *(continued)*

GENERAL INDICATIONS	GENERAL MECHANISM OF ACTION	GENERAL CONTRAINDICATIONS, PRECAUTIONS, AND ADVERSE EFFECTS
Opioids: oxycodone		
• Treatment of severe pain • Management of chronic severe pain in patients requiring around-the-clock long-term opioid management • Painful diabetic neuropathy • Restless legs syndrome	• Mu receptor agonist that changes pain perceptions at the spinal cord and into the CNS	• Medication is contraindicated in patients with significant respiratory depression and in patients with hypercarbia, GI obstruction, and paralytic ileus. • Use caution in opioid naïve patients, with abrupt discontinuation, and with CNS depression, head trauma, psychosis and increased ICP, cardiovascular disease, seizures, adrenal insufficiency, hypothyroidism, and myxedema. • Adverse effects include laryngospasm, seizure, ileus, bradycardia, GI obstruction, constipation, euphoria, dysphoria, confusion, blurred vision, dysuria, dyspnea, hypotension, hallucinations, nausea, drowsiness, vomiting, diarrhea, abdominal pain, or fatigue.
Opioids: tramadol		
• Moderate to moderately severe acute pain • Moderate chronic pain or moderately severe chronic pain in patients requiring continuous around-the-clock treatment for an extended period of time • Adjunctive treatment of osteoarthritis • Diabetic neuropathy • Postherpetic neuralgia • Postoperative shivering	• Agonistic activity at the central opiate receptor	• There are no direct contraindications. • Use caution in polysorbate 80 hypersensitivity, CNS depression, head trauma, seizure and increased ICP, severe pulmonary disease, biliary disease, GI obstruction or GI disease, substance abuse, renal or hepatic impairments, geriatric populations, adrenal insufficiency, hypothyroidism, and myxedema. • Adverse effects include hepatic failure, pancreatitis, bradycardia, seizures, pulmonary edema, arrhythmia, bronchospasm, constipation, hallucinations, hypertension, hypertonia, dyspnea, urinary retention, peripheral edema, blurred vision, withdrawal with abrupt discontinuation, hepatitis, amnesia, confusion, nausea, dizziness, headache, vomiting, drowsiness, agitation, and pruritus.

(continued)

TABLE A.2 Common Pain and Sedation Medications for Certified Emergency Nursing *(continued)*

GENERAL INDICATIONS	GENERAL MECHANISM OF ACTION	GENERAL CONTRAINDICATIONS, PRECAUTIONS, AND ADVERSE EFFECTS
Sedatives: benzodiazepines (midazolam)		
<ul><li>Procedural sedation</li><li>Amnesia induction</li><li>Control of preoperative anxiety</li><li>General anesthesia induction and maintenance</li><li>Seizures</li><li>Sedation maintenance in mechanically ventilated patients</li><li>Relief of agitation and/or anxiety</li><li>Treatment of status epilepticus refractory to standard therapy</li><li>Sedation during RSI</li><li>Treatment of alcohol withdrawal including delirium tremens</li></ul>	<ul><li>Act on the hypothalamic, thalamic, and limbic regions to produce CNS depression</li></ul>	<ul><li>Medication is contraindicated in sleep apnea or severe respiratory insufficiency/failure that is not mechanically ventilated, and in acute closed-angle glaucoma.</li><li>Use caution in geriatric populations; psychiatric conditions including bipolar, depression, mania, psychosis or suicidal ideation; CNS depression; hepatic disease; substance use; and dementia.</li><li>Adverse effects include coma, seizure, apnea, pneumothorax, arrhythmia, bradycardia, delirium, confusion, hypotension, hallucinations, memory impairment, constipation, respiratory depression, tolerance, psychological dependence, withdrawal if abruptly discontinued, drowsiness, dizziness, weakness, headache, and tremor.</li></ul>
Sedatives: dexmedetomidine		
<ul><li>Sedation induction and maintenance of mechanically ventilated ICU patients</li><li>Procedural sedation of nonintubated patients undergoing surgical procedures</li><li>Preanesthetic sedation</li></ul>	<ul><li>Centrally act as agonist to alpha-2-adrenoceptors, resulting in sedation and analgesia without significant ventilatory effects</li></ul>	<ul><li>There are no direct contraindications.</li><li>Use caution in patients with hypovolemia, diabetes, bradycardia, hypotension, uncontrolled hypertension, hepatic disease, and renal failure.</li><li>Adverse effects include hypotension and bradycardia (may require decreased dose or discontinuation), arrhythmia, hyperkalemia, renal failure, apnea, respiratory depression, hypoxia, hypovolemia, anemia, nausea, anxiety, fever, vomiting, diaphoresis, dizziness, headache, and diarrhea.</li></ul>

ALS, amyotrophic lateral sclerosis; CNS, central nervous system; COX, cyclooxygenase; GABA, gamma-aminobutyric acid; GI, gastrointestinal; G6PD, glucose-6-phosphate dehydrogenase; ICP, intracranial pressure; IV, intravenous; MAOI, monoamine oxidase inhibitor; MS, multiple sclerosis; NMDA, N-methyl-D-aspartate; RSI, rapid sequence intubation; SIADH, syndrome of inappropriate antidiuretic hormone secretion; TBI, traumatic brain injury.

TABLE A.3 Common Intravenous Fluids for Certified Emergency Nursing

GENERAL INDICATIONS	GENERAL MECHANISM OF ACTION	GENERAL CONTRAINDICATIONS, PRECAUTIONS, AND ADVERSE EFFECTS
D5NS		
• Parenteral (IV) treatment for hypoglycemia and hyperkalemia • Nutritional and parenteral nutrition	• Replaces and supplements glucose • Supplies energy to cells	• Medication is contraindicated in hyperglycemia and severe dehydration. Dextrose solutions can worsen the patient's hyperosmolar state. • Use caution in hypernatremia, hyperchloremia, metabolic acidosis, infection, diabetes, hepatic disease, HF with fluid overload, and electrolyte imbalance. • Adverse effects include hyperglycemia.
D5W		
• Parenteral (IV) treatment for hypoglycemia and hyperkalemia • Nutritional and parenteral nutrition • Oral glucose tolerance test	• Replaces and supplements glucose • Supplies energy to cells	• Medication is contraindicated in hyperglycemia and severe dehydration. Dextrose solutions can worsen the patient's hyperosmolar state. • Use caution in infection, diabetes, hepatic disease, HF with fluid overload, and electrolyte imbalance. • Adverse effects include hyperglycemia.
Normal saline (sodium chloride, 3%, 0.9%, 0.45%)		
• Dehydration or hypovolemia, including during diabetic ketoacidosis and shock • Hyponatremia • Mucolysis and sputum induction in patients with cystic fibrosis • Treatment of nasal congestion and dryness • Nutritional supplementation • Temporary relief of corneal edema • Treatment of increased ICP (3% hypertonic solution) • Inpatient management of viral bronchiolitis	• Regulates membrane potential of cells to help maintain water/sodium balance and homeostatic function	• There are no direct contraindications. • Use caution in hypernatremia, hyperchloremia, HF with fluid overload, and metabolic acidosis. • Adverse effects include HF, encephalopathy, hypernatremia, and sodium retention.
Lactated Ringer's solution		
• Any condition requiring volume repletion or electrolyte supplementation • Hypotension • Any condition requiring an increase in pH level	• Regulates homeostasis by supplementing water and electrolyte balance	• There are no true contraindications. • Use caution in alkalosis; diabetes; metabolic disturbances (hypokalemia, hypercalcemia, or metabolic acidosis); arrhythmia; hypoxemia; and pulmonary, cardiovascular, and hepatic disease • Adverse effects include change in taste, weight gain, vomiting, stomach pain, seizures, nausea, dizziness, faintness, nervousness, confusion, blurred vision, or edema.

D5NS, dextrose 5% in normal saline; D5W, dextrose 5% in water; HF, heart failure; ICP, intracranial pressure; IV, intravenous.

TABLE A.4   Common Steroids for Certified Emergency Nursing

GENERAL INDICATIONS	GENERAL MECHANISM OF ACTION	GENERAL CONTRAINDICATIONS, PRECAUTIONS, AND ADVERSE EFFECTS
Corticosteroids (prednisone, methylprednisolone, hydrocortisone)		
<ul><li>Maintenance therapy of primary or secondary adrenocortical insufficiency</li><li>Congenital adrenal hyperplasia</li><li>Kidney transplant rejection prophylaxis</li><li>Chronic graft-versus-host disease</li><li>Acute lymphocytic leukemia</li><li>Chronic lymphocytic leukemia</li><li>Short-term treatment of hypercalcemia secondary disease</li><li>Inflammatory bowel disease</li><li>Crohn's disease</li><li>Ulcerative colitis</li><li>Rheumatic conditions</li><li>Systemic autoimmune conditions</li><li>Hemolytic anemia</li><li>Asthma exacerbation</li><li>Thrombocytopenia or ITP</li><li>Myasthenia gravis</li><li>Psoriatic arthritis</li><li>Proteinuria in nephrotic syndrome</li><li>Severe erythema multiforme or Stevens–Johnson syndrome</li><li>Treatment of ACE inhibitor-induced angioedema</li><li>Allergic disorders including anaphylaxis</li><li>ARDS</li><li>Pneumonia</li><li>Hodgkin lymphoma</li><li>Multiple myeloma</li><li>Duchenne muscular dystrophy</li><li>Carpal tunnel syndrome</li><li>Autoimmune hepatitis</li><li>Primary amyloidosis</li><li>Exacerbation of COPD</li><li>Idiopathic or viral pericarditis</li><li>Interstitial nephritis</li><li>Bell's palsy</li><li>Transplant rejection</li></ul>	<ul><li>Inhibit steps in the inflammatory pathway to prevent systemic infection and inflammation of the lungs and to reduce mucus production</li></ul>	<ul><li>Patients receiving corticosteroids for an extended time or in high doses are at increased risk of immunosuppression, making them more prone to infection.</li><li>Avoid using in patients with Cushing syndrome</li><li>Use caution in untreated infection, diabetes, glaucoma, immunodepression, and liver disease.</li><li>Adverse effects include growth inhibition, osteoporosis, osteopenia, impaired wound healing, immunosuppression, candidiasis, fluid retention, hypernatremia, euphoria, hallucinations, hyperglycemia, nausea, weight gain, fluid retention, emotional lability, headache, hoarseness, diaphoresis, and bronchospasm.</li><li>Medication may reduce glucose tolerance, causing hyperglycemia in patients with diabetes.</li></ul>

ACE, angiotensin-converting enzyme; ARDS, acute respiratory distress syndrome; COPD, chronic obstructive pulmonary disease; ITP, immune thrombocytopenic purpura.

RESOURCES

Hooper, D. C. (2022). Fluroquinolones. *UpToDate*. https://www.uptodate.com/contents/fluoroquinolones

Mayo Foundation for Medical Education and Research. (2022). *Lactated Ringer's (intravenous route): Side effects*. https://www.mayoclinic.org/drugs-supplements/lactated-ringers-intravenous-route/side-effects/drg-20489612?p=1

Prescribers' Digital Reference. (n.d.-a). *Acetaminophen* [Drug information]. https://www.pdr.net/drug-summary/Ofirmev-acetaminophen-1346

Prescribers' Digital Reference. (n.d.-b). *Amidate (etomidate)* [Drug information]. https://www.pdr.net/drug-summary/Amidate-etomidate-675

Prescribers' Digital Reference. (n.d.-c). *Amikacin sulfate* [Drug information]. https://www.pdr.net/drug-summary/Amikacin-Sulfate-amikacin-sulfate-676

Prescribers' Digital Reference. (n.d.-d). *Ampicillin* [Drug information]. https://www.pdr.net/drug-summary/Ampicillin-for-Injection-ampicillin-677

Prescribers' Digital Reference. (n.d.-e). *Ativan injection (lorazepam)* [Drug information]. https://www.pdr.net/drug-summary/Ativan-Injection-lorazepam-996

Prescribers' Digital Reference. (n.d.-f). *Azithromycin* [Drug information]. https://www.pdr.net/drug-summary/Azithromycin-azithromycin-24249

Prescribers' Digital Reference. (n.d.-g). *Bactrim (sulfamethoxazole/trimethoprim)* [Drug information]. https://www.pdr.net/drug-summary/Bactrim-Bactrim-DS-sulfamethoxazole-trimethoprim-686

Prescribers' Digital Reference. (n.d.-h). *Cefazolin sodium* [Drug information]. https://www.pdr.net/drug-summary/Cefazolin-Sodium-cefazolin-sodium-1193

Prescribers' Digital Reference. (n.d.-i). *Cefepime hydrochloride (Maxipime)* [Drug information]. https://www.pdr.net/drug-summary/Maxipime-cefepime-hydrochloride-3215.5755

Prescribers' Digital Reference. (n.d.-j). *Ceftriaxone* [Drug information]. https://www.pdr.net/drug-summary/Ceftriaxone-ceftriaxone-1723

Prescribers' Digital Reference. (n.d.-k). *Cefuroxime* [Drug information]. https://www.pdr.net/drug-summary/Zinacef-cefuroxime-242

Prescribers' Digital Reference. (n.d.-l). *Ciprofloxacin* [Drug information]. https://www.pdr.net/drug-summary/Ciprofloxacin-Injection-ciprofloxacin-3255

Prescribers' Digital Reference. (n.d.-m). *Clindamycin* [Drug information]. https://www.pdr.net/drug-summary/Cleocin-Phosphate-Injection-clindamycin-1865

Prescribers' Digital Reference. (n.d.-n). *Dexmedetomidine hydrochloride* [Drug information]. https://www.pdr.net/drug-summary/Precedex-dexmedetomidine-hydrochloride-1271

Prescribers' Digital Reference. (n.d.-o). *Dextrose monohydrate* [Drug information]. https://www.pdr.net/drug-summary/5--Dextrose-dextrose-monohydrate-24283

Prescribers' Digital Reference. (n.d.-p). *Dilaudid (hydromorphone hydrochloride)* [Drug information]. https://www.pdr.net/drug-summary/Dilaudid-Injection-and-HP-Injection-hydromorphone-hydrochloride-490

Prescribers' Digital Reference. (n.d.-q). *Diprivan (propofol)* [Drug information]. https://www.pdr.net/drug-summary/Diprivan-propofol-1719

Prescribers' Digital Reference. (n.d.-r). *Doxycycline* [Drug information]. https://www.pdr.net/drug-summary/Doxycycline-doxycycline-24308

Prescribers' Digital Reference. (n.d.-s). *Ertapenem* [Drug information]. https://www.pdr.net/drug-summary/Invanz-ertapenem-359

Prescribers' Digital Reference. (n.d.-t). *Fentanyl citrate (fentanyl citrate)* [Drug information]. https://www.pdr.net/drug-summary/Fentanyl-Citrate-fentanyl-citrate-2474

Prescribers' Digital Reference. (n.d.-u). *Fluconazole* [Drug information]. https://www.pdr.net/drug-summary/Diflucan-fluconazole-1847

Prescribers' Digital Reference. (n.d.-v). *Gentamicin sulfate* [Drug information]. https://www.pdr.net/drug-summary/Gentamicin-Injection-40-mg-mL-gentamicin-sulfate-3299

Prescribers' Digital Reference. (n.d.-w). *Ketamine* [Drug information]. https://www.pdr.net/drug-summary/ Ketalar-ketamine-hydrochloride-1999#10

Prescribers' Digital Reference. (n.d.-x). *Merrem (meropenem)* [Drug information]. https://www.pdr.net/drug -summary/Merrem-meropenem-2055

Prescribers' Digital Reference. (n.d.-y). *Morphine sulfate* [Drug information]. https://www.pdr.net/drug-summary/ Morphine-Sulfate-Tablets-morphine-sulfate-1520

Prescribers' Digital Reference. (n.d.-z). *Neomycin sulfate* [Drug information]. https://www.pdr.net/drug-summary/ Neomycin-Sulfate-neomycin-sulfate-819

Prescribers' Digital Reference. (n.d.-aa). *Neurontin* [Drug information]. https://www.pdr.net/drug-summary/ Neurontin-gabapentin-2477.4218

Prescribers' Digital Reference. (n.d.-ab). *Oxycodone* [Drug information]. https://www.pdr.net/drug-summary/ Oxycodone-HCl-oxycodone-hydrochloride-24333

Prescribers' Digital Reference. (n.d.-ac). *Pentamidine* [Drug information]. https://www.pdr.net/drug-summary/ NebuPent-pentamidine-isethionate-1408

Prescribers' Digital Reference. (n.d.-ad). *Phenobarbital* [Drug information]. https://www.pdr.net/drug-summary/ Phenobarbital-Elixir-phenobarbital-2669#10

Prescribers' Digital Reference. (n.d.-ae). *Prednisone* [Drug information]. https://www.pdr.net/drug-summary/ Prednisone-Prednisone-Intensol-prednisone-2575

Prescribers' Digital Reference. (n.d.-af). *Sodium chloride* [Drug information]. https://www.pdr.net/drug-summary/ Sodium-Chloride-sodium-chloride-24245

Prescribers' Digital Reference. (n.d.-ag). *Streptomycin* [Drug information]. https://www.pdr.net/drug-summary/ Streptomycin-streptomycin-1600

Prescribers' Digital Reference. (n.d.-ah). *Teflaro (ceftaroline fosamil)* [Drug information]. https://www.pdr.net/ drug-summary/Teflaro-ceftaroline-fosamil-158

Prescribers' Digital Reference. (n.d.-ai). *Tobramycin* [Drug information]. https://www.pdr.net/drug-summary/ Tobramycin-tobramycin-916

Prescribers' Digital Reference. (n.d.-aj). *Vancomycin hydrochloride* [Drug information]. https://www.pdr.net/ drug-summary/Vancocin-vancomycin-hydrochloride-802

Prescribers' Digital Reference. (n.d.-ak). *Zohydro-ER (hydrocodone bitartrate)* [Drug information]. https://www.pdr. net/drug-summary/Zohydro-ER-hydrocodone-bitartrate-3389

Prescribers' Digital Reference. (n.d.-al). *Zyvox (linezolid)* [Drug information]. https://www.pdr.net/drug-summary/ Zyvox-linezolid-2341

INDEX

Page entries that appear in italics refer to content in the practice test and practice test answer chapters.

ABBREVIATIONS

AAA	abdominal aortic aneurysm
ABG	arterial blood gas
ABI	ankle-brachial index
AC	alternating current
ACE	angiotensin-converting enzyme
ACLS	advanced cardiovascular life support
ACS	acute coronary syndrome
ADH	antidiuretic hormone
ADL	activity of daily living
AICDs	automatic implantable cardioverter-defibrillator
AKI	acute kidney injury
ALS	amyotrophic lateral sclerosis
ALT	alanine aminotransferase
AMA	against medical advice
AMI	acute myocardial infarction
AMS	altered mental status
ANA	antinuclear antibody
ANA	American Nurses Association
ARF	acute renal failure
AST	aspartate aminotransferase
APRN	advanced practice registered nurse
aPTT	activated partial thromboplastin time
ARDS	acute respiratory distress syndrome
ARS	acute retroviral syndrome
ATP	adenosine triphosphate
AUDIT-C	alcohol use disorders identification test
AV	atrioventricular
BCEN	Board of Certification for Emergency Nursing
BIPAP	bilevel positive airway pressure
BLS	basic life support
BMP	basic metabolic panel
BNP	brain natriuretic peptide
BPH	benign prostatic hyperplasia
BPPV	benign paroxysmal positional vertigo
BRAO	branch retinal artery occlusion
BRAT	bananas, rice, applesauce, and toast
BSATD	Brief Screener for Alcohol, Tobacco, and Other Drugs
BUN	blood urea nitrogen
BVM	bag-valve-mask
CAD	coronary artery disease
CAP	community-acquired pneumonia
CAUTI	catheter-associated urinary tract infections
CBC	complete blood count
CDC	Centers for Disease Control and Prevention
CHF	congestive heart failure
CHG	chlorhexidine gluconate
CIWA	Clinical Institute Withdrawal Assessment
CI	crush injury
CK	creatine kinase
CKD	chronic kidney disease
CK-MB	creatine kinase–myoglobin binding
CLABSI	central line–associated bloodstream infection
CMP	comprehensive metabolic panel
CMV	cytomegalovirus
CN	cranial nerve
CNS	central nervous system
CO	carbon monoxide
COWS	clinical opioid withdrawal scale
COPD	chronic obstructive pulmonary disease
COX	cyclooxygenase
CPAP	continuous positive airway pressure
CPK	creatine phosphokinase
CPP	cerebral perfusion pressure
CPR	cardiopulmonary resuscitation
CRAO	central retinal artery occlusion

CRE	carbapenem-resistant Enterobacteriaceae
CRP	C-reactive protein
CRRT	continuous renal replacement therapy
CSF	cerebrospinal fluid
CTA	computed tomography angiography
CVA	cerebrovascular accident
CXR	chest x-ray
DC	direct current
DI	diabetes insipidus
DKA	diabetic ketoacidosis
DM	diabetes mellitus
DMARDs	disease-modifying antirheumatic drugs
DPL	diagnostic peritoneal lavage
DTaP	diphtheria, tetanus, and pertussis vaccine, pediatric formulation
DVT	deep vein thrombosis
EBV	Epstein-Barr virus
ECMO	extracorporeal membrane oxygenation
ED	emergency department
EEG	electroencephalogram
EIA	enzyme immunoassay
EKG	electrocardiogram
EMG	electromyography
EMS	Emergency Medical Services
EMTALA	Emergency Medical Treatment and Labor Act
ENA	Emergency Nurses Association
ENT	ear, nose, throat
ERCP	endoscopic retrograde cholangiopancreatography
ESI	Emergency Severity Index
ESI	epidural steroid injection
ESR	erythrocyte sedimentation rate
ESRD	end-stage renal disease
ETOH	ethyl alcohol
ETT	endotracheal tube
FAST	focused assessment with examination sonography in trauma
FFP	fresh frozen plasma
fFN	fetal fibronectin
FHT	fetal heart tones
FOB	fecal occult blood
GABA	gamma-aminobutyric acid
GBS	Guillain–Barré syndrome
GCS	Glasgow Coma Scale
GERD	gastroesophageal reflux disease
GFR	glomerular filtration rate
GHB	gamma hydroxybutyrate
GI	gastrointestinal
GSW	gunshot wound
GU	genitourinary
H&H	hemoglobin and hematocrit
hCG	human chorionic gonadotropin
HEENT	head, eyes, ears, nose, and throat
HELLP	hemolysis, elevated liver enzymes, and low platelets
HEPA	high efficiency particulate air
HF	heart failure
HHS	hyperglycemic hyperosmolar syndrome
HINTS	head impulse-nystagmus-test of skew
HIPAA	Health Insurance Portability and Accountability Act of 1996
HIT	heparin-induced thrombocytopenia
HIV	human immunodeficiency virus
HLA	human leukocyte antigen
HOB	head of bed
HSV	herpes simplex virus
HZO	herpes zoster ophthalmicus
I&D	incision and drainage
IBS	irritable bowel syndrome

ICD	implantable cardioverter-defibrillator
ICP	intracranial pressure
ICU	intensive care unit
IgE	immunoglobulin E
IgF	insulin-like growth factor
IM	intramuscular
INR	international normalized ratio
IOP	intraocular pressure
I/O	intake/output
IUD	intrauterine device
IS	incentive spirometry
ITP	immune thrombocytopenic purpura
IV	intravenous
IVC	inferior vena cava
IVF	intravenous fluid
IVIG	intravenous immunoglobin
JVD	jugular vein distention
LDH	lactate dehydrogenase
LET	leukocyte esterase test
LFT	liver function test
LMP	last menstrual period
LOC	level of consciousness
LP	lumbar puncture
LPN	licensed practical nurse
LRI	lower respiratory infection
LSD	lysergic acid diethylamide
LVN	licensed vocational nurse
MAP	mean arterial pressure
MAOI	monoamine oxidase inhibitor
MB	myoglobin binding
MCI	mass casualty incident
MDIs	metered dose inhalers
MDMA	3,4-methylenedioxy-methamphetamine
MDRO	multidrug-resistant organism
MHC	major histocompatibility complex
MODS	multiple organ dysfunction syndrome
MOI	mechanism of injury
MRA	magnetic resonance angiography
MRI	magnetic resonance imaging
MRSA	methicillin-resistant *Staphylococcus aureus*
MSSA	methicillin-sensitive *Staphylococcus aureus*
MS	multiple sclerosis
MTP	massive transfusion protocol
MTP	medical termination of pregnancy
MVC	motor vehicle crash
NAAT	nucleic acid amplification test
NC	nasal cannula
NG	nasogastric
NIH	National Institutes of Health
NIHSS	National Institutes of Health Stroke Scale
NIPPV	nasal intermittent positive pressure ventilation
NMDA	*N*-methyl-D-aspartate
NMS	neuroleptic malignant syndrome
NPO	nothing by mouth
NRB	non-rebreather mask
NSAIDs	nonsteroidal anti-inflammatory drugs
NSTEMI	non-STEMI
OB	obstetrics
OB/GYN	obstetrics/gynecology
OE	otitis externa
OM	otitis media
OPTN	organ procurement and transplant network
OSHA	Occupational Safety and Health Administration
OTC	over-the-counter
PAC	premature atrial contractions
PCC	prothrombin complex concentrate
PAD	peripheral arterial disease